D

Nutrition Policy in Public Health

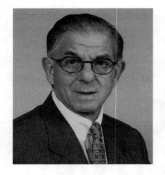

Felix Bronner, PhD, is professor emeritus of BioStructure and Function and of Nutritional Sciences at the University of Connecticut. A graduate of the University of California at Berkeley and Davis, with a graduate degree from the Massachusetts Institute of Technology, and the recipient of an honorary doctorate from France, Dr. Bronner has worked in the general area of calcium nutrition and metabolism for the past 40 years. He was among the first to study the kinetics of ^{45}Ca in humans, he has done detailed kinetic and balance studies in rats, and, in the past decade, has used these data, along with published information, to develop a quantitative analysis of calcium transport in the intestine and kidney, and of calcium homeostasis. His interest in calcium and mineral nutrition has spurred an interest in nutrition policy.

Dr. Bronner has published 93 research articles, has contributed 64 chapters to texts and symposia volumes, and has edited 57 volumes of texts and symposia. He was founding editor of *Current Topics in Membranes and Transport* and first chair of the Gordon Research Conference on Bones and Teeth. He has served on the editorial boards of the *American Journal of Clinical Nutrition, The Journal of Nutrition,* and still serves on the editorial board of *The American Journal of Physiology.*

A member of numerous scientific societies, including a fellowship in the American Association for the Advancement of Science and the American Institute of Nutrition, Dr. Bronner was the 1974 recipient of the Andre Lichtwitz prize, awarded by the French National Institute of Medical Research (INSERM) for outstanding work in calcium and phosphorus metabolism, and the honoree of the 4th International Workshop on Calcium and Phosphate Transport Across BioMembranes, held in Lyon in 1989 under North Atlantic Treaty Organization (NATO) sponsorship. He has organized and chaired national and international symposia and workshops and trained graduate students and many postdoctoral fellows.

NUTRITION POLICY
IN PUBLIC HEALTH

Felix Bronner, PhD
Editor

Springer Publishing Company

Springer Publishing Company, Inc.
536 Broadway
New York, NY 10012–3955

Cover design by Margaret Dunin
Acquisition Editor: Matt Fenton
Production Editor: Pamela Lankas

97 98 99 00 01 / 5 4 3 2 1

Library of Congress Cataloging-in-Publication Data

Nutrition policy in public health / Felix Bronner, editor.
     p.   cm.
    Includes bibliographical references and index.
    ISBN 0-8261-9660-8
    1. Nutrition policy—United States.   2. Nutrition—United States.
  3. Public health—United States.   I. Bronner, Felix.
   TX360.U6N867   1997
363.8'5'0973—dc21   97-3392
                                          CIP

Printed in the United States of America

Contents

Preface

In the past nutrition policy has concerned itself largely with underdeveloped countries. There the development of cash crops, the decrease in subsistence farming, and the migration of rural populations to cities and shanty towns have led to poorly nourished populations, with the resulting need for policies that would sustain the poor in terms of their nutrition. This is another way of saying that the development of nutrition policy received its impetus from the absence or shortage of foods, that is, from undernutrition.

In a highly developed country like the United States, however, it is the plethora of food choices that has led to the need for developing a nutrition policy to ensure that food intake by the population is neither excessive, nor restricted to few foods with limited nutrient content. Thus it is overnutrition, or at least the threat of it, that may be considered a major impetus for the formulation of U.S. nutrition policy. Another major factor is the increasing recognition that better health and longer life can result if people become aware of the benefits of restricted fat intake, of antioxidants, of increased calcium intake, or get to know the factors in foods that can bring about or exacerbate cancer, to name only some nutritional recommendations with public health relevance. At the same time, social and economic divisions in the U.S. population have led to the need, recognized in various ways during the past 50 years, but especially since the White House Conference in 1969, for government programs to help provide adequate nutrition for the millions of the U.S. population who, in terms of their family income, are designated as "poor," or who require special assistance.

Groups that have been recognized as needing nutritional assistance include pregnant women and children, school children, and those in the U.S. population entitled to food stamps. In all of those programs, an attempt is made to provide or encourage the consumption of health-promoting foods, that is, foods that help provide the nutrients needed by the various population groups. In addition, government agencies have publicized recommendations relating to the consumption of vegetables and fruit, to limitations on fat intake, and dietary allowances in general. The question immediately arises as to who will acquaint the public and specific target groups with these policy recommendations.

Public health officers, preferably with special nutrition training, have a significant task in making policy known and helping to enforce it where possible and appropriate. Above all, they must inform the health profession and the public about existing nutrition policies and, through education, with the help of literature and via media, make the population as a whole aware of the need to practice these policies. If people practice healthful nutrition and demand as consumers that appropriate foods be available to them, then processors, suppliers, and public officials will make sure such foods are widely available and reasonably priced.

The need to acquaint public health officials with existing nutrition policy and to help trained personnel to function as nutrition policy officers in public health settings—whether at the municipal, state, or federal level—has led to the writing of this book. This material is the result of several sequences of a group-taught course in the *University of Connecticut Public Health Program* and of input by colleagues and editors.

The book is divided into four sections. Section I deals in five chapters with General Aspects of Nutrition Policy. The first of these, by C. Peter Timmer of Harvard University, deals with the rationale and approaches to nutrition policy in public health and outlines some of the major policy problems that will need resolution in the future, notably the question of coercive versus free food choices.

Because food intake is very much a behavioral issue, my colleague David Gregorio raises the question in Chapter 2 of how people can be motivated to eat more health-promoting foods, particularly if this involves significant changes in eating habits. Several approaches are outlined, some of which are particularly suited to the educational role of the public health nutrition officer. Joseph F. Borzelleca of the Medical College of Virginia outlines in Chapter 3 the health risks that food additives, pesticides, and microbial infection may pose and how existing legislation, listed and summarized in historical perspective, has contributed to minimizing these risks. In Chapter 4, Barbara Blechner and Stephen Fontana discuss in detail U.S. legislation as it pertains to food and nutrition. These two chapters provide the background information for the practicing nutrition officer on existing laws and legal structures safeguarding the U.S. food supply.

In Chapter 5, Paul Lachance of Rutgers University informs the reader of basic food-processing technology and what changes food may undergo from field to consumer. This also is essential background for nutrition officers, particularly in light of the enormous choice of foods available to consumers in U.S. retail outlets.

Part II of the book, consisting of Chapters 6 through 12, identifies a variety of nutritional or nutrition-based conditions of public health concern. Eileen Kennedy, of the U.S. Department of Agriculture Center of Nutrition Policy, discusses undernutrition in Chapter 6 and the means to minimize incidence and severity. In Chapter 7, Barbara Moore, C. Everett Koop, and Judith Stern deal with overnutrition, which, on a population basis, has become a major scourge for the U.S. and populations in other developed countries. The chapter contains a number of useful recommendations on how to keep energy expenditures and food intake in balance. Aryeh Stein of Michigan State University deals with coronary heart disease and the necessity and difficulties of minimizing fat intake in Chapter 8, inasmuch as high fat intake has been identified as the principal cause of coronary heart disease in the U.S. population. The role of nutrition in the prevention, control, and treatment of cancer is discussed in Chapter 9, by Carole Palmer and Johanna Dwyer of Tufts University. They discuss how nutrition practices, such as low fat intake, can minimize the incidence of some cancers, how important nutrition is in the care of cancer patients, and what public health initiatives are proposed in the effort to combat cancers.

As people live longer, thinning of their bone structure has become a common ailment, affecting both men and women. Chapter 10 discusses osteoporosis and the role calcium nutrition can play in minimizing the occurrence of this condition. Dental health is readily improved when drinking-water supplies are fluoridated. Martin Giniger of the University of Medicine and Dentistry of New Jersey discusses dental caries in Chapter 11, the evidence that fluoridation of drinking water provides an essential nutrient and how it counteracts dental caries. He also describes the public policy issues raised by foes of water fluoridation. Chapter 12 identifies selected disease entities that particularly profit from nutrition intervention, with folic acid supplementation an outstanding example of the prevention of neural tube defects.

Part III of the book deals with nutrition policies and approaches targeted at populations at risk and comprises three chapters. Chapter 13, by Alma Cain of the Connecticut Department of Public Health, discusses the nutritional needs of pregnant mothers and their young children, with emphasis on the Special Supplemental Food Program for Woman, Infants and Children (WIC), the major U.S. program in that field. She provides historical information on the growth of the WIC program, how it helps women and children with limited income, and describes other programs designed to provide food aid. Aryeh Stein, in Chapter 14, deals with nutrition policy for preschool and school children, placing emphasis on the need to develop appropriate nutrition habits early so as to minimize nutrition-related conditions like obesity in later life. In Chapter 15, David Rush, Robert Russell, and Irwin Rosenberg, from the Human Nutrition Research Center on Aging in Boston, discuss nutrition policy for the elderly. They evaluate the needs for the different groups of elderly, those living alone, and those in assisted living arrangements and discuss what needs to be done for this growing segment of the population.

In Part IV, Nutrition Policy Perspective, Nancy Milio of the University of North Carolina, building on experience in Norway and Finland, develops in detail what Peter Timmer alluded to in the first chapter, namely, how national nutrition recommendations can be made into effective policy. This is indeed a major concern for nutrition policy formulation and execution in the United States. One of the significant take-home points from her chapter is the necessity for all social structures to work together if nutrition policy is to be more than preaching in the wilderness.

Cooperation is also a necessity in a multiauthored book. I want to thank the contributors for their chapters, their willingness to make changes and to adapt their material to the multiple audience at whom this book is directed: nutrition officers in a public health setting, public health officers interested in nutrition policy and students aspiring to these positions. Thanks must also go to the publisher for recognizing the need for this book, the first to deal comprehensively with nutrition policy in the public health of the United States.

Farmington, Connecticut   FELIX BRONNER
Editor

Contributors

Barbara Blechner, JD
Assistant Professor
Department of Community
  Medicine and Health Care
University of Connecticut Health
  Center
Farmington, CT 06030-1910

Joseph F. Borzelleca, PhD
Professor
Department of Pharmacology and
  Toxicology
Medical College of Virginia
P.O. Box 980613
Richmond, VA 23298-0613

Alma W. Cain, MS
State WIC Director
State of Connecticut
Department of Public Health and
  Addiction Services
150 Washington Street
Hartford, CT 06106

Johanna T. Dwyer, DSc
Director
Frances Stern Nutrition Center
NE Medical Center Hospitals
750 Washington Street, Box 783
Boston, MA 02111

Stephen Fontana, JD
Department of Community
  Medicine and Health Care
University of Connecticut Health
  Center
Farmington, CT 06030-1910

Martin S. Giniger, DMD, PhD
Director
Division of Diagnostic Sciences
University of Medicine and
  Dentistry of New Jersey
110 Bergen Street, Room C-827
Newark, NJ 07103

David I. Gregorio, PhD
Assistant Professor
Department of Community
  Medicine and Health Care
University of Connecticut Health
  Center
Farmington, CT 06030-1910

Eileen T. Kennedy, DSc
Center for Nutrition Policy and
  Promotion
USDA
1120 20th Street NW, Suite 200
Washington, DC 20036

C. Everett Koop, MD
Chairman, Shape Up America
6707 Democracy Boulevard,
  Suite 107
Bethesda, MD 20817-1129

Paul A. Lachance, PhD, DSc
Professor and Chair
Department of Food Science
Rutgers, the State University of
  New Jersey
New Brunswick, NJ 08903-0231

Nancy Milio, PhD
Professor
Health Policy Administration
University of North Carolina at
  Chapel Hill
Carrington Hall-CB 740
Chapel Hill, NC 27599-7460

Barbara J. Moore, PhD
President, Shape Up America
6707 Democracy Boulevard,
  Suite 107
Bethesda, MD 20817-1129

Carole A. Palmer, EdD
Professor
Division of Nutrition and
  Preventive Dentistry
Tufts University School of Dental
  Medicine
1 Kneeland Street
Boston, MA 02111

Irwin Rosenberg, MD
Director, Jean Mayer USDA
  Human Nutrition Center on
  Aging at Tufts University
711 Washington Street
Boston, MA 02111

David Rush, MD
Jean Mayer USDA Human
  Nutrition Center on Aging at
  Tufts University
711 Washington Street
Boston, MA 02111

Robert Russell, MD
Jean Mayer USDA Human
  Nutrition Center on Aging at
  Tufts University
711 Washington Street
Boston, MA 02111

Aryeh D. Stein, PhD
Assistant Professor
Program in Epidemiology
Michigan State University
A214 East Fee Hall
East Lansing, MI 48824-1316

Judith S. Stern, ScD
Professor
Departments of Nutrition and
  Internal Medicine
University of California at Davis
3150 B Meyer Hall
Davis, CA 95616

C. Peter Timmer, PhD
Thomas D. Cabot Professor of
  Development Studies At-Large
Harvard University
One Eliot Street
Cambridge, MA 02138

General Aspects of Nutrition Policy

Part I

General Aspects of
Nutrition Policy

CHAPTER 1

Nutrition Policy in Public Health: Rationale and Approaches

C. Peter Timmer

W hat are the dimensions of a nutrition policy in the field of public health? Why should public policy intervene in private decisions about food and nutrition? This chapter examines these questions in order to build the foundations for the chapters that follow, chapters that provide details on what a public health nutritionist, for example, needs to know to be informed about the major policy debates involving nutrition and health.

Virtually none of these debates involves food availability per se, at least not in the context of the United States and other rich countries. Although nutritionists at all levels need to understand basic trends in the world food economy and the evolving balance between global food production and increasing demands for that food, the long-run trends have been quite favorable. Since 1950, the trend in food availability per capita has been rising, prices for staple grains in world markets have trended downward under the weight of chronic surpluses, and average calorie intake per capita per day reaches new records almost every year. If everyone on the globe had equal access to these food resources, there would be no hunger or famine.

And yet problems of hunger and famine continue to exist in many countries of the world, and most nutritionists are concerned about these problems, if for no other reason than that their clientele is also concerned and seeks information from experts who should understand the solutions to such problems. It should be apparent, however, that the continuing problems of hunger and famine are not nutritional problems. Instead, they are caused by deep-seated political, ethnic, and economic divisions that often hold the nutritional status of entire populations hostage to bitter disputes. Nutritionists do need to understand the complexities of these situations, but their professional skills are no more relevant to solving them than are the skills of the agronomist, the engineer, or the baker.

This book focuses on what nutritionists can do, and the knowledge they need to do it. As this introductory chapter explains, much complexity and controversy remains even when the role is narrowed to such obvious topics as the relationship between nutrition and disease and what counsel an informed nutritionist can provide to a concerned public. The complexity stems from the multiple forces impinging on the nutrition–disease relationship, as is illustrated in Figure 1.1, which is taken from *Food Policy Analysis* (Timmer, Falcon, & Pearson, 1983), the standard reference in the field. Many of the dimensions of this relationship are treated in detail in this volume.

The controversy stems from two highly emotional components of every American's life: the appeal and safety of the daily diet and the freedom to make private decisions without government interference. When these two elements are in conflict, as they are almost every day for every citizen, public controversy and political heat are sure to be generated. Public health nutritionists find themselves squarely in the middle of the controversy because they seek mechanisms to improve people's daily diets.

NUTRITION POLICY IN PUBLIC HEALTH: AN ECONOMIC PERSPECTIVE

The American supermarket is the envy of the world. Other societies, rich and poor alike, marvel at the amount, diversity, quality, convenience, and relative cost of the items available at literally thousands of neighborhood food stores across the United States.[1] No other major society spends such a

---

1. A cook recently marveled to the *Boston Globe* that he could buy fresh habanero chili peppers in Williamstown, Massachusetts, in January.

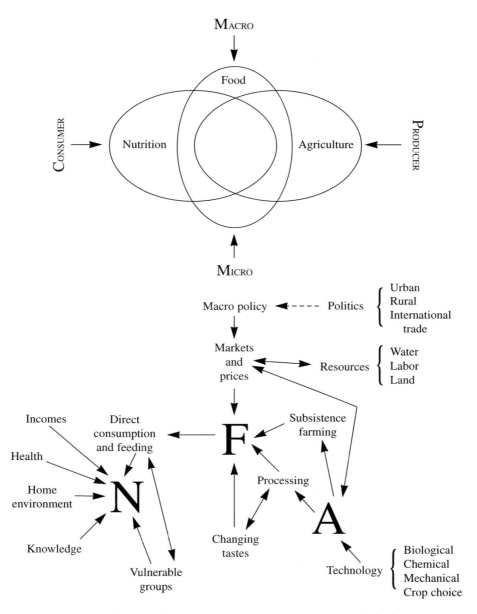

Figure 1.1 Linkages among agriculture (A), food (F), and nutrition (N).

Source: C. Peter Timmer, Walter P. Falcon, and Scott R. Pearson, *Food Policy Analysis*, Baltimore: Johns Hopkins University Press for the World Bank, 1983, p. 8. Reproduced with permission.

small fraction of its income on food, and the sheer availability and appeal of the American food supply offer a substantial bonus to consumer welfare.

At the same time that the modern supermarket and the 10,000 or so items that stock it were evolving to their present state, the American diet and health care system were contributing to longer life expectancies and larger physiques. Since 1900 the major gains in life expectancy have been among the younger and nonwhite parts of the population, but those are precisely the groups likely to benefit from better nutrition, control of infectious diseases, and improved maternal care.

With such an outstanding record of progress, the American public might well be expected to show great satisfaction with their food system, content in the knowledge that the diet is healthy and safe. And indeed, there are many satisfied consumers who use the great variety and quality of foods available in the United States to choose a diet of excellent nutritional quality, high taste appeal, and moderate cost. To the consumer who has the *motivation, knowledge, and financial means*, the American food system offers a diet as healthy, safe, and appetizing as any in history.

Despite this potential for great consumer satisfaction and excellent nutritional status, there is a disturbing mood in America's supermarkets and kitchens. An undercurrent of uncertainty, frustration, and outright fear of much of the food in the American food supply has caught much of the public. Heart disease, cancer, diabetes, "tired blood," and reduced sexual vigor, we are told, may be caused by the ingredients that we put into our foods, take out of our foods, or both. At the same time, certain foods or food components are held in almost magical awe. For example, vitamins A, C, and E, brewer's yeast, rose hips, and almost anything "organic" are thought by some to cure disease and prevent aging, cancer, and the common cold.

In this atmosphere of disbelief, uncertainty, and fear, many in the American population are looking for reassurance and direction in the form of simple rules. Which foods are unsafe? How much vitamin A? Will a pill work, or must it come from broccoli? Are eggs good or bad? In scientific and public-policy forums government, industry, and university experts have attempted to respond by describing the complexity of the scientific evidence and the range of statistical uncertainty, but to many this smacks of cover-up or self-serving propaganda. The nutrition messiahs, with their instant dietary salvation, have found a massive audience by playing off the public's fears against the imperfect scientific evidence.

This book attempts to present the scientific evidence in a format and at a level that makes it useful to nutritional professionals to grapple with these issues. In reviewing the scientific evidence, however, it is important to recognize the distinction between scientific debate and policy debate. Inherent in the distinction is a fundamental dilemma for the American democratic system. When private choices, even when fully informed, lead to public health problems, who shall decide on the nature and extent of remedies? When the remedies involve substantial economic dislocation for farmers and food processors, who shall bear the costs? When the remedies involve substantial exercise and dietary adjustments, how will the population be motivated to make the changes?

DEALING WITH COMPLEXITY AND TRADE-OFFS

Most of the chapters in this book stress the complex interactions among nutrients, lifestyle, genetic makeup, and health. Life expectancy, for example, depends on a large number of variables, only some of which can be consciously controlled by the individual. Moreover, over a certain significant range some choice variables can substitute for others in a manner illustrated in Figure 1.2. It must be emphasized that Figure 1.2 shows a hypothetical relationship only. Medical evidence is not yet as precise as the diagram would indicate (although it was first introduced 20 years ago). But the direction of interaction of dietary restrictions and physical exercise is well accepted by the medical community even if the extent of synergism between the two (and smoking, another very important variable in the relationship) is not well understood.

Figure 1.2 illustrates both the individual and the policy dilemmas inherent in the likely link between diet and disease. A "good" lifestyle includes sufficient physical exercise to maintain an "excellent" rating for aerobic capacity as well as significant dietary restrictions to maintain low risk levels of serum cholesterol and other blood lipids (and other restrictions on total caloric intake, simple carbohydrates, and highly processed foods). This particular example also includes no smoking as a lifestyle element. The years of freedom from chronic disease at age 40 that can be anticipated with this lifestyle combination can also be achieved, however, with somewhat less exercise and more stringent dietary restrictions or by more exercise and fewer dietary restrictions. A greater risk of chronic disease is likely with reductions along both of the axes.

The private dilemma is the cost an individual is willing to pay now

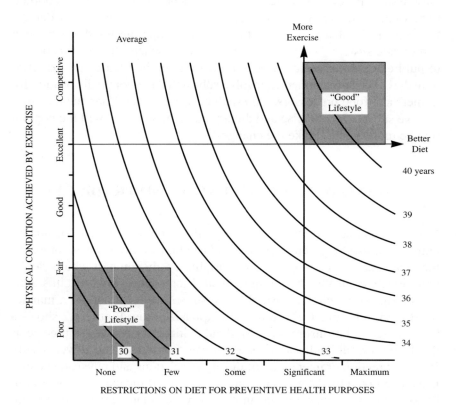

Figure 1.2 The role of diet and exercise in living longer: The hypothetical relationship between physical condition from exercise, diet restrictions, and expected number of years free from chronic disease for a 40-year-old nonsmoking adult.

SOURCE: C. Peter Timmer and Malden C. Nesheim, Nutrition, Product Quality, and Safety. In Bruce L. Gardner & James W. Richardson, (Eds.), *Consensus and conflict in U.S. agriculture.* College Station, Texas: Texas A & M University Press, 1979, p. 167.

(e.g., at age 40) for an uncertain, but probably higher, quality of life 30 to 40 years in the future. Are the "pleasures" of the "poor" lifestyle subset in Figure 1.2 worth the likely, but by no means certain, price that may be paid from heart disease or other chronic illness in later years? It would seem extremely difficult for society to make this choice for the individual, and yet extremely important on humanitarian grounds that the choice be informed by the best scientific evidence available.

But society's interest in this decision extends beyond humanitarian concern. Even if sufficient information were available to indicate the probable benefits of the "good" lifestyle, many in society will continue to choose the "poor" lifestyle for a variety of personal reasons. Although the individual who chooses the "poor" lifestyle pays part of the costs through more chronic disease and higher medical costs, not all of such costs are private. Society pays an important share of such costs through losses in productivity of workers and through partial public financing of medical costs. There is a strong social investment in the individual's lifestyle decision, and some mechanism is needed to reconcile the difference between private and public costs and benefits to alternative dietary/lifestyle decisions.

It is here that the substitution possibilities inherent in Figure 1.2 present enormous policy implications. Health may be improved through various combinations of lifestyle changes, including exercise, diet, and smoking. To some individuals, alteration of one component of lifestyle, for example, exercise, may be much more acceptable than alterations in other components. The opportunity exists for individuals to substitute movement along the "more exercise" direction in Figure 1.2 for movement along the "better diet" direction, while still maintaining a personally satisfying expectation of future health.

What should society do when faced with such a dilemma? An economist is tempted to answer that society should spend its educational and regulatory money where it will bring the greatest marginal gain, and scientists should do the research to determine if that is in exercise, diet, smoking, or other factors. Such an answer would be naive in three ways. First, our society may not have mechanisms for making sound decisions in such scientifically controversial areas. Second, scientists are not able to quantify these relationships with sufficient precision for public policymaking to take the "facts" as given. Third, lifestyle, including dietary practices, is immersed in and grows out of a complex American social and political economy. The American food system, in particular, has a very large stake in policy decisions aimed at altering the composition of the American diet for health and safety reasons. Many citizens, including many knowledgeable consumers, would feel much more comfortable achieving significant health gains through improved private lifestyles than through increased regulation of the American food system and greater restrictions on what may be eaten with good conscience.

FUTURE PATHS FOR NUTRITION POLICY: SHOULD THE GOVERNMENT DO MORE OR LESS?

Whatever the merit of the scientific evidence linking diet to health problems, consumers will pressure their elected representatives and food producers to make foods safer and the diet healthier. The chapters in this book present a balanced perspective that emphasizes the significance of the link. The issue of changing dietary patterns for health purposes is not restricted to a few vegetarians and health-food enthusiasts, but has entered the consciousness of the mainstream American consumer. This consumer votes both at the ballot box *and* in the marketplace. Both votes are likely to call forth a response from food suppliers and their lobbyists and directly from legislators seeking to respond to a mandate that says "keep our foods safe and healthy!" But should government regulators and policymakers be doing more or less to satisfy that demand? There is a range of possibilities.

Less Regulation of the Food Industry

Many farmers and representatives of food processors and distributors feel that *less* regulation of the U.S. food system would improve welfare of both producers and consumers. A key complaint is the Delaney amendment, which prohibits the addition to the food supply of any material known to cause cancer in man or animals. The Delaney amendment was enacted in an era when analytical methods were far less sensitive than those in use today. A logical case exists for modifying the Delaney amendment so that the tolerance is not zero, but some very small amount. Basic food and drug legislation requires that all additives be "safe," however. Even in the absence of the Delaney amendment it would be extremely difficult to show that a known carcinogen is safe.

Further, however, the prohibitive approach to regulating safety does not permit a cost–benefit assessment of whether certain chemicals might cause more good than harm, nor does it permit the consumer to make that decision on an informed, individual basis. The cases of saccharin, cyclamates, nitrites, and other commercially important additives, coloring agents, and so on illustrate how real and difficult the issues are. Despite the fact that it seems silly to ban the use of a chemical whose social benefits outweigh its social costs, present scientific evidence on health costs and benefits is so slippery that even technical assessments of the issue are almost impossible.

For example, a technical report by the National Academy of Sciences found any claims for benefits from saccharin were unsubstantiated. But from an economist's perspective, the availability of a sugar-free product expands the range of consumer choice, especially where to "spend" one's calories, and this contributes to enhanced consumer welfare. The controversy is over any association of medical benefits, such as weight loss, with such consumer benefits. In general, there is no recognized decision-making process for deciding fairly when costs outweigh benefits, and vice versa. Historically, Congress has legislated waivers to the Delaney amendment on a chemical-by-chemical (and producer-lobby-by-producer-lobby) basis. Such ad hoc tinkering with the safety of the nation's food supply is probably inevitable without better mechanisms for resolving disputes that arise when food safety, freedom of choice for consumers, and the profitability of the food industry are in conflict.

Keep the Same Approach to Food Regulation

A second alternative is to leave the food system to find its own path in the context of changing technology, consumer tastes, and present regulations and standards. This path emphasizes the extremely wide choice of foods available to most American consumers and their ability to enjoy the safest and highest quality food supply in the world. But this approach also recognizes that the American food system is not static, and mere failure to enact new public regulations will not result in a status quo situation. It is possible to outline the broad trends of where the American food system is headed even without significant changes in how it is regulated.

The most visible trend is toward more processed foods using a wide range of substitutes, especially for natural foods thought to cause health problems, such as eggs, whole milk, butter, and cheese, and certain vegetable oils. Part of this trend involves the use of manufactured or synthetic products to make convenience or "instant" foods, such as soups or liquid meals. As this trend continues, existing product identity standards come under pressure from manufacturers to permit substitutes and synthetics, in order to manufacture a product similar in nutritional quality (or appearance) to the original.

The concern of nutritional scientists is that a trend toward more highly processed foods created from mixtures of ingredients unique to human evolutionary experience may cause long-run health problems. This concern is distinct from a prior worry that the "natural" diet consumed by affluent Americans since World War II, emphasizing red meat, eggs, dairy products, and increasing amounts of sugar and fats, also presents long-term health problems. Leaving the current regulatory approach intact does virtually nothing to allay either concern. New initiatives will be needed to do that.

Increased Emphasis on Nutrition Education

In a society that values freedom of choice by consumers, concerns about the safety and nutritional value of an individual's diet can be addressed in an unintrusive manner through nutrition education. Indeed, nearly all participants in the food system, from farmers to consumers to food processors and distributors, feel that providing nutrition education is an appropriate role for government, and that programs could be improved and expanded.

The appeal of more and better nutrition education stems from several sources. First, as noted, it does not intervene in the freedom of choice of individuals, either directly or indirectly, as do regulations and pricing interventions. If both the public and concerned policymakers are assured that consumers are truly well informed about current nutritional issues, including the public health dimensions of private dietary decisions, then food choice can and should be left to the individual consumer. The $5 to $10 billion spent annually for food advertising significantly influences what we want and choose. Yet, few would argue that the major thrust of this advertising is to improve our diets and nutritional status.

The second reason for the appeal of programs to improve nutrition education is that sufficient knowledge now exists to recommend healthy diets, but the knowledge is inadequate (or too controversial) to justify more massive interventions into the food system to force substantial changes in current dietary practices. Many people in the United States are now in excellent nutritional health, and if others simply emulated these role models, they could enjoy similar nutritional benefits. No major breakthroughs in scientific understanding would be necessary, although understanding the epidemiology of such good lifestyle patterns would be extremely important. Such understanding is needed to clarify the trade-offs and substitutions among the various dimensions of chronic disease. Accurate information of the sort hypothesized and modeled in Figure 1.2 would be an important component of a nutrition education program because it deals specifically with the critical question for such programs: What is the message?

The controversial aspect of this approach is how to bring about behavioral change. Even with agreement on a message (and this is not easy), and the example of good nutritional role models, our understanding of how to make nutrition education *effective* is seriously inadequate.

The third reason for widespread support for nutrition education is that, at least as traditionally conducted, the programs are relatively inexpensive. Probably not even $100 million is spent each year by governments and nutrition groups to improve nutritional understanding, whereas food advertising budgets may be a hundred times larger. Even major expansions in nutrition-education programs that are meant to improve the public's understanding of good nutritional practices and strengthen the motivation of consumers would use only a tiny fraction of the money that is spent to persuade them to buy specific food products.

There may well be a fourth reason for the widespread support enjoyed by nutrition-education initiatives. As traditionally conducted, these programs do not threaten anyone's vital economic interests because they do not in fact change food-consumption behavior in any significant way. The objective of much nutrition education has been to ensure consumption of a variety of foods that provide the required nutrients in adequate amounts. When nutritional educators begin to mount programs aimed specifically at reducing the intake of foods thought to be associated with major public health problems, such as coronary heart disease, cancer, and diabetes, then opposition and widespread controversy erupts quickly.

Thus significant expansion of nutritional education, especially attempts to focus on diet-related health issues, will be controversial. Again, part of the controversy revolves around the debate over appropriate roles for the public and private sectors, but a major part stems from the distinction between the nutritional and health risks associated with a dietary recommendation (which are usually exceedingly low), and the economic risks and costs to the food industry associated with adoption of a recommendation by consumers. These costs can be large.

For example, most nutritionists, including several represented in this volume, feel that most Americans should move toward consuming a diet with fewer highly refined, processed foods, with more fruits, vegetables, and whole grains, less saturated fats, dietary cholesterol, sugar, and fewer calories. These directions for dietary improvement are not intended as an individually prescribed diet, and they would not be satisfactory for millions of Americans with specific nutritional problems who require specialized medical attention. However, if the focus is on a population-wide average into which individuals are free to fit their knowledge, preferences, needs, and doctor's advice, such dietary changes in aggregate are likely to cause significant health improvements at relatively little health or nutritional risk.

Advocating such dietary changes as the basis of an expanded nutritional education program is controversial, not because of widespread fears of substantial health risks associated with the new diets, but because of the economic costs and dislocations to farmers and the food industry should these changes be widely adopted. In short, the critical issue for nutrition education is the content of the message and whether the private sector can agree on a message that makes public health sense, as well as economic sense.

More Activist Interventions

Many consumer activists are frustrated by what they see as industry intransigence in cleaning up America's food supply, eliminating potentially dangerous chemicals as additives, preservatives, or ingredients in processed foods, and reducing fat and sugar content in packaged cereals and meals. Monthly press releases attack each popular ethnic cuisine as "time bombs filled with saturated fat," with calls to regulate the nutritional quality of the nation's restaurants as well as its grocery stores. When children die from contaminated hamburgers in a fast-food restaurant, public concern rises and support is mobilized for more aggressive efforts to guarantee the safety of the nation's food supply.

Even the antigovernment mood prevailing in the mid-1990s cannot stem the desire of the American population for a risk-free environment and a deep-seated belief that the government should provide it. Consumer activists are tapping into this desire and using it as a political force in efforts to create a safer and healthier diet, at least as they understand the scientific evidence. If disputes between these activists and representatives from the food industry are settled in the political arena, then political solutions will be imposed, whatever the scientific evidence says. This is not necessarily a reassuring outcome; everyone is a food consumer, but only a relative few are food producers.

Consequently, a new mechanism for resolution of food issues is urgently needed. The most important aspect of such a mechanism would be the ability to engage in dialogue without the fear of economic disaster, on one hand, or of widespread and immediate health risks, on the other. Both parties, but especially those groups responsible for generating and evaluating scientific evidence with respect to health risks and safety of our food, must show great restraint in how their positions are presented. The press is constantly looking for sensational stories and much economic damage can be done by creating unjustified fears in the public mind and subsequent pressure for ill-considered public-policy interventions.

THE CHALLENGE OF NUTRITION
IN PUBLIC HEALTH

As scientific knowledge about the role of nutrition in the nation's public health increases, and the risks from various dietary choices are quantified, the challenge of who will bear those risks will be sharpened. In a litigious society such as the United States, the public seems to want all risks shifted from the individual to the manufacturer or the government (that is, to society as a whole). But food choices are highly individualistic, and no diet, no matter how "natural," is without some risk. Mustard, for example, contains naturally exactly the same carcinogen (3-amino, 1,2,3-triazole) that caused the "cranberry cancer scare" in the late 1950s.

A spectrum of approaches, from more to less coercive, is available for coping with this challenge. The most restrictive approach in terms of freedom of choice is simply to ban "risky" foods or food components. As already noted, the Delaney Amendment uses this approach with respect to known carcinogens, but when the economic impact is large, or when there is a public outcry over loss of a favorite food item, for example, noncaloric sweeteners and "diet" soft drinks, Congress has accommodated freedom of choice rather than the intent or the letter of the law.

A second approach is to hold manufacturers liable for any health consequences of the food they sell. When beef or chicken is contaminated with deadly bacteria and individuals die from specific episodes, the case for legal recourse is clear. But can manufacturers of butter, or dairy farmers, be held liable for the heart disease and premature deaths caused by "excessive" intake of saturated fats by individuals? If manufacturers of tobacco are ultimately held responsible for deaths from lung cancer among heavy smokers of cigarettes, as U. S. district courts are now ruling, can a class-action suit against a variety of food processors be far behind?

What seems little appreciated in this debate is how coercive food choices will be if the public continues to abdicate all willingness to accept individual responsibility for the risks presented by lifestyle choices over diet and exercise. If manufacturers are forced to assume the costs of these risks, only "safe" food will appear in the marketplace, and the array of choices presently available will narrow considerably. If government somehow accepts the costs of these risks, perhaps through full funding of medical costs and "damages" from poor choice of diet, the tax burden will be truly burdensome.

Faced with these dilemmas, the populations of the most wealthy nations, including the United States, might wish to rethink how they value their freedom of choice in matters so intensely personal as lifestyle and diet. As the philosophy of the welfare state is challenged on both economic and social grounds, a reassertion of the role of informed personal responsibility takes on political respectability. But this respectability also comes with a price: the cost to both society and the individual of becoming truly informed about the health consequences of alternative dietary choices and lifestyles. It is hoped that this book can contribute to making many individuals more informed about those choices, and at a modest cost!

REFERENCE

Timmer, C. P., Falcon, W. P., & Pearson, S. P. (1983). *Food policy analysis.* Baltimore, MD: Johns Hopkins University Press for the World Bank.

CHAPTER 2

Behavior and Food Intake: What Constitutes Effective Policy?

David I. Gregorio

One would be hard pressed to exaggerate the relevance of diet to the well-being of the public. Both the composition and quantity of the foods that individuals consume have been implicated in at least 5 of the 10 leading causes of death for Americans—coronary heart disease, several cancers, cerebrovascular disease, diabetes mellitus, and atherosclerosis (United States Public Health Service [USPHS], 1990.) Current estimates hold that 300,000 deaths per year, or roughly one of every seven deaths in the United States, are "caused" by what we eat (McGinnis & Foege, 1993). If the concept of diet is broadened to include the use of tobacco and alcohol, the number of "diet-induced" deaths approaches 800,000 annually. Indeed, the effects of eating, drinking, and smoking affect the mortality profile of our population to a considerably greater extent than the combined effects of our physical environment, biological agents, sexual practices, illicit drug use, injury, and deficiencies of our health care delivery system. According to *The U.S. Surgeon General's Report on Nutrition and Health* (USPHS, 1988), dietary patterns, more so than any other personal choice including the use of tobacco and/or alcohol, will influence the health of Americans. To paraphrase Mark Twain, "After you've eliminated all the eatables, drinkables and smokables, what you are left with is health." (Twain, 1924, p. 214).

It is understandable that our nation's disease prevention/health promotion initiative stresses the importance of dietary change in modifying the illness and mortality experience of our population. National health promotion and disease prevention objectives of *Healthy People 2000* (USPHS, 1990) call for significant reduction of coronary heart disease and cancer death rates, as well as reductions in the prevalence of obesity, growth retardation, anemia, and osteoporosis via the pursuit of the following risk-reduction objectives:

- Decrease the intake of saturated fat from 36% to no more than 30% of all calories consumed;
- double the consumption of complex carbohydrates and fiber-containing foods to five or more daily servings of fruits and vegetables and six or more daily servings of grain products;
- increase by as much as fivefold the proportion of adults consuming two or more servings of calcium-rich foods each day;
- decrease by one-quarter the proportion of food preparers who add salt to food during preparation, and by one-third the proportion of individuals who add salt to foods that they eat;
- cut by two-thirds the proportion of children with iron deficiencies; and
- nearly double (+80%) the proportion of overweight persons seeking to attain an appropriate body weight through sound dietary practices combined with regular physical activity.

How to achieve such ends remains a key public health challenge. Prevailing models of health promotion at our disposal emphasize the psychosocial functioning of individuals, and, as such, may have limited utility. Data on the efficacy of clinical interventions and self-help initiatives to modify long-term dietary habits suggest that the probability of reaching national health promotion/disease prevention objectives by the Year 2000, or at any time within our life span, is low. Long-term behavior modification is rarely achieved by more than 1 in 10 of persons, yet all of the Year 2000 objectives call for change by a much greater proportion of the population. Moreover, risks posed by poor nutrition are not uniformly distributed among the population but cluster among disadvantaged persons—the poor, racial/ethnic minorities, the very young, and the elderly (USPHS, 1991). Health-promotion efforts aimed at these groups with messages about long-term behavior change have had only mixed success.

Although there should be full commitment to encourage healthy lifestyles among all individuals, there is ample reason for public health leaders to consider paradigms for dietary change that emphasize institutions and social systems, rather than only individuals and their psyches. Many people working in health promotion have understood for some time that social circumstances are often at the root of at-risk behavior (Waitzkin, 1983). Along with initiatives to modify the beliefs and behaviors of individuals, attention should therefore be placed on interventions that tend to change dietary policies/practices of communities as a whole. This involves analysis of the social order that bears on the production and distribution of foods. The challenge to the health care system is to recognize and pursue efficacious "upstream" approaches that will change the environments that put individuals at risk because of poor nutrition (McLeroy, Bibeau, Steckler, Glanz, 1988). At the very least, such effort to bring about new structures and policies can facilitate health-promoting actions by individuals.

Fortunately, considerable groundwork has been laid by sociologists and political scientists who have monitored social change movements for political and cultural reform. This chapter encourages health promoters to reflect on those accumulated experiences and consider the varied opportunities available to promote system-wide changes in food consumption practices.

THE CHALLENGE OF SECURING COLLECTIVE HEALTH OUTCOMES

In his provocative essay of more than 20 years ago, "A Case For Refocusing Upstream," John McKinlay (1979) exhorted public health leaders to resist taking up transitory clinical interventions that respond to the immediate health problems encountered by individuals in favor of more deliberate efforts that address broader policy issues about how the population at large is exposed to harm.

> A clear majority of our resources and activities in the health field are devoted to what I term "downstream endeavors"—in the form of superficial, categorical tinkering in response to almost perennial shifts from one health issue to the next, without really solving anything. . . . Clearly, people and groups have important immediate needs which must be recognized and attended to. Nevertheless, one must be wary of the *short-term nature* and *ultimate futility* of such down-stream endeavors. (p. 9)

The salience of his message has not diminished with time. Health promoters are again discouraged from engaging in "categorical tinkering," but
rather, are encouraged to look upstream "away from those individuals and
groups who are mistakenly held to be responsible for their condition,
toward a range of broader political and economic forces" (McKinlay,
1974, p. 10).

In the spirit of McKinlay's treatise, we can differentiate health-promotion
initiatives according to whether the intended beneficiary of the intervention is the individual (which are essentially downstream endeavors that I
will subsequently refer to as "personal health initiatives") or the larger
community within which individuals interact (which I consider to be
upstream initiatives that will subsequently be referred to as "collective
health initiatives") (see Table 2.1). Typically, health promotion focusing
on individuals is intended, like McKinlay's notion of a downstream
endeavor, to remove/modify the risks confronting individuals in need. As
such, they strive for disease prevention through lifestyle change and/or the
use of efficacious health care technologies. Health-promotion efforts
which emphasize the collective well-being of groups, on the other hand,
reflect an upstream orientation to modify environments within which individual exposures occur.

This distinction between personal and collective health initiatives does
not rest on the number of individuals that a program affects. Community-
wide interventions such as the cardiovascular-risk-reduction efforts of the
Stanford 5-community study (Farquahar et al., 1977) or the Minnesota
Heart Health Program (Luepker, Murray, Jacobs, Mittlemark, Bracht,
1994) are intended to induce change in the health practices of substantial
numbers of individuals, but can still be classified as falling within the
domain of personal health initiatives, because their target is the individual.
What identifies personal health initiatives is that they apply exclusively to
the parties who undertake a prescribed course of action, such as avoiding
saturated fats, restricting caloric intake, moderating use of alcohol, supplementing vitamins, and the like.

Collective health outcomes, on the other hand, are like any public good.
Whatever benefit is to be accrued through intervention will be available to
all members, whether or not a particular individual expresses commitment,
invests resources, or takes action necessary to secure the desired outcome.
Put another way, collective health outcomes are indivisible—they cannot
readily be withheld from a particular member of the group. "They must be
available to everyone if they are available to anyone" (Olson, 1982, p. 14).

Table 2.1 Typology of Health-Promotion Initiatives According to the Focus of Action and Intended Beneficiaries

Intended beneficiary	Focus of action		
	Prevention	Detection	Treatment
The individual (Personal health initiatives)	Minimize personal exposure to pathogens (e.g., Diet control, exercise)	Use available modalities for screening, diagnosis, treatment, and surveillance of disease (e.g., Periodic health examination)	
The community (Collective health initiatives)	Control public hazards (e.g., Food inspection, Marketplace restrictions)	Develop, disseminate, and adopt promising health care innovations (e. g., Medical education reform, Health care financing)	

Numerous comparisons can be suggested to illustrate this distinction between personal and collective health initiatives. The consequences of a worksite-based smoking-cessation program are of a personal health nature in that they tend to reduce the risk of cardiovascular disease and cancer for individuals who chose to avoid/discontinue the use of tobacco. Initiatives to regulate the advertising and sale of cigarettes, on the other hand, connote a collective health outcome inasmuch as all members of the community, smokers and nonsmokers, proponents and opponents of a smoke-free environment alike, stand to gain from limiting access of the population to tobacco products. In a like manner, self-help efforts at weight control or at limiting consumption of saturated fat can attenuate the risk of illness only for individuals who undertake such action, whereas mandatory labeling of the nutritional content of foodstuffs has the potential to protect all individuals. It does so, among other things, by making food distributors aware of the commercial benefits of limiting the amount of fat in their products. Community-wide cholesterol screening programs will detect hypercholesteremia only in those individuals who are examined, whereas reforms in medical education to improve the counseling skills of physicians regarding nutrition will tend to benefit all patients.

At the beginning of this century our public health movement enjoyed unparalleled success in bringing about system-wide reform to protect, and indeed, improve our environment, the workplace, and the health care delivery system (Starr, 1983). Over recent decades, however, public health activists increasingly have shifted attention to education and clinical intervention programs that disproportionately emphasize personal health and its psychosocial determinants. Current focus for conceptualizing health behavior and health promotion strategies has been through intrapersonal paradigms like the Health Belief Model (Kirscht, 1988), Social Learning Theory (Perry, Baranowski, & Parcel, 1990), Self-Efficacy (Bandura, 1977), Self-Regulation Theory (Leventhal, Leventhal, Zimmer- man, & Gutmann, 1983), and the like. According to such perspectives, individuals are presumed to act on the basis of informed self-interest to change behavior in ways that will enhance their personal health. In turn, when such effort is multiplied repeatedly within a population, the collective well-being of the community is thought to be advanced.

The Health Belief Model, shown in Figure 2.1, is typical of this viewpoint. It holds that individuals are more likely to undertake measures to prevent or minimize illness whenever they judge themselves to be vulnerable to disease, injury, or disability; consider the condition in question to be serious; are convinced of their capacity to undertake necessary action to ameliorate the problem, and see few barriers to taking action; and, ultimately, are induced to action by some external cue or stimulus (Kirscht, 1988). Accordingly, health-promotion efforts to enhance dietary habits of individuals have focused attention on (a) *informing* the public of the health consequences of personal behavior (e.g., the effects of saturated fats or sugar on health, the importance of periodic health examinations, the value of prompt clinical intervention, and the like); (b) *reducing* barriers, whether real or perceived, that are thought to inhibit desired individual behavior (e.g., offering low-cost, accessible cholesterol screening, providing culturally appropriate educational materials, and the like); and (c) *triggering action* through media and educational campaigns (e.g., the annual American Cancer Society's "Great American Smoke Out," the "Five-a-day for Life" program, and the like).

Many commentators question whether the early success of public health has been adequately sustained. We presently know considerably more about how individuals perceive their responsibility for promoting their own good health than we do about the social causes of disease (Tesh, 1981). Critics of this intrapersonal health-promotion paradigm have noted that in essence, individuals are blamed for health practices and outcomes that may be largely beyond their control (Crawford, 1979; Freudenberg,

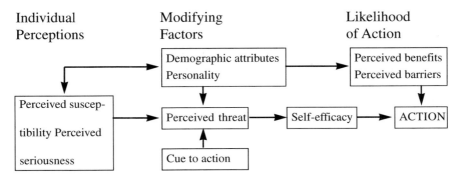

Figure 2.1 The Health Belief Model.

1978; Tesh, 1981). Absent from explanations of poor health or health practices are the larger societal forces that determine life chances and experiences of individuals (e.g., educational and occupational mobility of a population) and control the availability of preventive and therapeutic modalities (e.g., principles of insurability that determine the scope of covered medical services).

More important for our present interests, such psychosocial reasoning may not be readily applicable to circumstances in which the health outcomes at stake pertain to the community as a whole rather than to individual persons. Whenever a personal health concern, such as the risk of hyperglycemia, is considered, it is recognized that risks to individuals tend to be differentially distributed according to one's background and lifestyle. By contrast, a collective health concern such as the desire to regulate commodities in order to reduce per capita sugar consumption, assumes that group members are characterized by nondifferential risks. That is, the health of the public as a whole is thought to be at stake because of overexposure to sucrose.

Whether the issue pertains to persons who are exposed to unknown environmental hazards, employment at an unsafe worksite, residence within a medically underserved area, the need for an emerging technology/ service, and the like, such "collective health threats" typically are shared in roughly equal measure by all persons who are part of the target community. Under such conditions, a given individual may be at a loss to gauge accurately personal vulnerability or assess the hazard that such an exposure may connote. For one thing, ubiquitous exposure may be difficult to quantify at the individual level (e.g., passive inhalation of tobacco smoke, exposures from groundwater contamination, and the like). For another thing, definitions of serious health outcomes (e.g., impaired lung function vs. frank respiratory disease, morbid obesity vs. cardiovascular disease) may be blurred by socially derived judgments about what constitutes "acceptable," "minimal" and "avoidable" risks. Thus, educational appeals to encourage risk-reduction behavior may not be considered realistic or necessary by the target audience.

Achieving collective health outcomes typically requires interest groups to invest time, capital, material resources, and labor power in pursuit of payoffs that eventually must be shared with all other group members. In fact, the direct "benefit" that is due to an individual who chooses to take action is likely to be greatly overshadowed by the "cost" to the individual in bringing about the desired result. Because members of a community will share the product of efforts to resolve a collective health problem, even if they do not share in the investment to achieve that end, many self-interested parties may opt to "ride free" on the efforts of others.

Consider the dilemma confronting a hypothetical population with a problem of groundwater contamination. Various solutions could be offered—exploration for new water sources, treatment of contaminated supplies, regulation of contaminants, and the like. Each strategy, however, requires deliberate effort by parties, individuals, and interest groups. Many of these activists will, in fact, be acting against their self-interest for the sake of community responsibility. It is within such a context that the conflict between personal ambition to maximize private gain and one's public obligation to enhance the community's well-being is apparent.

For one thing, all members of the community stand to benefit from whatever action is undertaken to assure an adequate water supply. It would be practically impossible to withhold from anyone the tangible benefits of a cleaner, healthier environment. Any health payoff that does result from collective action must necessarily be extended to all community members—those who endorse and actively contribute to the process as well as to those opposing the effort!

For another, whatever action the solitary individual or group does undertake, no matter how thorough and effective, may not be sufficient to produce a discernible impact. Similarly, a decision to withhold commitment or effort toward a common solution is unlikely to jeopardize the effort of others committed to such a goal.

From such a vantage point then, the individual has relatively little reason to work toward a collective goal and considerable reason to withhold participation. In short, a decision to involve oneself in collective action is risky; the effort that one makes will be significant in terms of the individual, but minimal in terms of the collective. Whereas it may have a significant effect on the quality of one's life by committing finite physical and material resources to the cause, it is not likely to have a recognizable effect on the fate of the collective effort. Hence, to do nothing with respect to groundwater safety is a safe strategy for preserving the individual assets without significantly undermining the interests of the larger community. This contrast between definite personal costs and indefinite and uncertain collective outcomes generally weighs heavily in favor of inactivity.

Under most circumstances where personal preferences must be weighed against collective wishes, individual self-interests are likely to be favored. This classic principle, known as "the tragedy of the common" (Hardin, 1968, p. 1243), aptly describes the dilemma that arises whenever an individual's obligations to work toward a collective goal conflicts with a personal desire to maximize private gain through minimal effort. Adaptations of this concept have been used to explain why such diverse collective initiatives as movements for nuclear disarmament, population control, environmental protection, or political change are often internally thwarted. Put simply, for the majority of issues confronting communities as wholes, many persons can be expected to consider particular practices/strategies for achieving collective objectives to be inconsistent with their personal needs and aspirations.

OPTIONS FOR MOTIVATING INDIVIDUAL PURSUIT OF COLLECTIVE HEALTH INITIATIVES

The effort to promote action by individuals on behalf of *the group* through informational appeals that stress the magnitude of a problem, one's vulnerability to the situation, or the efficacy of proposed remedies may be insufficient to mobilize persons. That is because most persons will not see themselves as vulnerable enough to justify the expenditure of their scarce, personal resources for the benefit of others. It also follows that when collective concerns are taken up by individuals, their participation in goal-directed behavior may be less than optimal. At least in the short run, the well-being of the collective tends to be overlooked or at least shortchanged by the individual. At the same time, as we seek to minimize our own investment, we tend to count on maximum responsible effort by others.

Unfortunately, in the absence of a well-intended, activist State that can be counted on to regulate circumstances that are harmful to the larger group or that can coerce individual effort on behalf of the community at large, health promoters have relatively few options for motivating individuals to secure collective health initiatives. Nonetheless, lessons from community mobilization efforts on behalf of sociopolitical reform (Alinsky, 1972; Ross, 1955) suggest several approaches that can be enumerated that are likely to enhance one's prospects for achieving collective goals.

Scan the Landscape

Health-promotion efforts rarely proceed unfettered. Judgments about appropriate health goals and promotion strategies can pit interest groups against one another. In that competition, it is not necessarily the party with superior ideals but the one that commands and uses essential resources effectively that is likely to succeed.

It is important for health promoters to assess their environment care-fully in search of other parties and interest groups with whom they share certain affinities. Whenever feasible, the perception of community should be broadened beyond geographic and temporal limits to embrace whatever parties share common interests because of identity (e.g., race, age, and the like) or experience (e.g., occupational groups, and the like). The objective here is to build on the interdependencies that exist among interest groups. In doing so, the "reconstituted community" grows in its capacity to mar-tial resources for goal attainment, while gaining stature in terms of its sense of purpose and meaning. These notions are captured in the princi-ples of community competence and empowerment (Minkler, 1990).

Limit Demands

Successful community action is likely to require considerable coordina-tion of individuals who join the effort with disparate interests and variable talents. Organizational pressures can readily distract these heterogeneous groups from their intended foci. The result often is that participants may be required to contribute additional "managerial" resources to the group and/or function in inappropriate or undesired roles (e.g., supervisor, recruiter, etc.). In essence, the "cost" to participate in an initiative has been raised and the appeal of engaging in collective action further diminished.

Whenever feasible, calls to action should be explicit regarding the number and range of demands that are to be placed on prospective constituents. Ideally, the elements of a group's division of labor, chain of command, and the like should be clearly presented at the time a party or group is recruited for action. In this way, individuals can more realistically judge the value of their involvement in relation to probable demands and outcomes.

Recruit Serially, Yet Selectively

Without question, the most important resource that can be brought to bear in pursuit of any collective health initiative is individuals. With their participation in the activity come the physical, material, intellectual, and emotional resources that are essential for goal attainment. It does not necessarily follow, however, that successful health-promotion efforts are marked by intensive efforts to mobilize activists. Indeed, considerable effort can be dissipated by leaders who seek to identify and mobilize constituents but have given no consideration to the role recruits would play and the costs of soliciting their participation. In short, if too much effort is spent attracting supports, too few resources may be available for pursuing objectives.

Health promoters should recognize that support of their efforts can exist at various levels and that multiple strategies for mobilizing the public are needed to reach these. Adherents represent the minimal level of support; they may be easiest to recruit, but may be very difficult to use. Adherents are persons and groups who, while endorsing the goals and strategies of an effort, fall short of committing other resources to the cause. Constituents, on the other hand, are involved in more than a symbolic fashion. They are persons or groups who commit tangible resources to pursuing a collective goal. Activists, in turn, are a subset of constituents who contribute to the cause through their labor power.

Collective health efforts will benefit from participants at all three levels. Hence, it is important that leaders accurately judge the kind and extent of commitment that they will require of others. In doing so, they can better determine those organizational demands that ultimately may detract from their goal-directed activities. Adherents can be efficiently involved in a collective effort through generalized mass appeals in the media. Dissemination of information or staging of media events are often sufficient to reach nonadherents and arouse interest, but may not be enough to encourage donations and volunteers. Typically, it requires significant effort to move individuals from the category of adherents to that of constituents, often requiring extended face-to-face interaction. Depending on the issue and the organization pursuing it, there may be little need to recruit additional activists, but there is considerable value in attracting additional adherents who reflect public sentiment favoring particular change. Only in those instances in which the need for tangible resources and individuals is apparent should an effort be made to solicit constituents from the pool of adherents or to mobilize additional activists from among the movement's constituents.

In itself, the recruitment of solitary individuals in support of collective health initiatives adds to the organization demands that confront leaders. Maintaining an adequate supply of talent and sustaining motivation over time can be difficult under the best of circumstances. Targeted recruitment of previously organized interest groups, rather than of solitary individuals may be preferred. Attracting voluntary associations[1] to an initiative offers health promoters several significant advantages over recruiting the sum of individuals of which the association is comprised.

• Associations are predisposed to pursue collective goals. Many voluntary associations are already committed to securing some change of political, economic, or cultural institutions. In their efforts, these associations are often exposed to innovative ideas and ideals well before others within the community. They also may be more willing to embrace promising initiatives before the efficacy of the innovation is firmly established. Moreover, voluntary associations offer their participants a setting for achieving expressive and substantive objectives. In essence, an enhanced payoff that is important to encouraging participation of individuals is available to those already participating in the association.

---

[1] Voluntary associations are intermediate structures within the social order, linking individuals to broader social institutions. They are distinguished, on the one hand, from primary groups such as kinship and friendship groups, which provide intimate interaction between individuals, and, on the other hand, from formal organizations such as governmental or educational institutions that form the social structure of a society (Lauman, 1973). Voluntary associations serve many functions for the individual and society—distributing differential power and prestige among the populace, segregating individuals on the basis of their background and interests, facilitating the dissemination of new ideas and practices, reinforcing important community values (Kornhauser, 1959). Examples of common voluntary associations in our society include professional and trade groups, veteran and patriotic organizations, sports clubs, political-action groups, neighborhood associations, community development organizations, hobby clubs, fraternities/sororities, health/self-help groups, charity, and welfare organizations.

• Associations have a functioning structure to direct group activities. Preexisting mechanisms for distributing responsibility among the rank-and-file, as well as mechanisms for coordinating individuals according to their backgrounds and interests are likely to be in place. Matters of leadership and cooperation, decision making and delegation of authority, and the like, typically have been previously worked out. Thus, the organizational demands placed on individuals who participate are clearly set in advance. Moreover, communication among association members is likely to reinforce shared concerns/ambitions (Granovetter, 1973). The accumulated experience of the group, unlike fads or solitary individuals, supports its ability to perpetuate itself. Thus it can be expected to endure over time.

• Their are practically unlimited opportunities for mobilizing voluntary associations. Analysts have long noted that "Americans of all ages, all conditions and all dispositions constantly form associations" (deTocqueville, 1835/1945, p. 114). Our involvement in voluntary associations is of a magnitude that exceeds that reported for other industrialized nations. On average, persons belong to one to three associations, other than their organized church. Estimates for the number of associations operating within typical communities range from 10 to 60 groups per 1,000 persons.

Enhance Payoffs

A final option which, although most effective, often is difficult to put into place, utilizes supplemental rewards for individuals who take the recommended action. Offers of monetary compensation, enhanced social position and prestige, increased power and authority over specified domains, are among the inducements that may persuade individuals to take the recommended action or to adopt the desired behavior.

Such offers often provide the needed inducements for persons to work actively (and effectively) toward realizing collective outcomes. In fact, it is not unreasonable that rank-and-file workers of organizations advocating change may not embrace the philosophies of the organizations for which they work. "Issue entrepreneurs" are common to many collective efforts that can draw on a stable resource base to supplement the compensation owed to participants. These activists-for-hire frequently can be seen moving freely from one "cause" to another in search of more ample compensation. Indeed, the cost of such expertise is more likely to be determined by prior experience and success than the importance or rightness of the case at hand.

SUMMARY

In spite of compelling justification, it is unreasonable to expect that many people can be motivated to consume more healthful diets if it involves a significant change in their eating habits. Moreover, prevailing health-promotion models that emphasize the psychosocial functioning of individuals may be inadequate in encouraging the public to work together toward collective nutritional health goals. Health promoters are cautioned that motivational appeals stressing the seriousness of health concerns or the individual's vulnerability to situations are likely to be ineffective in these situations.

Collective health initiatives can dramatically improve the well-being of individuals. Notwithstanding the difficulties inherent in encouraging individuals to work toward collective interests, health promoters should be mindful of the importance of including collective health initiatives in a comprehensive health-promotion/disease-prevention strategy. Will Rogers once noted "Even if you're on the right track, you'll eventually get run over if you just sit there" (Rogers, 1993, p. 169).

Appropriate planning can avoid or at least diminish the many difficulties inherent in getting individuals to take on the collective good. Targeted campaigns to organized groups, rather than single individuals, are likely to yield the greatest return and should constitute the major effort of health officials concerned with nutrition and nutrition policy.

REFERENCES

Alinsky, S. D. (1972). *Rules for radicals.* New York: Random House.

Bandura, A. (1977). Self-efficacy: Toward a unifying theory of behavior change. *Psychological Review, 84,* 191–215.

Crawford, R. (1979). Individual responsibility and health politics in the 1970's. In S. Reverby & D. Rosner (Eds.), *Health care in America: Essays in social history.* Philadelphia: Temple University Press.

de Tocqueville, A. (1945). *Democracy in America* (Vol. 2), New York: Knopf. (Original work published 1835)

Farquhar, J., Maccoby, N., Wood, P. D., Bretrose, H., Brown, B. W., Alexander, J. K., Haskell, W. L., McAlister, A. L., Meyer, A. J., Nash, J. D., & Stern, M. P. (1977). Community education for cardiovascular health. *Lancet, 1,* 1192–1195.

Freudenberg, N. (1978). Shaping the future of health education: From behavior change to social change. *Health Education Monographs, 6,* 372–377.

Granovetter, M. S., (1973). The strength of weak ties. *American Journal of Sociology, 78,* 37–45.

Hardin, G. (1968). The tragedy of the common. *Science, 162,* 1243–1248.

Kirscht, J. (1988). The Health Belief Model and predictions of health action. In D. Gotchman (Ed.), *Health behavior: Emerging research perspective.* New York: Plenum Press.

Kornhauser, W. (1940). *The politics of mass society.* New York: Harcourt, Brace & World.

Lauman, E. O. (1973). *Bonds of pluralism.* New York: Wiley.

Leventhal, H., Zimmerman, R., & Gutmann, M. (1984). Compliance: A self-regulation perspective. In D. Gentry (Ed.), *Handbook of behavioral medicine.* New York: Guilford Press.

Luepker, R. V., Murray, D. M., Jacobs, D. R., Mittlemark, M. B., Bracht, N., Carlaw, R., Crow, R., Elmer, D., Finnegan, J., Folsom, A. R., Grim, R., Hannan, P. J., Jeffery, R., Lando, H., McGovern, P., Mullis, R., Perry, C. L., Pechacek, J., Pirie, P., Sprafka, J. M., Weisbrod, R., & Blackburn, H. (1994). Community education for cardiovascular disease prevention: Risk factor changes in the Minnesota Heart Health Program. *American Journal of Public Health, 84,* 1383–1393.

McGinnis, M., & Foege, W. H. (1993). Actual causes of death in the United States. *Journal of the American Medical Association, 270,* 2207–2212.

McKinlay, J. B. (1979). A case for refocusing upstream: The political economy of illness. In E. Garity Jaco (Ed.), *Patients, physicians and illness* (3rd ed., pp. 9–24). New York: Free Press.

McLeroy, K. B., Bibeau, D., Steckler, A., & Glanz, K. (1988). An ecological perspective on health promotion programs. *Health Education Quarterly, 15,* 351–377.

Minkler, M. (1990). Improving health through community organization. In Glanz, Lewis, & Rimer (Eds.), *Health behavior and health education* (pp. 257–287). San Francisco: Jossey-Bass.

Olson, M. (1968). *The logic of collective action: Public goods and the theory of groups.* Cambridge, MA: Harvard University Press.

Perry, C. L., Baranowski, T., & Parcel, G. S. (1990). How individuals, environments and health behavior interact: Social learning theory. In Glanz, Lewis, & Rimer (Eds.), *Health behavior and health education* (pp. 161–186). San Francisco: Jossey-Bass.

Rogers, W. (1993). In R. Collins (Ed.), *Will Rogers says. . . .: Favorite quotes selected by the Will Rogers memorial staff.* Oklahoma City, OK: Neighbors and Quaid.

Ross, M. (1955). *Community organization: Theory and principles.* New York: Harper & Row.

Starr, P. (1983). The boundaries of public health. In *The social transformation of American medicine* (pp. 180–197). New York: Basic Books.

Tesh, S. (1981). Disease causality and politics. *Journal of Health Politics, Policy and Law, 6,* 369–390.

Twain, M. (1924). In C. Nieder (Ed.), *Mark Twain's autobiography.* New York: Harper.

United States Public Health Service. (1988). *The surgeon general's report on nutrition and health.* DHHS Pub. No. (PHS) 88-50210. Washington, DC: U.S. Department of Health and Human Services.

United States Department of Health and Human Services, Public Health Service. (1990). *Health people 2000: National health promotion and disease prevention objectives.* DHHS Pub. No. (PHS) 91-50213. Washington, DC: U.S. Department of Health and Human Services.

Waitzkin, H. (1983). The social origins of illness: A neglected history. In *The second sickness, contradictions of capitalist health care* (pp. 65–86). New York: The Free Press.

CHAPTER 3

Food-Borne Health Risks: Food Additives, Pesticides, and Microbes

Joseph F. Borzelleca

I t may be stating the obvious but the food supply in the United States is one of the safest, if not the safest, in the world. This is due in great measure to the cooperative efforts of the food-producing, food-processing, and food-distribution industries and the appropriate federal regulatory agencies including the U.S. Department of Agriculture (USDA), the U.S. Food and Drug Administration (USFDA), and the U.S. Environmental Protection Agency (USEPA), as well as state and local regulatory agencies. To further ensure the safety of food consumed in the United States (and elsewhere), the government cooperates with other countries to establish international policies and standards for identification and safety. For example, the United Nation's Codex Alimentarius Commission (the Codex) establishes codes and standards involving technical specification, good manufacturing practice, and safety issues. There have been no serious problems and certainly no epidemics related to the chemicals involved in the production and/or processing of foods. Food-related adverse health effects have been microbiological in origin. Microbiological contamination continues to be a problem with the food supply in the United States.

It has been estimated that the average American consumes approximately 1200 pounds of food per year at an average cost of approximately

$1600.00. Approximately 14 cents of every consumer dollar is spent on food.

CLASSIFICATION OF CHEMICALLY BASED AGENTS FOUND IN FOOD

Chemicals found in foods include those that are naturally occurring, are intrinsic to the food, and help to define the food, those that are intentionally added to food for specific purposes (direct food additives), those nonintentionally found in food (indirect food additives), and substances that usually occur naturally with the food, but are not an intrinsic part of the food (contaminants).

Intentional or direct food additives are agents added to foods for specific purposes. There are approximately 2800 approved direct food additives. These are usually classified on the basis of their functionality and include processing aids, texturizing agents, preservatives, flavoring and appearance agents, and nutritional supplements. Processing aids are agents used during production and processing including further processing by the consumer. Processing aids include anticaking agents, dough conditioners, drying agents, emulsifiers, enzymes, flour-treating agents, formulation aids, humectants, leavening agents, lubricants, solvents and vehicles, surface-active agents, and synergists. Texturizing agents are used to provide consistency and texture to foods and include aerating agents, bulking agents, enzymes, firming agents, formulation aids and binders, stabilizers and thickeners, and texturizers. Preservatives are added to foods to decrease the rate of degradation and spoilage during processing and storage. Chemical preservatives include antibacterials, antioxidants, curing and pickling agents, gases, sequestrants, and miscellaneous agents. Radiation and drying are also effective methods of preservation. Flavoring and appearance include Food Drug and Cosmetic (F D & C) colors; flavors and flavoring agents; flavor enhancers; surface-finishing agents; and nutritive and nonnutritive sweeteners. Nutritional supplements are micronutrients and macronutrients that are added to foods to replace nutrients lost during processing or to supplement levels in the food.

Nonintentional or indirect food additives are ingredients found in foods that are not directly added to foods and are not natural constituents of foods. These agents occur in foods as a result of production, processing, packaging, and/or storage. Indirect food additives that occur in foods as a result of production include antibiotics and other agents used to prevent and/or treat disease, growth-promoting agents, microorganisms and their toxic metabolites, parasites, pesticide residues, metals and metallic compounds, and radioactive substances. Agents that occur as a result of processing include foreign materials, microorganisms and their toxic metabolites, processing residues, and radionuclides. Indirect food additives that occur as a result of packaging and storage include identification materials, microorganisms and their toxic metabolites, migrants and leachates from packaging materials, and miscellaneous materials from external sources.

Pesticides

The Federal Insecticide, Fungicide, and Rodenticide Act (FIFRA) defines a pesticide as "any substance or mixture of substances intended for preventing, destroying, repelling, or mitigating any insects, rodents, nematodes, fungi, or weeds or any other forms of life declared to be pests; a substance or mixture of substances intended for use as a plant regulator, defoliant or desiccant." There are about 1,400 active chemical ingredients used as pesticides and these are marketed in about 60,000 formulations; however, only several hundred are used in the production of food. The U.S. pesticide industry produces about 1 billion pounds of pesticides per year. The total value of the pesticides used in the United States is in excess of $5 billion annually. It has been reported that the United States uses 35%–45% of the total pesticides used throughout the world. Herbicides constitute more than 50% of all pesticides used in the United States. Commercial agriculture uses about 90% of the pesticides produced. It should be noted that the term pesticide may refer to the active ingredient or to the mixture of the active ingredient and the inert ingredient (inert means nonpesticidal and not necessarily nontoxic and includes solvents, propellants, surfactants, diluents, carriers, and synergists). Efficacy and safety of pesticides must be established by the manufacturer. Guidelines for the proper safety evaluation of pesticides have been established by the USEPA.

There are several methods for classifying pesticides.

1. *Target pests.* These include avicides (birds), insecticides (insects), rodenticides (rodents), and herbicides (weeds).

2. *Source or origin.* These include naturally occurring chemicals or botanicals such as nicotine, pyrethrum, rotenone, hellebore, and camphor

and synthetic chemicals including inorganic chemicals, such as metals and metallic salts, and organic chemicals, such as organophosphates, carbamates, and halogenated hydrocarbons.

3. *Method of exposure to the pest.* These include stomach poisons where entry is by ingestion of treated food and absorption is from the gut. Target species are chewing insects, such as ants, flies, grasshoppers, and crickets. In contact poisons entry is through the cuticle and the trachea following application to the body surface. Target species are insects with piercing-sucking mouth parts, such as aphids, mosquitoes, and bed bugs. Fumigants are used as vapors in enclosed spaces and entry is through the trachea. Target species include all insects. Residual poisons are applied to the surfaces of insects and entry is through the cuticle, especially of the tarsi. Target species include all insects.

4. *Mechanisms of action.* These include neurotoxins such as the organophosphates, carbamates, and pyrethrin; metabolic inhibitors such as hydrogen cyanide and rotenone; mixed function oxidase (MFO) inhibitors such as propyl isome; hormonmimetics such as juvenile hormone analogues; cytoplasmic poisons such as mercuric chloride, and physical poisons such as sulfur, lime, and mineral.

5. *Chemical class.* Included are aliphatic and aromatic compounds, hydrocarbons, metals, and metallic salts.

Most pesticides are not selective; that is, they usually affect the same target organ(s) in the target species, the pest, and the nontarget species. Rapid knock-down pesticides usually affect the nervous system primarily; longer acting pesticides affect other tissues, but may also affect the nervous system.

Exposure and/or intoxication to pesticides may be acute, as in suicides and following spills or improper application; or chronic, usually involving exposure to low or very low levels for long periods of time. Signs and symptoms of pesticide intoxication depend on the chemical nature of the pesticide, its pharmacological/toxicological properties, and the conditions of exposure including level and duration. Specific antidotes are available for certain pesticides.

Public health issues surrounding the use of pesticides include (1) a critical evaluation of the need for their use; (2) the safety of production workers and applicators; (3) the safety of consumers of agricultural products, including potentially sensitive subsegments of the population; (4) interactions of pesticides with other chemicals including drugs, nutrients, other food chemicals, and environmental chemicals; (5) environmental and ecological concerns including groundwater and surface-water pollution, effects on wildlife, persistence, bioaccumulation, and altering the balance of nature; and (6) risk/benefit considerations including economic aspects, increasing food production per acre, decreasing food losses during storage, and destroying vectors of disease. The proper use of pesticides contributes significantly to increasing potential life expectancy.

Tolerance is the concentration of a pesticide and/or its breakdown products permitted by the USEPA on agricultural products. The USEPA regulates the use of pesticides in conjunction with the USFDA. The level of pesticide permitted on raw agricultural commodities is determined following a critical evaluation of a large body of toxicological or safety data, field trials, and economic considerations. Tolerances for processed foods are determined following a critical evaluation of toxicological/safety data and information concerning the fate of the pesticide during processing (e.g., does it concentrate or break down?). For processed foods, economic impact is rarely considered by regulatory agencies. Monitoring for pesticide residues in domestic and imported raw and processed foods is performed by the USFDA and in meat and poultry by the USDA. The USFDA uses incidence/level monitoring and Total Diet Study, a measure of consumption of various foods, to assist it in determining compliance. Both domestic and imported food must meet the same residue standards. The food industry very carefully monitors pesticide residues to ensure that they are at or below the level approved by the USEPA.

The occurrence of pesticides in consumed foods is very low and is usually below tolerance levels. For example, a study of 6,970 samples of 81 types of fruits and vegetables for 111 pesticides was conducted by H.E.B. Stores in Texas. It was reported that 2.4% of the commodities tested had pesticide residues higher than EPA tolerances or were cases in which the EPA had not established a tolerance. None of the approximately 3,200 samples of milk-based and soy-based infant formulas had detectable levels of pesticides. Pesticide levels are often reduced during processing, refining, and storage. Pesticide residues are not a health problem for the consumer when the pesticides are used properly, that is, in accordance with good agricultural practice and the appropriate regulations, and the food is properly processed and prepared for consumption. No valid human epidemiological studies have been reported that establish a positive correlation between the consumption of pesticide residues in food and adverse health effects. Improper use of pesticides could result in higher residue levels than approved by the USEPA. This could occur as a result of ignorance on the part of the applicator or the improper use could be deliberate. In either event, the residue, although higher than acceptable, would probably not constitute a health hazard to the consumer because of the wide margin of safety that is used in establishing safe residue levels. The improper use of pesticides applied commercially is probably rare for a number of reasons. All commercial applicators are now licensed following an intensive training program. This minimizes, but does not completely eliminate, improper application. If crops are identified with higher than approved residue levels, the crops are usually destroyed and the producer sustains a severe financial loss unless the residue level can be effectively lowered. The improper use of pesticides commercially can be controlled or eliminated by more extensive monitoring.

Contaminants are organisms, parts of organisms or chemicals naturally associated with food but not an intrinsic part of food. Biological and microbiological contaminants include animal and insect parts, filth, bacteria, molds, viruses, and parasites and their toxic metabolites. Chemical contaminants include pesticides, growth-promoting agents, and metals. Physical contaminants include radionuclides.

SAFETY OF FOOD INGREDIENTS

The safety of food additives is based on safety/toxicological data and/or history of safe use and is assured by compliance with the appropriate food safety regulations and proper handling by the consumer.

Safety Evaluation

Safety evaluation is a scientific process of assessing the potential toxicity, that is, the potential adverse health effects of a chemical or physical agent. Initially, this occurs in nonhuman (usually animal) systems and then in humans, when the animal data are adequate and support human testing. A safety-evaluation program is a scientific study designed to identify safe exposure conditions for humans. As such, it must conform to the rigorous principles of scientific experimentation. The data generated from these studies are then critically evaluated and extrapolated to human exposure conditions. Safety is not an inherent biological property of an agent. Safety is a relative term and refers to dose or concentration, route, and duration of exposure to an agent that will not elicit adverse health effects.

Safety-evaluation programs are necessary for societal, regulatory, and economic reasons and are intended to protect the health of the consuming public and involved workers. The societal need is based on moral and ethical obligations for the safety and well-being of fellow humans. Compliance with regulations is mandatory if regulated products are to be marketed. The regulatory agencies are charged with protecting public health and this involves monitoring to ensure compliance with appropriate regulations. Economic reasons to ensure safe products include maintaining market share and preventing litigation.

The single most important factor in the proper design of safety evaluation studies is that the *experimental conditions, including dose, route, and duration of exposure, must simulate anticipated human exposure conditions.* This facilitates extrapolation of animal data to humans. Other considerations include minimizing the use of animals by maximizing the amount of information gleaned from each animal and by identifying critical decision points to determine the need for further experimentation, selecting the appropriate animal model, and proper statistical analysis of the data. *Each agent should be considered unique and testing should be designed for the specific agent* (case-by-case approach). Guidelines from the appropriate regulatory agencies are helpful in the design and implementation of safety studies, however.

The initial step in a safety evaluation program is a clear and succinct statement of the problem or issue to be addressed; for example, how much of a color additive can be added to beverages that will be consumed by adults and children; what is an acceptable residue of a pesticide on apples.

In order to develop an appropriate experimental design, certain background information is necessary. This includes a statement of need for the particular agent, the potential benefits to be derived from its introduction into the marketplace, a thorough search of the scientific literature on the agent and chemically related ones, chemical and physical characterization of the agent, other identifying nomenclature such as the Chemical Abstracts Number (CAS number), structure–activity relationships (SAR), analytical methods, manufacturing practices, and fate during processing. Reliable anticipated human exposure data are essential and these should include nature, conditions, levels, and duration of exposure. If necessary, 100% replacement may be assumed. This information will be used in the experimental design to estimate dose and other conditions of exposure. All the data are critically evaluated by competent toxicologists and adequacy of the data to establish safe exposure conditions for humans is determined. If the data are adequate, testing may not be necessary, safe exposure conditions are defined, and an Acceptable Daily Intake (ADI) is established. Inadequacies are identified and addressed to ensure adequate safety data.

The first test to be conducted is the *acute toxicity test*. Acute exposure refers to a single exposure or dose or the dose may be divided into several doses over the course of the day. This test is designed to evaluate potential toxicity following a single exposure to a chemical or physical agent, to develop an acute toxicity profile, to establish a dose–response relationship, to identify probable sites and mechanisms of toxicity, to assist in dosage selection for further toxicity testing, to identify gender and species differences, and to provide information that could be helpful in managing cases of acute human intoxication to the agent. Exposure conditions must simulate human exposure conditions. Adequate numbers of male and female rodents and nonrodents are used. Parameters evaluated include changes in behavior, motor activity, reflexes, gastrointestinal activity, respiration, skin, food consumption, body weight, morbidity, and mortality. Animals are observed for at least 14 days postdosing. All animals that die during the study and those that survive the postdosing period are necropsied.

Short-term tests for genetic toxicity are conducted at this time. These tests measure the ability of a chemical agent to cause changes in deoxyribonucleic acid (DNA) or in chromosomes and to assess the potential mutagenicity/carcinogenicity of the chemical. The major classes of genetic toxicity tests include those that measure forward and reverse mutations, such as point or deletion mutations, clastogenic or chromosomal changes, such as chromosome aberrations, and micronuclear and DNA damage, such as strand breaks and unscheduled DNA synthesis.

Comparative biodisposition studies, often referred to as absorption, distribution, biotransformation, excretion, and kinetic (ADMEK) studies, are conducted to determine the fate of the chemical in various animal species (in vitro using isolated organs or tissues, cell cultures, or suspensions or in vivo using the intact animal), to identify the appropriate species for further testing, and to provide data to establish appropriate dosing regimens for further toxicity testing. Appropriate animal species often means that the biotransformation of the chemical in that species is the same as in the intact human.

Repeated dosing tests involve exposing adequate numbers of male and female rodents and/or nonrodents to a chemical or physical agent under appropriate experimental conditions for 14–28 consecutive days. These studies are designed to develop a repeated dosing-toxicity profile, to establish dose–response relationships, to identify target organs of toxicity and probable mechanisms of action, and to provide data to establish doses for further animal testing. Parameters evaluated include body weight, food consumption, food efficiency, morbidity and mortality, behavior, signs of intoxication, hematology (blood cells and clotting), clinical chemistry (chemical constituents in the serum), urinalysis (chemicals and cells in the urine), organ weights and their appearance, and gross and histopathological tissue changes. All animals that die during the exposure period and those that survive the treatment (and recovery) period are necropsied and selected tissues examined histopathologically.

Subchronic toxicity tests may be viewed as the most critical studies in a safety-evaluation program because many of the toxic effects seen in longer term studies are usually seen within 3 months, except for cancer and delayed neurotoxicity. Appropriate numbers of young adult male and female rodents and nonrodents are used. Again, exposure conditions must simulate human exposure conditions. Parameters evaluated include body weight, food consumption, food efficiency, morbidity and mortality, behavior, signs of intoxication, ophthalmology (detailed examination of the eye), hematology and clinical chemistry, urinalysis, organ weights and appearance, and gross and histopathological tissue changes. Animals are observed at least twice daily during the study. All animals that die during the exposure period and those that survive the treatment (and recovery) period are necropsied and selected tissues examined histopathologically.

Reproductive toxicity tests are designed to assess the adverse effects of the chemical on most aspects of reproduction, including gonadal function, estrous cycles, mating behavior, conception, gestation, parturition, neonatal morbidity and mortality, lactation, weaning, growth and development of the offspring, and the reproductive capacity of the offspring. Adequate numbers of male and female rodents are used. The initial test is usually a Segment I study, a one-generation test that is approved by the USFDA. A subsequent test is a multigeneration reproduction study (MGR) involving at least two generations, which is also conducted in rodents, usually the rat. Parameters evaluated include those related to reproductive performance and outcome and body weight, food consumption, behavior, signs of intoxication, morbidity, and mortality. Parents and offspring may be necropsied and selected tissues evaluated histopathologically.

Developmental toxicity tests are designed to assess the adverse effects of the test material on the developing organism, when either or both parents are exposed to the test material prior to conception, or when the female is exposed during gestation and/or postnatally. Usually the pregnant female receives the test material during the period of organogenesis, which is the period of heightened sensitivity of the developing organism to adverse influences; it usually occurs during the first trimester. Depending on the stage of development, a chemical may be termed an embrytoxin, fetotoxin, or a teratogen. Adequate numbers of pregnant female rodents and nonrodents (usually the rabbit) are used. The parameters evaluated include body weight, food and water consumption, behavior, signs of intoxication, gross examination of the uterus of the dams, and size, sex, weight and gross and microscopic morphology of the offspring. A Segment II, USFDA protocol may be used.

Long-term toxicity tests usually involve 6–24 months of continuous exposure to the test material. Adequate numbers of young adult male and female rodents and nonrodents are used. These tests are designed to develop a long-term toxicity profile in several species for comparative purposes, to identify target organs and mechanisms of toxicity, to establish dose–response relationships, to provide data on cumulative effects and on reversibility of effects, to assess carcinogenic potential, and to identify the "no observed adverse effect level" (NOAEL) and the "lowest observed adverse effect level" (LOAEL) for extrapolation to humans. Parameters evaluated include body weight, food consumption, food efficiency, morbidity and mortality, behavior, signs of intoxication, ophthalmology, hematology and clinical chemistry, urinalysis, organ weights and their appearance, and gross and histopathological tissue changes. All animals that die during the exposure period, those that are sacrificed at selected intervals, and those that survive the treatment (and recovery) period are necropsied and selected tissues examined histopathologically.

Chronic toxicity or lifetime tests are conducted to assess the toxic effects of the test material during a lifetime of exposure (that may include in utero exposure), to develop a chronic toxicity profile, to establish dose–response relationships, to identify target organs and mechanisms of toxicity, to provide data on cumulative effects, to assess the reversibility of compound-related effects, to assess definitively the carcinogenicity of the test material, and to identify the no observed adverse effect level and the lowest observed adverse effect level for extrapolation to humans. Parameters evaluated are similar to those described under long-term toxicity tests. All animals that die during the exposure period and those that survive the treatment (and recovery) period are necropsied and selected tissues examined histopathologically.

Carcinogenicity or oncogenicity studies are definitive tests designed to assess the carcinogenicity of the test material. These tests are usually conducted in the mouse and rat. These tests are considered definitive because the exposure is very long, usually 18–24 months of continuous exposure, and the doses are very high, often orders of magnitude higher than anticipated human exposure. It should be noted that at these very high doses, the biodisposition of the test material may be significantly different from that observed at lower doses, thereby making these studies less appropriate for extrapolation to humans who are usually exposed to low doses. Parameters evaluated include signs of intoxication, morbidity, and mortality. All animals that die during the exposure period and those that survive the treatment period are necropsied and selected tissues examined histopathologically. To conserve resources, carcinogenicity/ oncogenicity studies can be combined with the chronic toxicity study (chronic toxicity/ carcinogenicity study).

The extent of testing necessary to establish safe conditions of exposure/ consumption is dependent on the chemical and physical nature of the ingredient and the extent of exposure (how much, by whom, and for how long). A comprehensive safety-evaluation program for a direct food additive or a pesticide is very expensive and time-consuming; it may take 5–10 years to complete and the costs could exceed $3 to $5 million. Although the expense is justified by the benefits that will accrue to the consuming public, the extent of testing can be reduced without compromising human safety by incorporating a tiered approach to testing, by the use of appropriate nonstandardized tests, and by the use of human data. There have been no recorded outbreaks of adverse health effects directly attributable to the use of approved direct and indirect food additives in the United States. This is due in great measure to the cooperative efforts of the USFDA, USDA, and USEPA to regulate and monitor the use of these chemicals and to the dedication of the food industry to provide wholesome and safe foods. However, this was not always the case. Regulations were necessary because at one time some elements of the food industry were not as committed to protecting public health as is often the case today.

A BRIEF HISTORY OF THE REGULATION OF FOOD ADDITIVES IN THE UNITED STATES

The first food inspection law was enacted in 1890, not to protect American consumers but to convince foreign companies that American food was safe and wholesome. The situation at that time was shocking. For example, it was not uncommon to add floor sweepings to pepper, lead salts to candy and cheese, copper salts to peas and pickles, acorns to coffee, and brick dust to cocoa. Some 80 colors were used in food processing. Often these were the same dyes used in the textile industry. It has been reported that dyes that were not acceptable to the textile industry were sometimes used in foods. Only 2 of the 80 colors used then are still used today, FD & C Red No. 3 and FD & C Blue No. 2. It was the confectioners of America who first introduced industry-wide standards of purity for colors used in their products shortly after the turn of the century.

The Tea Importation Act of 1897 made it unlawful to import tea that was "inferior in purity, quality, and fitness for consumption to the standards provided in section 43 of this title."

Upton Sinclair's book, *The Jungle*, describes vividly the situation that prevailed in the meat industry in Chicago. It had a significant impact on the American public and on its representatives in Washington. In 1883, a young physician and chemist, Dr. Harvey Washington Wiley, was hired by the U.S. Department of Agriculture as head of the Bureau of Chemistry. His charge was to protect the consuming public from unsafe food ingredients. To accomplish this, he evaluated the safety of commonly used food ingredients by feeding them to healthy young male employees of the Department of Agriculture, the "poison squad," who were required to take all their specially prepared meals in the kitchen of the Bureau of Chemistry. Dr. Wiley carefully observed their responses to the various ingredients. He issued a number of bulletins that summarized his studies on the safety of food ingredients. His efforts and Sinclair's book led to the enactment of the Pure Food and Drug Law or the Food and Drugs Act of 1906 (FDA, Public Law 59-384 and its amendments). This six-page document was the first law to address the issue of food safety. It was enacted "for preventing the manufacture, sale, or transportation of adulterated or misbranded or poisonous or deleterious foods, drugs, medicines, and liquors, and for regulating traffic therein, and for other purposes." It required a label identifying the contents but not the weight or volume. The Bureau of Chemistry was responsible for enforcing the Food and Drugs Act.

The Federal Meat Inspection Act was approved in 1907 (Public Law 59-242) and was enforced by the USDA. The provisions of this Act were completely revised by the Wholesome Meat Act, which was approved in 1967. The Act provided for meat and meat food products to be "wholesome, not adulterated, and properly marked, labeled, and packaged."

The Insecticide Act of 1910 was the government's first attempt to regulate pesticides.

The Gould Amendment of the FDA (1913) required the declaration of the net contents on the label.

The Federal Trade Commission Act of 1914 empowered the Federal Trade Commission (FTC) to monitor food advertising.

The Filled Milk Act of 1923 prohibited the sale of milk to which fat or oil other than milk fat had been added.

The Federal Import Milk Act of 1927 (Public Law 69-625) established regulations for the importation of milk and cream into the United States to protect the public health.

The Food, Drug, and Insecticide Administration (FDIA) was established by Congress in 1927 to enforce the Food and Drugs Act; the FDIA became the Food and Drug Administration in 1931.

The Federal Food, Drug, and Cosmetic Act of 1938 (FDCA, Public Law No. 75-717) was the result of the sulfonamide elixir incident in which diethylene glycol was used and resulted in a number of deaths, especially of children. Under the Act, the FDA was given authority to perform plant inspections, to establish standards of identity for individual food products, to certify colors (it created three categories of colors: colors approved for use in foods, drugs, and cosmetics (FD&C colors), colors approved for use in drugs and cosmetics only (D&C colors), and colors approved for external use only (external D&C colors), and to obtain injunctions (in federal court) against violators of the law. In 1940, the FDA became part of what is now known as the Department of Health and Human Services.

The Agriculture Marketing Act was passed in 1946.

The Federal Insecticide, Fungicide, and Rodenticide Act (FIFRA) was passed in 1947. FIFRA established criteria for evaluating the safety of pesticides.

The Miller Amendment of the FDCA (Public Law 83-518), passed in 1954, empowered the FDA to establish tolerances for "economic poisons" or pesticides in or on fruits, vegetables, and agricultural produce.

Food Additives Amendment of 1958 (Public Law No. 85-929) empowered the FDA "to prohibit the use in foods of additives which have not been adequately tested to establish their safety." The term *food additive* was officially defined as

> any substance the intended use of which results or may reasonably be expected to result, directly or indirectly, in its becoming a component

or otherwise affecting the characteristics of any food (including any substance intended for use in producing, manufacturing, packing, processing, preparing, treating, packaging, transporting or holding food; and
including any source of radiation intended for any such use), if such substance is not generally recognized as safe [GRAS] among experts qualified by scientific training and experience to evaluate its safety, as having
been adequately shown through scientific procedures (or in the case of a
substance used in food prior to January 1, 1958, through either scientific
procedures, or experience based on common use in food) to be safe
under the conditions of its intended use.

A food was considered adulterated unless a regulation was issued
describing the conditions under which the additive could be used.

Section 409 described procedures for submitting a petition to the FDA
for approval of a specific ingredient for specific applications. This submis-
sion was to include data to prove the efficacy of the ingredient, the amount
needed to produce the desired effect, analytical methods for detecting the
ingredient and other substances formed as a result of the addition of the
ingredient, and safety information. The petition would be approved or
denied within 90–180 days of filing.

Food ingredients were to be regulated as food additives, generally recognized as safe ingredients [GRAS], or prior-sanctioned ingredients. The
latter category includes those ingredients that the USFDA approved on an
individual basis by way of letter to the petitioners. Some of the letters have
apparently disappeared from the files of the FDA, but not from company
files. The USFDA no longer approves ingredients as prior sanctioned. The Act
required that food additives be adequately tested to establish their safety.

GRAS was a separate status, distinct from food additives. It was the intent
of Congress that GRAS substances would not have to undergo mandatory
premarket approval by the FDA. GRAS substances had to satisfy the following criteria, however:

- general recognition of safety by qualified experts;
- the experts must be qualified by scientific training and experience;
- the experts must base their determination of safety on scientific procedures;
- for substances used in foods prior to 1958, determination of safety
  could be made on the basis of scientific procedures or established
  safe use (common use) in food;

- the intended uses of the GRAS substance must be considered as part of the determination of general recognition of safety.

It was the intent of Congress for the private sector to have the right to make GRAS determinations. This was supported in 1988 when the FDA issued a final rule and declared that "persons have the right to make independent GRAS determinations."

Safety is defined in the Code of Federal Regulations (CFR) (21 CFR Sec. 170.3 (i), 1994) to mean "that there is a reasonable certainty in the views of competent scientists that the substance is not harmful under the intended conditions of use;" that is, reasonable certainty of no harm. With respect to *absolute safety* (that no harm will occur under any conditions of exposure/use), the FDA has stated:

It is impossible in the present state of scientific knowledge to establish with complete certainty the absolute harmlessness of the use of any substance. Safety may be determined by scientific procedures or by general recognition of safety. In determining safety, the following factors shall be considered: (1) The probable consumption of the substance and of a substance formed in or on food because of its use. (2) The cumulative effect of the substance in the diet, taking into account any chemically or pharmacologically related substance or substances in such diet. (3) Safety factors which, in the opinion of experts qualified by scientific training and experience to evaluate the safety of food and food ingredients, are generally recognized as appropriate.

GRAS status depends on general recognition or common knowledge throughout the scientific community that is knowledgeable about the safety of food or of ingredients added to foods and not on safety per se. FDA has declared that "a substance may not be determined to be GRAS when its characteristics are known only to a few experts." FDA has further stated that "general recognition of safety requires not only the general availability of appropriate evidence on the substance but also general agreement on the interpretation of evidence. FDA believes that this general agreement can occur only when similarly qualified experts share an understanding of the concept of safety." The term general has been interpreted to mean "extensively, though not universally; most frequently, but not without exception."

The Delaney Clause stated "that no additive shall be deemed safe if it is found to induce cancer when ingested by man or animal, or, if it is found, after tests which are appropriate for the evaluation of the safety of food additives, to induce cancer in man or animal." The Delaney Clause applies to the additive as a whole and not to de minimis amounts of carcinogenic constituents (FDA's constituent policy of 1982). The Delaney Clause does not apply to GRAS substances; Congress intended GRAS substances to be exempt from the Delaney Clause. It is possible that carcinogens that pose a trivial risk for humans and are therefore safe could be classified as GRAS.

With respect to scientific procedures, the FDA has stated:

> General recognition of safety based upon scientific procedures shall require the same quantity and quality of scientific evidence as is required to obtain approval of a food additive regulation for the ingredient. General recognition of safety through scientific procedures shall ordinarily be based upon published studies which may be corroborated by unpublished studies and other data and information.

The FDA has further stated that:

> General recognition of safety through scientific procedures does require that the scientific evidence . . . has been published in the literature or otherwise widely disseminated throughout the scientific community knowledgeable about the safety of food ingredients. . . . Accordingly, there will be at least some gap between the gathering of the scientific knowledge necessary to provide the toxicological underpinning for general recognition of safety and the dissemination to and assimilation by the scientific community of this material that is necessary for general recognition of safety to exist.

The courts have ruled that the complete absence of published information on a substance precludes a determination of GRAS. The data need not come from its use in food only; for example, if the substance is an ingredient of a drug formulation and a food, then the drug data can also be considered.

With respect to common use in food (prior to 1958), the FDA opined that:

> General recognition of safety through experience based on common use in food prior to January 1, 1958 may be determined without the quantity or quality of scientific procedures required for the approval of a food

additive regulation. General recognition . . . shall ordinarily be based on generally available data and information.

If the food has been consumed for many years, it is presumed safe. Common has been defined as "a substantial history of consumption of a substance by a number of consumers." Common use is not limited to the United States. Common use as a drug may not satisfy the common-use-in-food requirement.

With respect to conditions of intended use, the FDA has stated: "It has been too often assumed that the GRAS substance may be used in any food, at any level, for any purpose. As a result, the uses of some GRAS food ingredients have proliferated to the point where the GRAS status was brought into serious question." Conditions of intended use is a limitation for GRAS substances and is intended to prevent GRAS status in one category from being automatically transferred to another.

As a result of this amendment to the Federal Food, Drug, and Cosmetic Act (FDCA), the petitioner is required to establish the safety of the food additive and must petition for premarket approval .

The Color Additive Amendments of 1960 (CAA) (Public Law No. 86-618) was enacted "to protect the public health by amending the Federal Food, Drug, and Cosmetic Act so as to authorize the use of suitable color additives in or on foods, drugs, and cosmetics, in accordance with regulations prescribing the conditions (including maximum tolerances) under which such additives may be safely used." Late in 1958 the Supreme Court ruled that the FDA did not have the authority to set tolerances or limits on colors used in foods. There was some concern about color safety because of 3 instances of diarrhea in children presumed to be caused by FD&C Orange No. 1 and FD&C Red No. 32 (used in candy and popcorn). Shortly after this, and based on animal toxicity data, the FDA delisted FD & C Orange No. 2 and FD&C Red No. 32. Late in 1958 and early 1959, FD&C Yellow Nos. 1, 2, 3, and 4 were delisted and this left no approved oil-soluble colors. Lakes were introduced. Lakes are defined as "straight color extended on a substratum by adsorption, coprecipitation, or chemical combination that does not include any combinations of ingredients made by a simple mixing process." A lake is a certified water-soluble FD&C color on a substrate of aluminum hydrate or aluminum hydroxide. The lakes are used to color oils or other products where water is not desirable. The lakes themselves must be certified by the FDA. Colors are now referred to as color additives and not food additives.

Title I of the Color Additive Amendment describes procedures for dealing with permitted certified and noncertified colors. It states that all colors, natural and synthetic, are to be treated in the same manner (equally). Pretesting requirements for all color additives were made uniform. The FDA was empowered to prescribe conditions of use, set specifications and tolerance limitations, and labeling and packaging requirements for the color and the foods that contain the color. In establishing safe conditions of use, the FDA is to consider the probable consumption of the color, and substance formed as a result of the consumption of the color, cumulative effects, analytical methods for detection and quantification of the color, safety factors, and potential carcinogenicity (Delaney-like clause). If the use of the color in foods promotes deception of the consumer, it cannot be listed.

In 1957, prior to passage of the Color Additives Amendment, the FDA began feeding studies in several animal species for all colors used in foods at that time. The data helped to establish acceptable daily intakes of color additives.

Title II of the Color Additives Amendment deals with provisional listing of color additives that were in use as of 12 July 1960. Provisional listing was to extend for $2^1/2$ years after the amendment was passed to permit scientific/safety studies on these colors to be completed. The USFDA was empowered to extend this time, and did. All colors in use at the time the CAA was passed were provisionally listed. Subsequently, the Certified Colors Manufacturers Association (now the International Association of Color Manufacturers) conducted a multimillion dollar safety evaluation of all certified colors to reaffirm their safety.

Most flavor ingredients are GRAS. In a remarkably effective and efficient cooperative venture between the Flavor and Extract Manufacturers Association (FEMA) and the FDA, the safety data on flavors and extracts are reviewed by an expert panel; and, if certain rigorous criteria are met, the material is determined to be GRAS. The procedures used are consistent with the intent of Congress when it passed the Amendments to the Food, Drug, and Cosmetic Act in 1958.

The Poultry Products Inspection Act of 1957 (Public Law 85-172) was enacted to ensure "that the health and welfare of consumers be protected by assuring that poultry products distributed to them are wholesome, not adulterated, and properly marked, labeled, and packaged."

Two additional Acts that were passed around this time were the Fair Packaging and Labeling Act of 1960 and the Animal Welfare Act of 1960.

The Wholesome Meat Act (Federal Meat Inspection Act) of 1967

(Public Law 59-242) was a complete revision of the Meat Inspection Act of 1907 (Public Law 59-242).

The Egg Products Inspection Act of 1970 (Public Law 91-597) was enacted to ensure "that the health and welfare of consumers be protected by the adoption of measures prescribed herein for assuring that eggs and egg products distributed to them and used in products consumed by them are wholesome, otherwise not adulterated, and properly labeled and packaged."

The 1970s saw the passage of three more Acts: The Federal Environmental Pesticide Control Act of 1972 (revision of FIFRA); The Safe Drinking Water Act of 1974; and The Fishery Conservation and Management Act of 1976.

The Saccharin Study and Labeling Act of 1977 (Public Law 95-203) prohibited the FDA from amending or revoking the interim food additive regulation applicable to saccharin. Under the provisions of the Delaney Amendment, the FDA must ban the use of any food additive found to cause cancer in laboratory animals or in humans. Because there were no other approved nonnutritive sweeteners, the public outcry to the banning of saccharin was such that Congress responded by passing this law.

The Pesticide Monitoring and Improvements Act of 1988 (Public Law 100-418) required the Secretary of Health and Human Services to

> place in effect computerized data management systems for the Food and Drug Administration under which the Administration will (A) record, summarize, and evaluate the results of its program for monitoring food products for pesticide residues . . . and provide information to assist the Environmental Protection Agency in carrying out its responsibilities under the Federal Insecticide, Fungicide, and Rodenticide Act and the Federal Food, Drug, and Cosmetic Act.

The Sanitary Food Transportation Act of 1990 (Public Law 101-500) was enacted "to prohibit certain food transportation practices and to provide for regulation by the Secretary of Transportation that will safeguard food and certain other products from contamination during motor or rail transportation, and for other purposes."

The Nutrition Labeling and Education Act of 1990 (NLEA, Public Law 101-535) mandated a Nutrition Facts label that includes standardized serving size; servings per container; calories per serving; calories from fat; percentage of daily value of total fat, saturated fat, cholesterol, sodium, total carbohydrate, dietary fiber, sugars, protein, selected vitamins (A, C, D), iron, and calcium based on a 2,000-calorie diet. This comprehensive and readily comprehensible label should enable consumers to know what they are eating and to permit comparisons among similar products. The order in which ingredients are listed is dependent on the level in the food; the ingredient present in the highest concentration is listed first and the others in decreasing order.

National Nutrition Monitoring and Related Research Act of 1990 (Public Law 101-445) was enacted:

> To strengthen national nutrition monitoring by requiring the Secretary of Agriculture and the Secretary of Health and Human Services to prepare and implement a ten-year plan to assess the dietary and nutritional status of the United States population, to support research on, and development of, nutrition monitoring, to foster national nutrition education, to establish dietary guidelines, and for other purposes.

Enforcement of these food regulations and monitoring by the appropriate regulatory agencies, coupled with cooperative interaction between these agencies and the producers, processors, and distributors of food, have resulted in making the American food supply among the finest and safest in the world. The history of food safety regulations in the United States parallelled advances in toxicology and other biomedical sciences, food production, and food technology. A serious public health problem due to the use of regulated chemicals in food has never occurred. Based on this history, it seems highly unlikely that there ever will be a problem caused by the use of regulated chemicals in food. The use of genetic engineering and biotechnology has resulted in the introduction of unique, more nutritious, more appealing, and less expensive foods. Here, also, the regulatory agencies and the food industry have cooperated to insure that these new foods are wholesome and safe.

From the public-health perspective, there is little need for concern for the safety of regulated chemicals used in the production, processing, or packaging of food. Attention should be directed to educating the consuming public and to continued and improved monitoring. Postmarketing surveillance (PMS) of approved food ingredients should be considered an essential component of a food-safety program. PMS should provide reliable data on consumption patterns, daily intake of the particular food chemical, and beneficial and adverse effects associated with the consumption of the new food or food ingredient. This continuing effort should provide continued assurance to the consumer, the regulator, and the producer that the material is safe. The consumer has a right to know the composition of processed foods and their nutritional value. The new label is informative but more information is needed. Appropriate health claims that are approved by the FDA should be included because many foods are considered functional foods; that is, they can prevent or modify the course of disease. The major issue today is proper utilization of available foods, not the safety of prepared or processed foods.

MICROBIAL AGENTS FOUND IN FOOD

Food-borne pathogens, which cause microbiological contamination of foods, continue to be a significant public health problem worldwide. This problem has been with humans since the beginning of time. In most instances, food-borne microbial diseases can be prevented by proper preparation and proper handling of cooked food. In the United States, the Centers for Disease Control and Prevention (CDC) tracks public health problems and has reported that food-borne pathogens may cause 6½ million acute sicknesses a year in the United States. Food-borne pathogens may be responsible for about 9,000 deaths annually. Most cases of food-borne illnesses are not reported because they are usually not life-threatening. The number of food-borne illnesses is increasing and this may result from ecological and social changes resulting in overcrowded and unsanitary conditions in developing countries and in countries at war; increases in foreign travel; importation of food from developing countries; changes in consumption habits, such as increased consumption of unprocessed foods; a growing population of individuals at risk including the chronically ill, the elderly, and the immunocompromised, and the introduction of new and/or novel food ingredients, such as macronutrient substitutes (for fat and sugar). It should be noted that virulence of an organism is dependent on many factors including the nature and number of the organism; growth conditions; the production of toxins (endo-, exo-); the nature, quantity, and conditions of consumption of the contaminated food; and the health of the consumer (chronically ill, immunocompromised).

The major classes of bacterial pathogens found in food include Acinetobacter (*Acinetobacter johnsonii* and *A calcoaceticus*, *A baumannii*, *A lwofii*; cyanobacteria); Aeromonas (*Aeromonas hydrophila*); Bacillus (gram-positive rods: *Bacillus cereus* and *B megaterium, B anthracis, B thuringiensis, B subtilis, B cereus* var. *mycoides*); Brucella (*Brucella melitensis, B abortus,* and *B suis); Chlamydia (Chlamydia psittaci*); Cocci (Gram-positive: *Staphylococcus aureus; Streptococcus pyogenes*); Enterobacteriaceae (Gram negative, facultative anaerobic bacilli); *Escherichia coli* and *E coli* 0157:H7, *E coli* VTEC, *E coli* EHEC, *E coli* ETEC; *Yersinia enterocolitica* and *Y pseudotuberculosis; Salmonella typhimurium* and *S agona, S choleraesuis, S enteritidis, S infantis, S wangata, S virchow, S typhi, S paratyphi, S livingstone, S javiana, S mikawasima; Shigella sonnei, S dysenteriae, S boudii,* and *S flexneri; Klebsiella pneumoniae*); Helicobacter (helicobacter pylori); Lactobacillus (*Lactobacillus rhamnosus* and *L Plantarum, L casei, L salivarius, L acidophilus*); Legionella (*Legionella pneumophila*); listeria (Gram-positive bacillus that is beta-hemolytic): *Listeria monocytogenes, L innocua, L ivanovii, L seeligeri, L welshimeri, L murrayi,* and *L grayi*); Plesiomonas (*Plesiomonas shigelloides*); Proteus (*P vulgaris* and *P morgani*); Pseudomonas (*Pseudomonas aeruginosa*); spore-formers (*Clostridium botulinum* and *C perfringens*); Vibrionaceae (*Vibrio cholerae* and *V mimicus, V parahaemolyticus, V vulnificus, V hollisae, V fluvialis, V danseka, V metschnikovii; Campylobacter jejuni* and *C coli,* [Gram-negative rod]).

Food-borne pathogens may be controlled commercially by rigorous adherence to quality-control standards developed for individual organizations. The use of hazard analysis critical control point (HACCP) systems and the ISO 9000 series of standards would enhance the production of safe foods. Irradiation of foods would increase food safety because many pathogens are sensitive to radiation. Healthier and safer animals for human consumption could be produced by using better methods of production including the use of probiotics and biotechnology. Bacteriocins (antimicrobial polypeptides produced by bacteria) added to foods could also improve their safety. These agents enjoy a history of safe use and are "natural" and would appeal to consumers. The principle of controlling microbial growth by bacterial competition is well established. Other chemical agents could also be used to control the growth of food pathogens including the lactoperoxidase system, sodium lactate, and sulfhydryl-containing amino acids and peptides. The use of appropriate packaging materials may also serve as a barrier to pathogenic bacteria.

The signs and symptoms of food-borne pathogenic infections are usually referable to the gastrointestinal tract and may include nausea, vomiting, cramps, and diarrhea. Fever may or may not be a sign of infection. Other systems may be affected if the organism or the toxin it produced enters the blood stream leading to septicemia. Most food-borne infections are not fatal in otherwise healthy individuals. Populations at risk include individuals with preexisting (chronic) disease or those who are immunocompromised, the elderly, and the very young. Examples of some food-borne pathogenic infections follow.

Salmonella

There are 2,200 known serotypes of salmonella and these include those highly adapted to humans (including *S typhi, S paratyphi A, B, C,* and *S sendai*); those that cause diseases primarily in animals (*S gallinarum-pullorum* in chickens, *S abortus equi* in horses, *S abortus ovis* in sheep, *S cholerae suis* in pigs and *S dublin* in cattle, and two human pathogens, *S dublin* and *S cholerae suis*); and those that are unadapted to specific hosts (*S agona, S infantis,* and *S saint paul; S typhi murium* and *S enteritidis* pose a serious threat to humans). Most bacterial diarrheal diseases worldwide are caused by salmonella. The foods most commonly associated with salmonella include poultry, eggs and egg products, meat, smoked fish, yeast, and airline food. Infected animals, such as pet turtles, may also be a source of salmonella. Salmonellosis may be caused by most strains of salmonella, including *S enteritidis, S typhi murium, S virchow,* and *S paratyphi*. Salmonellosis may be associated with gastroenteritis, enteric fever, bacteremi, and infections at sites other than the gastrointestinal tract. At increased risk are children, persons with AIDS, and individuals being treated for peptic ulcers with H_2 antagonists and antibiotics. Outbreaks of salmonellosis have usually been associated with egg-related products and/or poultry.

Typhoid fever is caused by *S typhi*, which is associated with milk, shellfish, water, and other improperly handled cooked foods; it can also be transmitted by chronic carriers.

Shigella

There are more than 30 known serotypes of shigella and these are divided into subgroups A (*S dysenteriae*, virulent); B (*S flexneri*); C (*S boydii*); and D (*S sonnei*, the most common cause of shigellosis [bacillary dysentery] in the United States). Shigella is distributed worldwide. Some of the foods most frequently associated with shigellosis include moist salads, turkey, shrimp, milk, beans, and apple cider; the source is often infected carriers (fecal–oral route) and flies. Shigellosis is often associated with severe gastrointestinal signs and symptoms including pain, distention, diarrhea, and electrolyte imbalance. Infection with shigella does not usually impart immunity.

Escherichia coli

There are four groups of *E coli*: enterotoxigenic (ETEC), enteroinvasive (EIEC), enteropathogenic (EPEC), and enterohemorrhagic (EHEC). *E coli* normally inhabit the gastrointestinal tract, but may spread to other tissues if the protective barriers in the gut are disrupted. Because it is opportunistic, it may cause disease in patients with compromised immune systems (for example, cancer, cirrhosis, or diabetes) or those receiving steroids, radiation, or antibiotics. The signs and symptoms caused by *E coli* in the gut (enterotoxic) include vomiting, diarrhea (rice-water stools), and electrolyte imbalances. Signs and symptoms caused by the invasive type include fever, headache, myalgia, cramps, and diarrhea (profuse, watery).

E coli 0157:H7 (a verotoxigenic *E coli*) is one of the most virulent forms of *E coli* known. It ranks behind *Toxoplasma gondii*, salmonella, and campylobacter as a serious food-borne disease. It was first identified as a food-borne pathogen in 1982 as a result of minor outbreaks of bloody diarrhea in Oregon and Michigan. This was followed by outbreaks in Ontario, Canada in 1985, in Minnesota in 1986, in Washington state in 1988, in Cabool, MO in 1990 (the largest outbreak up to that time, which was caused by contaminated water), in Massachusetts in 1991 (due to contaminated apple cider), in Oregon in 1991 (due to fecal pollution of a lake used for swimming), and in Washington state in 1993 (due to undercooked hamburger meat). *E coli* 0157:H7 is also associated with Hemolytic Uremic Syndrome (HUS), and renal failure in children that usually follows bloody diarrhea. Most outbreaks have been associated with insufficiently cooked hamburger meat, although rare roast beef, raw milk, and contaminated water have also been shown to be the source of the organism.

Enterotoxigenic *E coli* was identified in two outbreaks in 1993. An outbreak in Rhode Island was associated with carrot/lettuce salad and one in New Hampshire was associated with tabouleh.

Yersinia

Yersinia is a psychrotrophic organism (that is, it can survive at temperatures of 5 degree C or less). Yersinosis is usually associated with gastrointestinal signs and symptoms including diarrhea. Foods involved include poultry, meats, and raw milk.

Staphylococcus

S aureus is found in the nose of humans, in and around the udders of lactating animals, in bruised tissues of poultry, skin infections such as furuncles, secretions from infected respiratory tract, and feces. Foods become contaminated by improper handling (transmission from wounds, storage at improper temperatures). Foods usually associated with staphyloccocal poisoning include meat and poultry products, sauces and gravies, cream-filled pastries, milk and dairy products, and salads. It is the staphylococcal enterotoxin and not the organisms per se that cause the following: nausea, vomiting, cramps, diarrhea, headache, and fever. The very young, the elderly, and the chronically ill are especially at risk.

Streptococcus

Contamination of food with *S pyogenes* usually results from handling by infected food handlers. *S faecalis* and *S faecium* are found in the intestinal tracts of animals and humans. Foods reported to be involved in adverse reactions caused by enterococci include meat dishes, fish, cheese, and sausage. The symptoms include nausea, vomiting, and diarrhea.

Bacillus anthracis

Intestinal anthracosis may result from ingesting meat contaminated with anthrax but it is uncommon.

Bacillus cereus

B cereus is associated with gastrointestinal signs and symptoms including vomiting and diarrhea. *B cereus* is found in water and soil and has been reported in rice, poultry, cereal and cereal products, vegetables, custards, and meat.

Brucella

Brucellosis is a rare disease and may be associated with *B abortus,* or *B melitensis.* Brucella may be found in meat, milk, and dairy products. Some of the signs and symptoms include undulating fever, headache, malaise, cervical pain, sweating, weakness, anemia, and constipation.

Campylobacter

Three species of campylobacter have been reported to be human pathogens: *C fetus fetus, C jejuni,* and *C coli.* Both *C jejuni* and *C coli* can cause severe gastroenteritis. Foods usually associated with campylobacteriosis include meat from infected animals, poultry, raw milk, and contaminated water. *C jejuni* may be associated with Guillain–Barré Syndrome.

Helicobacter

H pylori infection has been associated with duodenal ulcer, gastritis, and dyspepsia. Infection with *H pylori* may increase the risk of gastric cancer. Raw poultry may be a mechanical vector for *H pylori.* It has not been found in other foods.

Listeria

There are seven serotypes of *Listeria monocytogenes.* Listeriosis in the United States is caused mainly by types 4b, 1b, and 1a. Listeriosis is most likely to occur in neonates, and persons above 40; peak incidence is during July and August. Persons with a preëxisting disease or with immunodeficiencies are at greater risk. Listeriosis can occur through ingestion of contaminated dairy products and poultry products and by contact with infectious material (meat from infected animals). *L monocytogenes* survives in soil and water; it is found in sewage and in decaying vegetation, and in vegetables grown in contaminated soil. High-risk foods include dairy products, raw milk, meat, and ready-to-eat and refrigerated foods. The most common form in adults is meningitis. Listeriosis may be accompanied by fever, bacteremia, and lymph-node enlargement. Although three outbreaks occurred in the United States between 1981–1985, it is not a significant public health problem at this time.

Clostridia

These gram-positive, spore-forming anaerobic bacilli exist widely in nature and are found in soil, vegetation, and in the gastrointestinal tracts of humans and animals. About 100 species have been identified, and 10–12 are pathogenic in humans and animals.

C botulinum

C botulinum elaborates seven distinct toxins and humans are poisoned by Types A (seen west of the Mississippi River), B (seen in the Eastern states), E (seen in Alaska and the Great Lakes area), or F (rare). The neurotoxins interfere with the release of acetylcholine at the endings of peripheral nerves and are considered among the most potent poisons known. Most common sources of *C botulinum* include home-canned foods and improperly canned low-acid foods, vegetables, fish, fruits, condiments, honey, meat, poultry, dairy products, and seafood. Signs and symptoms are primarily neurological and may result in respiratory failure and paralysis. Mortality is high (35%–65%).

C perfringens

C perfringens is found in soil, water, air, and feces. The toxin elaborated by Strain A causes a mild gastroenteritis that is self-limiting but the toxin elaborated by Strain C usually causes a severe, fatal gastroenteritis characterized by severe diarrhea, distention with gas, and collapse. Foods associated with Clostridia disease include contaminated meat and milk.

Vibrios

Vibrios are found in water, milk, poultry, meat, oysters, and fish. They are usually associated with severe gastroenteritis that may be fatal.

Vibrio cholerae

V cholerae 01 Eltor was associated with the outbreak in Peru that spread to other countries in 1991 (seventh cholera pandemic). The eighth cholera pandemic occurred in 1993 and involved Bangladesh, India, Pakistan, Nepal, China, and Malaysia. The organism associated with this pandemic was *V cholerae* 0139 (Bengal).

V fulnificus is found in oysters. It rarely poses a severe health problem for individuals in good health. Especially sensitive are immunocompromised persons or those with achlorhydria, chronic liver disease, or hemochromatosis. *V parahaemolyticus* is associated with sea food and has been associated with reactive arthritis.

Aeromonas

Aeromonas occur in fish and other seafood, poultry, meat, and water and can produce enterotoxins, cytotoxins, and hemolysins.

Lactic Acid Bacteria

Lactic acid bacteria are found in most nonsterile parts of the body. These bacteria are used to produce fermented foods and their benefits to health have been well documented. Occasionally they may cause infections in humans, especially individuals who have serious illnesses. *L rhamnosus, L plantarum, L casei, L salivarius,* and *L acidophilus* have been associated with bacterial endocarditis. *L acidophilus, L rhamnosus,* and other unspecified strains have been associated with gastrointestinal infection. The continued use of lactic acid bacteria in the production of food does not pose any threat to health. Their beneficial effects have a long history.

Plesiomonas

P shigelloides has been found in some farmed freshwater fish. The significance for humans has not been clearly established, but diarrhea was reported in individuals whose stools were positive for the organism.

Pseudomonas

Pseudomonas have been isolated from fresh and spoiled fish. Pseudomonas infections usually occur in hospitals from contact with persons carrying the organism. Nausea, vomiting, cramps, and diarrhea are the signs and symptoms most often reported in patients. Some strains of pseudomonas have antibacterial properties.

Legionella

Legionella spp. have been found in water and their presence in food is usually the result of using contaminated water. It affects several target systems including the gastrointestinal tract.

Mycobacterium

M avium has been found in water and its presence in food is the result of using contaminated water.

Acinetobacter

Only a limited number of acinetobacter are capable of causing disease in humans; for example, *A calcoaceticus, A baumannii, A johnsonii,* and *A lwoffii.*

Cyanobacteria

Cyanobacteria produce neurotoxins (anatoxin-a and anatoxin-a(s), hepatotoxins, and cytotoxins.

Chlamydia

C psittaci was associated with chlamydiosis in workers at a duck farm and processing plant.

FOOD-BORNE VIRAL DISEASES

Hepatitis and gastrointestinal disorders including gastroenteritis and diarrhea may be caused by viruses found in water, seafood, raw milk from infected animals, and other foods (for example, fresh fruit).

FOOD-BORNE PARASITIC INFECTIONS

Parasitic intestinal disease is a serious health problem, especially in developing countries and in immunocompromised individuals. The pathogenic parasites may be ingested in contaminated food or water.

Pathogenic protozoa include *Cryptosporidium parvum, Toxoplasma gondii, Giardia lamblia, Deentamoeba fragilis, Blastocystis hominis, Balantidium coli, Isospora belli, Entamoeba spp, Sarcoystis spp,* and cyclospora. Pathogenic roundworms (nematodes) that may infect flesh food include

Ascaris lumbricoides, Trichuris trichiura, Capillaria philippinesis, Angiostrongylus costaricensis, Anisakis simplex, and *Trichinella spp.* Pathogenic flukes (trematodes) include *Fasciolopsis buski* (associated with contaminated raw water plants), *Heterophyes heterophyes* and *Metagonium yokogawai* associated with infected freshwater fish; and *Echinostoma spp* associated with raw infected snails, amphibians, or fish. The genus Taenia includes pathogenic tapeworms (cestodes).

The gastrointestinal diseases including diarrhea caused by protozoa usually follow the ingestion of contaminated water. Pathogenic nematodes are usually found in the flesh of the infected animals; for example, Anisakis in fish and Trichinella in pork. Infections with some tapeworms occur when animal tissue infected with the organism is ingested (for example, *Diphyllobothrium dendriticum* and *Diphyllobothrium latum* in fish). Other infections are the result of contact with human carriers (for example, taenia solium). Flukes, especially the liver fluke, *Fasciola hepatica,* create serious public health problems. Trematode or fluke infections usually occur following the ingestion of raw or improperly cooked freshwater fish, shellfish, frogs, snakes, and plants associated with contaminated seafood (aquatic vegetables).

Plankton

Bivalves including clams, mussels, cockles, oysters, and scallops may ingest toxic dinoflagellates (*Gonyaulax catenella, G acatenella, G tamarensis,* and *Pyrodinium phoneus*), "red tide," from June to October. These organisms produce saxitoxin, a potent neurotoxin that is resistant to cooking. The condition that results from ingesting contaminated bivalves, known as paralytic shellfish poisoning or dinoflagellate poisoning, is characterized by circumoral paresthesias, nausea, vomiting, cramps, muscle weakness, and peripheral paralysis including respiratory paralysis. Death is usually caused by respiratory failure.

Molds and Mycotoxins

Molds have been used in the production of various foods (for example, cheeses) for many years and may synthesize compounds that are beneficial or harmful (mycotoxins). Molds are usually associated with grains and grain products and occur in the field (during production) or during storage.

Aspergillus spp

Aspergillus flavus and *Aspergillus parasiticus* produce aflatoxins (AFB1, B2, G1, G2, and M1) that affect the liver; some are carcinogenic. Both strains of Aspergillus have been associated with corn and other grains, peanuts and legumes, spices, dairy products, meat, and fish. *Aspergillus ochraceus* produces ochratoxin, a nephrotoxin and a carcinogen. *Aspergillus terrus* (found on rice) produces territrem-B, a neurotoxin. Sterigmatocystin, which is produced by *Aspergillus versiolar*, is found on corn and is reported to be carcinogenic. Other mycotoxins produced by Aspergillus include kojic acid and cytochalasins E, B, F, and H.

Fusarium spp

Fusarium mycotoxins including zearalenones (ZEA, estrogenic), deoxynivalenol (DON, vomitoxin) and nivalenol (NIV), have been detected in corn and cereal grains. *Fusarium moniliforme* elaborates fumonisins B1, B2, B3, B4, A1 and A2 and fusarins A, C, and F; some of these have been reported to be carcinogenic. Trichothecenes including T-2 toxin (immunotoxin) have been reported on corn, cereal grains, and wheat and are elaborated by *Fusarium graminearum, Fusarium poae,* and *Fusarium sporotrichioides.*

Penicillium spp

Mycotoxins are elaborated by various species of Penicillium. *Penicillium verrucosum* elaborates ochratoxin A (nephrotoxin) and citrinin; *Penicillium viridicatum* elaborates ochratoxin; *Penicillium aurantiogriseum* elaborates xanthomegnin, viomellein, and vioxanthin; *Penicillium expansum* elaborates citrinin; *Penicillium citreoviride* elaborates citreoviridin; *penicillium cyclopium* elaborates penicillinic acid; *Penicillium rubrum* elaborates rubratoxins A and B (hepatotoxin and developmental toxin); and *Penicillium patulatum* elaborates patulin (developmental toxin). Other mycotoxins elaborated include cyclopizaonic acid (toxic to muscle, liver, spleen).

Ergot

Claviceps purpurea produces ergot alkaoids, which may cause ergotism. Ergot is found mostly on grains.

NATURALLY OCCURRING TOXICANTS IN FOOD

Probably the most renowned of the naturally occuring toxicants are those found in seafood. The seafood toxins include ciguatoxins, which are neurotoxins that affect many tissues and that are found in ciguatera that have ingested the dinoflagellate, *Gambierdiscus toxicus*.

Tetrodotoxin, a potent neurotoxin produced by marine microbes and accumulated by the reticulated blowfish (puffer fish); paralytic shellfish poisoning (PSP) due to accumulation in mussels, clams, and scallops of a neurotoxin, saxitoxin, produced by the dinoflagellates *Gymnodinium catenatum* (*Gonyaulax catenella*), *Alexandrium tomarense* (*G tamerensis*) and *A catenella* (*G acatenella*), *Pyrodinium phoneus*, and *Anabaena circinalis*; domoic acid (amnesic shellfish poisoning), a toxin found in shellfish that have ingested the diatoms, *Pseudonitzschia pungens* and *P australis*; diarrhetic shellfish poisoning (DSP) is due to a toxin containing okadaic acid, which is produced by *Dinophysis acuminata*, and these organisms are consumed by shellfish; palytoxin containing polycavernosides A and B is elaborated by the red alga; Caulerpa toxifolia, a green alga, produces a toxin that is found in the flesh of fish that have consumed the alga; hemotoxin is found in the blood of the moray eel and the conger but not in the flesh; hepatotoxins from the consumption of the livers of Japanese mackerel, sea bass, sandfish, porgy, abalone, sea turtles.

Biogenic amines are produced in certain foods such as meat, cheese, fish, sauerkraut, and alcoholic beverages. Some of the amines include histamine, tyramine, phenylethylamine, and spermine.

Toxic constituents have been identified in mushrooms (hydrazines, diazonium salts, ibotenic acid, phallotoxins, amatoxins); in comfrey (pyrrolizidine alkaloids); potatoes (glycoalkaloids); green peas (beta-N-oxalyl-L-alpha, beta-diaminopropionic acid, beta-ODAP); cycad fruits (beta-methylamino-L-alanine, BMAA); cassava (cyanogenic compounds including linamarin); soybeans (protease inhibitors); and certain Chinese herbal teas (aconitine). Other classes of potentially toxic chemicals found naturally in foods include alkaloids; phenols (flavonoids, coumarins, furocoumarins, tannins, gossypol); amino acids (domoic acid, shellfish toxin, acromelic acid from mushrooms, D-amino acids, which are hepatoxic and nephrotoxic); phytates from certain grains; saponins in legumes and grains; lectins from red kidney beans; phytoestrogens; and vicine and divicine from broad beans.

Food-borne pathogens usually result from improper production or processing of food, although some microbes and toxins are found naturally in certain foods. The usual target organ of toxicity is the gastrointestinal tract but other sites may also be involved. The most potent toxins are the neurotoxins. Food-borne pathogens can be controlled in commercial operations by strict adherence to quality-control standards. More difficult control is at the level of the consumer. This will require an intensive and extensive educational effort spearheaded by the appropriate governmental agencies with the cooperation of the food industry and academic institutions. Appropriate labels will provide invaluable guidance to the consumer at the critical point of preparation and storage. The enthusiastic cooperation of the media is absolutely essential if a program to eliminate food-borne pathogens is to be successful.

CONCLUSIONS

The production, processing, and distribution of food that is nutritious, safe, and affordable is a laudable public health goal. Economic progress is impossible in a population that is undernourished for whatever reason. If available resources including talents are expended exclusively to produce food, there will be no advances in technology or artistic pursuits. But merely increasing food production is not enough. Food that is produced must satisfy basic nutritional needs. In addition, it must be safe and available. Chemical and physical agents are used to improve the nutritional profile of foods, to modify organoleptic properties (for example, taste, smell, mouth-feel), to prolong shelf-life, and make the food affordable for the consuming public. Agents that are used in food processing are evaluated for safety prior to introduction into the marketplace. The extent of safety testing that is conducted is dependent on the chemical nature of the ingredient and the extent of exposure; less data are required for an indirect food additive than for a direct additive. There has never been an outbreak of adverse health effects caused by an approved food ingredient in the United States. This is due in great measure to the concerns and cooperative efforts of the food-producing, processing, and distribution industries and the appropriate regulatory agencies, both federal and state. Controlling food-borne pathogens presents a greater challenge because of the nature of the microbes, including their ubiquity and virulence. Strict adherence to appropriate quality–control guidelines in the production and processing of food will minimize or eliminate some of the hazards. The use of novel approaches to control microbes, for example, radiation, will also help to eliminate some of the dangers posed by microbial contamination. Multimedia education of the consumer and the use of appropriate labels will ultimately eliminate this hazard.

Public health officials and those concerned with the health and safety of the consuming public should actively and aggressively reassure the public that the current food supply is nutritious and safe and should be enjoyed. In addition, guidance on the proper handling of food should be offered.

REFERENCES

Berger, S., & Cwiek, K. (1987). Nutritional importance of pesticides. In J. N. Hathcock (Ed.), *Nutritional toxicology* (Vol. II, pp. 281–288). New York: Academic Press.

Borzelleca, J. F. (1992). Macronutrient substitutes: Safety evaluation. *Regulatory Toxicology and Pharmacology, 16,* 253–64.

Coats, J. R. (1987). Toxicology of pesticide residues in foods. In J. N. Hathcock (Ed.), *Nutritional toxicology* (Vol. II, pp. 249–279). New York: Academic Press.

Degnan, F. H. (1991). Rethinking the applicability and usefulness of the GRAS concept. *Food, Drug, Cosmetic Law Journal, 46,* 553–582.

Doyle, M. E., Steinhart, C. E., & Cochrane, B. A. (1994) *Food safety 1994.* New York: Marcel Dekker.

Food Research Institute. (1994). *Food safety 1994.* New York: Marcel Dekker.

Food Research Institute. (1995). *Food safety 1995.* New York: Marcel Dekker.

Hallagan, J. B., & Hall, R. L. (1995). FEMA-GRAS- A GRAS assessment program for flavor ingredients. *Regulatory Toxicology and Pharmacology, 21,* 422–430.

Hutt, P. B. (1978). Food regulation. *Food, Drug, Cosmetic Law Journal, 33,* 505–589.

Irving, G. W., Jr. (1982). Determination of the GRAS status of food ingredients in nutritional toxicology, In J. N. Hathcock (Ed.), *Nutritional toxicology* (Vol. 1, pp. 435–450). New York: Academic Press.

Kotsonis, F. N., Burdock, G. A., & Glamm, W. G. (1996). Food toxicology. In C. D. Klaassen (Ed.), *Casarett and Doull's toxicology, the basic science of poisons* (5th ed., pp. 909–949). New York: McGraw-Hill.

Lloyd, W. E. (1986). *Safety evaluation of drugs and chemicals.* New York: Hemisphere Publishing Co.

Miller, S. A. (1991). Food additives and contaminants. In M.O. Amdur, J. Doull, & C. D. Klaassen (Eds.), *Casarett and Doull's toxicology* (4th ed., pp. 819–853). New York: Pergamon.

Thayer, A. M. (1992, June 15). Food additives. *Chemical Engineering News*, pp. 26–44.

The Food and Drug Law Institute.(1993). *Compilation of food and drug laws.* Washington, DC: Author.

U.S. Food and Drug Administration, Center for Food Safety and Applied Nutrition. (1993). *Toxicological principles for the safety assessment of direct food additives and color additives used in food* ("Redbook II"). Washington, DC: U.S. Government Printing Office.

CHAPTER 4

Legal Aspects of Food Protection

Barbara Blechner and Stephen Fontana

L aws that encompass nutrition are part of a complex system of laws that concern food. The federal government, the 50 states, and the municipalities of the United States all promulgate laws that regulate the food we eat and influence our dietary choices. Federal and state constitutions, statutes, judicial opinions and local laws and regulations are included in the intricate web of laws that determine how we are fed.

Traditionally, laws have been developed to rectify onerous situations. The protective arm of the law initially focused on protecting the safety of its citizens from food contamination and safe food became synonymous with quality food. As food production and processing technology improved, and knowledge of nutritional science grew, however, people came to associate food quality with nutrition and general healthfulness as well as safety. In response, the law evolved not only to protect people, but also to serve the larger goal of enhancing the nutritional value of the food we eat.

Food-law development in the United States has relied on the generally accepted principle that society has the right to mandate conduct to ensure food quality. The Constitution of the United States, the source of this principle, allows federal regulation of all items that enter interstate commerce and therefore allows regulation of food. The Food and Drug Administration (FDA) bears the main responsibility for the safety of the nation's food supply and the main body of food law that pertains to it.

The Department of Agriculture (USDA) and the Federal Trade Commission (FTC), also contribute regulations to the larger body of food law and these regulations frequently mirror FDA regulations. The federal government also accepts some responsibility for improved nutrition to underserved populations by overseeing food-assistance programs. In addition, the Constitution mandates in the Tenth Amendment that all powers not delegated to the federal government by the Constitution are reserved by the states. The states, under their "police power" mandate, are responsible for the protection of the health, safety, and welfare of the population, and therefore may promulgate laws to ensure the quality and safety of the foods we eat. The states frequently either delegate these powers to the local health departments, or local departments of health exercise these powers concurrent with states (Christoffel, 1982). States and municipalities exercise inspection and licensing authority over food as it is manufactured, distributed, and sold in wholesale and retail outlets and restaurants.

This chapter looks at the legal issues of nutrition from a historic perspective and examines the evolution of U.S. food law from colonial times to the present (cf. Chapter 3). It concentrates on the development of federal food law in Congress, of food regulations at the FDA, and on court cases that tested both Congressional laws and FDA regulations. Finally, it discusses some potential directions U.S. food law may take in the future.

U.S. food law covers four areas: safety and quality assurance, nutrition labeling, vitamin and dietary supplement regulation, and health claims. Safety and quality assurance focus on the federal government's efforts to assess and guarantee food purity. Nutrition labeling encompasses the federal government's efforts to communicate important information about food content and healthfulness. Vitamin and dietary supplement regulation comprises the federal government's attempts to control both the health claims and labeling standards of these food products. Health claims regulation addresses the federal government's activities to monitor and verify the alleged benefits of foods.

Throughout the development of food law there have been constant checks and balances in the form of court cases that have attempted to settle controversies over legislation. These controversies have helped shape the laws about food and nutrition. The food law that has developed and continues to evolve is a consensus of societal opinion that has arrived at a balance between zealous protection of the health and safety of society on the one hand and industrial and corporate needs on the other hand.

U.S. FOOD LAW (1641 TO 1938)

Safety, Quality Assurance, and the FDA

People have always cared about food quality and safety. Since ancient times, different societies have assessed criminal and civil penalties for food adulteration (Hutt & Merrill, 1991). American food law dates back to colonial times. As colonists settled here, they found that they needed laws to deter food adulteration (Janssen, 1975). In 1641 Massachusetts passed the first American food law, requiring the "official inspection of beef and pork to determine 'that the best be not left out.'" (Hutt & Hutt, 1984, p. 35). Five years later, Massachusetts also passed the first bread law, mandating weight standards (Hutt & Hutt, 1984; Janssen, 1975). In 1720, after several tragic incidents, the Massachusetts colony rewrote this bread law to prohibit not only substituting grains in bread flour, but also to prevent the production of bread "found wanting either in the goodness of the stuff whereof the same shall be made, or in the due working or baking thereof" (Janssen, 1975, p. 667). Similar laws were enacted by other colonies (Lyons & Rumore, 1994).

In 1785 Massachusetts passed the first food-adulteration law in the new United States, the "Act against selling unwholesome Provisions." It carried penalties for selling "diseased, corrupted, contagious or unwholesome" food (Janssen, 1975, pp. 668–669; Nestle, 1994, p. 38). Many states and localities then passed similar laws in the 1800s that emphasized the prevention of food adulteration through weight standards and inspections.

By the end of the 19th century, however, local laws could not ensure the safety of foods shipped from other states or overseas. U.S. industrialization and urbanization generated growing demand for packaged foods, but state officials had neither the resources nor expertise to create and enforce standardized food laws.

Two events ultimately compelled national action. In 1903, Dr. Wiley, the Chief Chemist of the U.S. Department of Agriculture, created a volunteer "poison squad" of 12 of his subordinates to eat foods containing suspect ingredients to test their safety (Janssen, 1980; Lyons & Rumore, 1994). When the public learned of these tests, and then read Upton Sinclair's *The Jungle* in 1906, with its graphic depiction of poor U.S. food safety, their concerns about food safety exploded.

Congress responded by passing the Federal Pure Food and Drugs Act.[1]*

---

* Subscripts refer to Notes, where legal references are cited.

The Act defined "food" as "all articles used for food, drink, confectionery, or condiment by man." (Cooper, Frank, & O'Flaherty, 1990, p. 658). It also defined adulteration, and prohibited selling misbranded or adulterated foods. Third, it allowed the government to stop producers from making suspect health claims about their products. Fourth, it established the Bureau of Chemistry, which became the Food and Drug Administration in 1930, to monitor and enforce food safety within the USDA (Greenberg, 1990).

Although the Act gave the government powers over misbranded or adulterated foods, it severely limited these powers. The law did not require any form of product labeling (Lyons & Rumore, 1994), nor did it create any legal standards for foods (Hutt & Merrill, 1991). It also did not allow the federal government to demand proof of food-product safety or effectiveness before producers put a product on the market (Kassel, 1994).

Over the next 30 years, the Federal Pure Food and Drug Act prevented many adulterated foods from reaching consumers, but food producers still violated the law. For instance, "Certain products containing water, glucose, grass seed and artificial color continued to be marketed as 'fruit' jams" (Kassel, 1994, p. 250; Lyons & Rumore, 1994, p. 172). In 1938, after more than 100 people died from drinking a supposedly healthful "Elixir of Sulfanilamide" (Janssen, 1980; Wax, 1995), Congress passed the Federal Food, Drug and Cosmetic Act (FFD&CA).[2] This Act created the legal framework for nearly all of our current U.S. food law.

THE BIRTH AND GROWTH OF THE FDA

The passage of the FFD & CA permitted the government to expand its jurisdiction over food products by broadening the definitions of "food" and "label." It prohibited adulterated food containing "any poisonous or deleterious substance which may render it injurious to health"; limited the amount of harmful substances that food could contain; and established standards for special dietary foods, such as weight-control products, to address growing complaints about their safety. In addition, it prohibited producers from putting false or misleading statements on food labels, and required food labels to list "the name and address of the manufacturer, the net quantity of contents, the statement of ingredients, and the name of the food" (Hutt & Hutt, 1984, p. 67).

Most important, however, the law greatly expanded the FDA's ability to implement the provisions of the law giving the agency extensive power to regulate, investigate, enforce, and develop policy. The agency now could regulate any area of food commerce that it felt would benefit from regulation, or when it received a request from industry or public interest groups about a current problem. The agency was required to provide a period of review for new regulations, during which interested parties could comment and suggest revisions, and to publish the final regulations. These regulations, according to the law, had to be "reasonable" and "promote honesty and fair dealing in the interest of consumers" (Hutt & Hutt, 1984).

Finally, the FDA received investigative powers to inspect food production and shipping facilities, to analyze food samples, and to educate food producers and the public (Janssen, 1980). The enforcement powers of the FDA included bringing and supporting civil actions for injunctions against individual producers for misbranding. These actions were and continue to be litigated by the Justice Department. The law also authorized the FDA to seize foods that violated the law.

The FDA shares authority with the USDA and the FTC in the area of policy development. The USDA has exclusive authority to regulate meat, poultry, and egg products,[3] whereas the FTC maintains overlapping authority to regulate all food advertising.[4]

The Nutrilite Case and the Delaney Amendment

During and after World War II, the FDA used the FFD&CA to broaden its powers over producers. As it used these powers, however, the FDA soon determined that it did not have enough authority to reshape completely all questionable behavior on the part of food producers. To achieve larger reforms, the FDA needed the help of the courts or Congress.

The FDA first found help in the courts. The courts proved willing not only to allow the FDA to prosecute violators, but to use FDA prosecutions to set policy. Generally, "the FDA created policy by bringing legal action against persons or companies that it considered to be in violation of the law. If the agency's actions were supported [in court], this then constituted policy for future action" (Wodicka, 1990, pp. 60–61).

To fight suspect health claims, for instance, in the late 1940s the FDA prosecuted a vitamin and mineral producer for false or misleading claims. To dispose of this litigation, the producer eventually entered into an agreement with the federal government called the "Nutrilite Consent Decree."[5]

This agreement allowed the FDA to establish restrictive industry guidelines for legally acceptable vitamin and mineral labeling (Hutt, 1986). With court help, the FDA then extended this consent decree to the entire vitamin- and mineral-producing industry, thereby broadening the aspects of food production under its control.

The FDA also received help from Congress. Shortly after the "Nutrilite" case, Congress moved to supplement FDA authority by granting the FDA powers to investigate chemicals in food generally. Congress recommended passing laws to create preapproval procedures for various additives and to prohibit carcinogens (cancer-causing agents) from processed foods altogether. In 1958, Congress passed the Food Additives Amendment,[6] also known as the Delaney Clause or Delaney Amendment (Nestle, 1994), which bolstered and expanded the FDA's authority to monitor both food ingredients and the dietary or health claims that producers made for them (Hutt, 1986). The Amendment prohibited the federal government from allowing any proven carcinogens at any level into processed foods. This became known as the "zero-risk" standard.

The Delaney Amendment made two important changes in the law. First, it allowed the FDA to restrict or ban any additive or food ingredient that it deemed unsafe (Hutt, 1986). Second, it shifted the burden of proof onto food producers by forcing them to prove that the additives they used were safe, rather than requiring the FDA to prove that those additives were unsafe (Greenberg, 1990). This change improved the FDA's ability to safeguard the food supply. "Preventing violations through premarketing clearance procedures gave consumers immeasurably better protection than merely prosecuting the few violations which could be proved by investigating after injuries were reported" (Janssen, 1980, p. 137).

In the 1960s, Congress passed other laws to expand the FDA's powers. The Fair Packaging and Labeling Act (FPLA),[7] for instance, gave the FDA the authority to block misleading, deceptive, and unfair food packaging and labeling (Lyons & Rumore, 1994). It explicitly required foods "to bear a label specifying the identity of the product, the net quantity of contents, and the net quantity of each serving" (Hutt & Hutt, 1984, p. 63).

Food-Assistance Programs

During this time period, Congress also created several programs to *deliver* improved food nutrition to certain underserved populations. These programs, the Special Supplemental Food Program for Women, Infants, and

Children (WIC), the Food Stamp program, and the School Breakfast and School Lunch program, all subsidize the purchase and/or consumption of food by those people who do not have the resources to provide fully balanced meals for themselves or their families.

WIC (cf. Chapter 13) serves mothers and small children who are ineligible for food stamps or Medicaid, but whose family income does not exceed 185% of the federal poverty level. It "provides nutrition counseling and healthy foods for pregnant women, post-partum mothers and their children up to age 5." (Center, 1995, p. A19). Under WIC, eligible families receive numbered vouchers for specific amounts of food items that "increase iron, calcium, protein and Vitamins A and C in the diet" (Peterman, 1995, p. 6D), such as milk, cheese, eggs, cereal, juice, peanut butter, beans, baby food, infant formula, and tuna (McVicar, 1995). WIC serves roughly 7 million people, and costs more than $4 billion annually (Center, 1995, cf. Chapter 13).

The Food Stamp program provides 27 million people in low-income households with coupons or vouchers to purchase food of any kind except alcohol and tobacco. The program, initiated in 1964, currently costs about $27 billion per year (Bessonette, 1995). The School Breakfast and School Lunch programs give roughly 25 million children from low-income households breakfasts and/or lunches with specified nutrient content.

State Programs

After World War II, many states passed laws, often modeled after federal laws, to complement and cooperate with federal efforts, particularly in the areas of inspections, licensing, and permit requirements (Kirschbaum, 1983). States then delegated or shared duties in these areas with the municipalities. Connecticut passed laws, for instance, authorizing the commissioner of consumer protection to inspect any establishment where bread, bread products, or grains "are manufactured, processed, packed, sold or held,"[8] as well as generally any establishment that produces, transports, or holds foods.[9]

Today, states share food-safety responsibility with the federal government and municipalities by contracting with the FDA to perform food inspections and conducting these and other program activities with local health departments. States focus on inspections of dairy farms, dairy plants, restaurants, and food-service establishments, exercising greater control over foods such as milk and milk products (Kirschbaum, 1983). The FDA, on the other hand, focuses on food inspections of manufacturing operations and "health-risk" industries, "concentrat[ing] much of its food inspection work plan on manufacturing and wholesale operations" (Kirschbaum, 1983, p. 201).

As the 1960s ended, and as both Congress and the FDA consolidated their powers to ensure food safety, quality, and nutrition, various forces began to reshape the FDA's mission. In 1969 President Nixon convened a White House Conference on Food, Nutrition and Health. The report issued after this conference "emphasized the need for sound nutrition . . . and the use of increased public information about nutrition" (Hutt & Merrill, 1991, p. 42). The FDA recognized that, to address these and other food concerns (such as the health effects of dietary fat) (Hutt, 1986), it had to reassess its mission.

RECENT HISTORY (1970-1990): HEALTH CLAIMS, NUTRITION LABELING, AND DIETARY SUPPLEMENTS

During the 1970s, the FDA determined that one of its primary goals was the establishment of a national food policy that focused on emerging, large-scale issues, such as nutrition and nutrition labeling. To achieve this goal, the FDA decided that the most efficient way to construe the FFD&CA was to issue regulations that set forth FDA policy.

The courts, for the most part, endorsed the FDA's approach to extending its regulatory powers. An appeals court stated that this approach

> provides the agency with an opportunity first to receive a wide spectrum of views proffered by all segments affected by the proposed rule (e.g., manufacturers, vendors, doctors, consumers) and then in a legislative fashion to consider and choose from several alternatives or options rather than limiting its decisions to narrow issues controlling a particular case. (*National Nutritional Foods Association v. Weinberger*, 1975)

Nutrition Labeling

Until 1970 the FDA had prohibited all health claims for foods, and sued companies for "outright nutrition claims that it considered false or misleading"

(Hutt & Hutt, 1984, p. 67). Meanwhile, increasingly sophisticated food producers had found ways to manipulate the law and make questionable claims. In 1972, as a concession to food producers, the FDA decided to relax its restrictions, and even allow more health claims on food labels. In return for this concession, the FDA required food producers to provide nutrition information to consumers.

To deter questionable health claims and to communicate nutritional information more efficiently, the FDA wrote new regulations to toughened nutrition labeling requirements. Because the FDA wanted to focus less on the vitamins in foods and more on ingredients that might cause cancer or heart disease, its final nutrition labeling regulations mandated that there be "a format for declaring the percentage of saturated, monounsaturated, and polyunsaturated fatty acids in a product" (Wodicka, 1990, pp. 61–62). The FDA also "issued general principles governing the establishment of nutritional quality guidelines" (Hutt & Hutt, 1984, p. 69), guidelines that prescribed "the minimum level or range of nutrient composition appropriate for a given class of food" (Hutt, 1986).

The FDA continued to regulate nutrition labeling in the 1970s by requiring that food labels disclose all "material facts" relating to claims made for them. This approach meshed well with Congressional legislation in the 1970s, such as the National Consumer Health Information and Health Promotion Act,[10] which encouraged the federal government to expand nutrition-related education (Hutt, 1986). These regulations largely stood intact, both because the public supported them, and because no food company cared to challenge them in court (Wodicka, 1990).

Originally, the FFD&CA prohibited companies from modifying their products without an explicit and specific exception, but this requirement discouraged companies from improving the healthfulness of their products. To encourage companies to make their products healthful, the FDA decided to step back from efforts to regulate food identity standards (i.e., what constitutes a natural, "real" food, as opposed to an "imitation" or "substitute" food).

By 1973 the FDA also decided that "appropriate labeling would be sufficient to protect the interests of consumers" as long as labeling defined "the 'common or usual name' of foods" (Hutt & Hutt, 1984, p. 66). It therefore had drafted new food-standards regulations that "required the use of the word 'imitation' only when the product was nutritionally inferior to its [natural] counterpart" (Wodicka, 1990, p. 63), yet also required that a food bear "a descriptive name that adequately distinguishe[s] it" from the food it sought to imitate (Cooper et al., 1990, p. 661). In relaxing its regulatory role in this area, the FDA hoped to reallocate its resources to focus on nutritional labeling.

Public interest groups that opposed the FDA's plan to relax its regulatory role became concerned by these new food standards regulations, however. In *Federation of Homemakers v. Schmidt* (1976), a national consumer group claimed that the FDA's actions created regulations in an arbitrary and capricious manner, thus violating the FFD&CA and the procedural safeguards it established. The court held, however, that the FFD&CA entitled the FDA to define "imitation," and that the agency had not violated Congress's objectives when it passed the FFD&CA. The court also held that the old definition of "imitation" "unduly deterred the development of new food products" (*Federation of Homemakers v. Schmidt*, 1975, p. 774). The court concluded, "This regulation, directed at the laudable aims of encouraging manufacture of nutritional food products and of better informing consumers . . . , lies well within the bounds of discretion which the FDA may exercise [to advance the public's welfare]." (*Federation of Homemakers v. Schmidt*, 1975, p. 774).

This case affirmed the FDA's "imitation" labeling regulations (Cooper et al., 1990), and established rule-making as a part of the FDA's established regulatory powers. Courts continue to uphold the validity of the FDA's food-standards regulations, as well as the agency's right to enforce its regulations as it best determines.

As a result of this case, industry groups quickly realized that they needed to develop other approaches for challenging FDA regulations. Although industry groups could sue the FDA, to win they had to convince a court to overturn regulations applying the specialized expertise of the FDA by showing that the regulations were not based on a fair evaluation of the evidence (Wodicka, 1990). Industry groups therefore decided that their best approaches now lay in attempting to persuade Congress to place legal restrictions on the FDA.

Dietary Supplements

The dietary-supplement industry vigorously pursued this alternate approach. Dietary supplements comprise various substances, such as vitamins, minerals, amino acids, herbs, and enzymes. Dietary-supplement producers often claim that their products contain ingredients, missing or deficient in a normal diet, that offer a unique health or lifestyle benefit. Americans respond to these claims. According to one survey, 40% of American adults use dietary supplements hoping to improve their health (Kassel, 1994). Many Americans also abuse dietary supplements, however, creating health risks for themselves (Kassel, 1994).

The federal government has attempted to regulate dietary supplements since the early 1900s, when producers made medicinal claims for cod-liver oil (Hutt, 1986). As the consumption of dietary supplements has risen, the FDA increasingly has involved itself in testing these supplements and investigating their manufacturers' claims. The dietary supplement industry, in return, has resisted these efforts (Kassel, 1994).

In 1966, after years of a quieter, case-by-case enforcement approach, the FDA raised the intensity of its approach when it published proposed dietary supplement regulations that would "limit the number of vitamins and minerals that could be added to foods, the levels at which they could be added, and the foods to which they could be added" (Hutt & Hutt, 1984, p.67). Threatened, the industry fought to revise or delay these regulations by pursuing its options within the administrative review process (Sidak, 1993). This strategy postponed the issuance of final regulations until 1973.

When the industry learned that these regulations "limited the numbers of nutrients that could lawfully be included, established lower and upper limits for these permissible levels, and specified the permitted combinations" (Hutt, 1986, p. 62), it sued the FDA in 1974 over the agency's method of reviewing evidence and writing regulations. In *National Nutritional Foods Association v. FDA* (1974), an appeals court required the FDA to broaden its regulations to conform to statutory requirements and to reopen the administrative record for additional evidence before it could implement final regulations that prescribed identity standards and label statements for vitamins and minerals.

Fearing that this court decision might be only a temporary victory and that the FDA's regulations ultimately would stand, the dietary-supplement industry convinced Congress to pass the Vitamin-Mineral Amendments in 1976.[11] These laws limited the agency's regulatory authority and enforcement power in relation to vitamin and dietary supplements (Sidak, 1993), and brought to a halt the FDA's efforts to limit the strength of any vitamin or mineral or the number or combination of vitamins, minerals, or other food ingredients in food.

The FDA tried to modify its regulations to satisfy the industry, but the industry continued to challenge them. In *National Nutritional Foods Association v. Mathews* (1977), an appeals court ruled that the FDA could not declare that vitamins over a set dosage constitute drugs rather than foods. In *National Nutritional Foods Association v. Kennedy* (1978), the same appeals court found that the FDA's decision to finalize and publish regulations on vitamins and mineral labeling requirements without further public comment or rule-making proceedings was improper (Kassel, 1994).

Given these repeated setbacks and huge federal budget cuts in the early 1980s, the FDA decided that, rather than endlessly struggle with the industry over dietary-supplement regulations, it would revoke the regulations (Sidak, 1993). Although it continued to issue food-policy statements and regulations (Hutt, 1986), the FDA also decided to end its strategy of large-scale regulation to set forth FDA policy, and to return to a vigorous case-by-case enforcement approach (Kassel, 1994).

Health Claims

New controversies continued to arise, however, especially in the area of health claims. In 1984 Kellogg's promoted All-Bran, which contained a high level of natural dietary fiber, "as a way to reduce the risk of cancer" (Cooper et al., 1990, p. 662). Although the FDA complained to Kellogg's about this misleading promotion (Hutt, 1986), it failed to stop it, in part because the FTC approved of the same advertising claims that the FDA found misleading (Cooper et al., 1990). Other companies soon began similar health- related campaigns for their products (Taylor, 1988), and by the time the FDA proposed a new health-claims policy in 1987, many companies already were claiming that their products reduced the risk of disease through lower levels of fat, calories, or cholesterol (Cooper et al., 1990).

Because of the reduction in federal resources, the role of state agencies with jurisdiction over food safety and nutrition issues grew during the 1980s (Kirschbaum, 1983). Some states boosted regulatory activity and oversight, increased enforcement of health and nutrition claims requirements, and pursued even more restrictive policies. New York was the most active state in its attempts to thwart food labeling and advertising violations. For example, in 1984, New York succeeded in stopping Campbell's Soup from promoting its products as "health insurance." In 1985, it induced the Beef Industry Council to change its "Beef Gives Strength" ads, citing scientific evidence linking saturated fat in beef to an increased risk of heart attack, stroke, and cancer as arguments against the "Beef Gives Strength" claim. In 1986, New York influenced many fast-food companies to "provide consumers with point-of-purchase ingredient information on fast food items" (Cooper et al., 1990, p. 655).

Given the current environment of administrative deregulation and decentralization, states most likely will continue to share responsibility in many areas of food law. Indeed, FDA officials predict that the FDA will increase the number of cases that it brings jointly with other federal and state agencies.

LINKING PRODUCTS TO HEALTH BENEFITS: FOOD LABELING AND HEALTH CLAIMS IN THE 1990s

During the late 1980s, controversy resurfaced over what food producers could or could not do to link their products or product ingredients to potential health benefits. This debate centered on the FDA's mission, and on whether restricting specific health claims, as opposed to general nutritional claims, helps or hinders the public's health: Nutritional claims promote the general benefits of consuming a food or food ingredient, whereas health claims promote specific, alleged health benefits of consuming a particular food or food ingredient. The issue therefore became whether food companies should be allowed to make health claims for their specific products, and whether, despite the First Amendment, the government could prohibit or severely restrict truthful claims about diet and health (Cooper et al., 1990).

National Nutrition Monitoring and Related Research Act and National Labeling and Education Act

In 1990 Congress addressed the issue of food monitoring and labeling in two ways. First, to evaluate more precisely America's nutritional needs, Congress passed the National Nutrition Monitoring and Related Research Act (NNMRRA).[12] This Act assesses the dietary and nutritional status of the people of the United States on a continuing basis and provides scientific data for the maintenance and improvement of the population's nutritional status. It also directed the Secretaries of Agriculture and of Health and Human Services jointly to publish nutritional and dietary guidelines for the public every 5 years.

Second, to control nutrition labeling, Congress passed the Nutrition

Labeling and Education Act (NLEA).[13] Gaps in the FFD&CA didn't give the FDA clear legal guidance for regulating food nutrition, or even for requiring nutrition labeling. Since Congress had begun to view the food label as a public health and consumer information tool (Shank, 1990), and now wanted to "take credit for helping the American consumer" (Greenberg, 1990, p. 11), it sought to address this issue through new laws and regulations (Lyons & Rumore, 1994).

The NLEA, the first big legislative food labeling effort in 25 years, covered four areas: nutrition labeling, food description claims, disease-related claims, and preemption of nonidentical state laws. First, the Act created a standardized "Nutrition Facts" label that producers had to put on all food products over a certain size or amount. This label, which formerly listed mainly vitamin content, now required "information on cholesterol, saturated fat, complex carbohydrates, sugars, fiber, and calories from fat" (Lyons & Rumore, 1994, p. 181). Second, the Act also stated that producers had to describe food content fully to claim that products either contained beneficial ingredients (such as dietary fiber), or lacked potentially harmful ingredients (such as cholesterol or fat). Third, the Act established proof requirements that were necessary if producers claimed that their products related to any disease or health-related condition, such as heart disease or cancer. Lastly, the Act barred states from creating or maintaining state laws regarding nutrition labeling covered by this new law without express exemption by the FDA.

The NLEA had several immediate and noticeable effects on food law and policy. First, it required the FDA to improve the procedures by which it validated health claims, putting the initiative back into the hands of the FDA. The FDA now had to investigate and verify food-producer claims of any link between a specific nutrient and its ability to reduce the risk or severity of a specific disease. The FDA interpreted the NLEA to mean that legitimate health claims must have measurable and substantial, not merely incidental, benefits.

Second, the law empowered the FDA to determine when a food becomes a drug. The FDA determined that a food is a drug when it makes a medical claim for curing certain diseases.

Third, it lowered the FDA's burden for showing that a claim is "false or misleading." Prior to the passage of the NLEA, the FDA had to establish how a statement was interpreted by the consumer, and then that interpretation was false or misleading. Under the NLEA, however, the first part of the test—establishing the meaning of the statement to the consumer—became easier, and in many cases, it became unnecessary to show that the interpretation by the consumer was false and misleading (Levitt, 1993).

Fourth, it eased the burden of the FDA under both parts of the test by requiring that claims must be supported by numerical data. Requiring quantifiable results strengthened the FDA's ability to show that a producer's claim is "false or misleading."

Finally, it exempted restaurants, take-out establishments, and certain small businesses from these provisions (Greenberg, 1990; Lyons & Rumore, 1994). Special foods, such as infant formulas (Lyons & Rumore, 1994), were also exempted, as was the USDA jurisdiction over meat and poultry products (McCutcheon, 1994). The law also allowed producers of fresh fruits, vegetables, and fish to follow voluntary guidelines, as long as they demonstrated substantial compliance with the NLEA.

The FDA embraced the NLEA as a way to standardize regulations regarding nutrition and labeling information, particularly as related to vitamins and dietary supplements. Pursuant to the NLEA's strict requirements, the FDA drafted regulations that included all food constituents other than vitamins or minerals in the list of product ingredients. The agency wrote this regulation to prevent dietary-supplement labels that would tout benefits without scientific support.

Almost immediately the food industry questioned the agency's interpretation of the NLEA, as did public-interest groups that opposed the new regulations because they did not think they went far enough. In *Arent v. Shalala* (1994), two public-interest groups sought to invalidate the FDA's voluntary nutritional labeling guidelines for raw fruits, vegetables, and fish, and to require mandatory nutrition labeling for these products. The court, however, found that both the FDA's final regulations, and the process by which the agency created them under the NLEA, fell within the FDA's discretion. The court stated that this case presented the type of conflict that must be resolved politically rather than by a court.

Industry groups that believed that the regulations went too far also challenged them. The food industry particularly disliked the FDA's interpretation of the NLEA's quantitative standards for health claim validity; it felt that the FDA's interpretation of the need for quantitative data did not reflect Congressional intent (Iannarone, 1992). Ultimately, however, the vitamin- and dietary-supplement industry decided to challenge the FDA over the NLEA by demanding that Congress, not the courts, restrict the FDA's powers.

The dietary-supplement industry lobbied Congress to shield it in two ways. First, the industry sought to delay implementation of the new dietary-supplement health claims regulations. Second, the industry asked Congress to pass legislation that would force the FDA to make its regulations less restrictive.

In 1992 Congress responded by passing the Dietary Supplement Act (DSA).[14] This law allowed the dietary-supplement industry to reach its first goal: to delay the FDA's NLEA-derived regulations. First, it postponed FDA implementation of the new dietary-supplement regulations until the end of 1993. Second, it directed the FDA to conduct further studies on dietary-supplement regulation. Third, it directed the FDA to create new dietary-supplement labeling regulations. Fourth, it authorized the FDA to grant permission to producers to make specific health claims for products (Sidak, 1993).

Dietary Supplement Health and Education Act

In December 1993, the FDA proposed to treat labeling and nutrition information for foods and dietary supplements in the same way, issuing revised dietary-supplement regulations under the DSA. These regulations reflected the agency's concerns about the safety and health hazards inherent in the use of many dietary supplements. The industry vehemently disapproved of these new regulations. It responded by pressuring Congress to pass the Dietary Supplement Health and Education Act (DSHEA),[15] which helped the industry to achieve its second goal: to rewrite the FDA's statutory mandate as it applied to dietary supplements.

In 1994 Congress passed the DSHEA to establish new standards for dietary supplements. Stating in the DSHEA that "scientific studies" increasingly documented "the benefits of dietary supplements to health promotion and disease prevention" and that "there is a link between the ingestion of certain nutrients or dietary supplements and the prevention of chronic diseases."[16] Congress used the DSHEA to modify the NLEA and the FFD&CA and carve out a protective regulatory niche for vitamins and dietary supplements. By defining a "dietary supplement" as a food, not as a drug or related item under the DSHEA, the item is subject to less restrictive labeling regulations.

Second, the DSHEA establishes different burdens of proof for the FDA and industry members concerning health claims. The DSHEA requires the FDA to show, either in a published article or other proof, that a supplement claim is false or misleading. The DSHEA requires manufacturers, however, to prove only that a supplement's claims are substantiated and truthful, not misleading.

Third, the DSHEA protects dietary supplements from onerous NLEA proof provisions regarding proof of safety. The DSHEA exempts dietary supplements from the strict preclearance procedures formerly required for new food additives under the Delaney Amendment. The DSHEA also exempts dietary supplements from the health claims preclearance procedure required for foods under the NLEA.

Finally, the DSHEA requires the FDA affirmatively to prove that a dietary supplement is adulterated. The DSHEA thus effectively changes back the FDA's role from preclearing supplements prospectively to policing supplements retrospectively. Such conflicting legal developments guarantee that the FDA's mission and role will continue to evolve, particularly as new controversies arise.

THE FUTURE

As a result of both the achievements of the FDA and controversies over its regulations, public interest in the agency is extremely high. This interest should continue as the FDA faces rapidly evolving technological, legal, and cultural challenges in the future.

For instance, after years in the background, food safety has reëmerged as a major concern. "[T]he appearance of new microbial pathogens in food, the development of new food products through biotechnology, and continued consumer concerns about the risks of carcinogenic pesticides in the food supply" all have contributed to a renewed sense of awareness and urgency about maintaining food safety (Nestle, 1994, p. 38). This concern results from changing methods of food production. Centralized food production, processing, and distribution systems create an environment in which organisms that have not previously been widely encountered in processed foods can flourish. In addition, "[t]he development of new agricultural products through techniques of genetic engineering—and FDA's decision that such products are safe unless proven otherwise—have stimulated further demands for more stringent regulatory and enforcement policies" (Nestle, 1994, p. 38).

In response, federal agencies are pressing efforts to curb these emerging threats to food safety. The USDA has proposed tougher guidelines for meat and poultry inspection and safety that would require packers to perform microscopic testing for bacteria and the use of special rinses and temperature controls. The Environmental Protection Agency (EPA) still bans pesticides that do not meet the Delaney Clause's "zero-risk" tolerance standard.

The food industry, on the other hand, is actively campaigning for less government regulation. The biotechnology industry, for instance, "argues that excessive regulation inhibits research and development and that its techniques are inherently safe" (Nestle, 1994, p. 38). The National Food Processors Association claims that the Delaney Clause is obsolete and must be changed.

Congress has responded to many industry concerns. On pesticide restriction, it has introduced a measure that would create a "negligible risk" standard for pesticide residues on raw and processed foods. That standard would allow producers to use a pesticide that poses a greater than negligible risk, if the pesticide's benefits outweigh the risk to consumers. On meat inspection, Congress has passed a 1-year freeze on new meat regulations.

Some within government, however, oppose these measures: they support strengthening food safety by instituting a "common sense test" for setting pesticide tolerances. The Clinton Administration similarly favors "a health-based standard" that would involve a "reasonable certainty of no harm" to consumers. (*Daily Report for Executives,* June 8, 1995, p. 110).

Although some FDA insiders believe that many labeling issues are settled, the food industry continues to question whether the FDA's "total ban or unduly stringent regulation of health claims on food labels [are] consistent with recent Supreme Court decisions according a significant degree of First Amendment protection to commercial speech" (Dunkel-berger & Taylor, 1993, pp. 631–632). The FDA maintains that its regulations affect only *unapproved* health claims, which do not receive First Amendment protection because "particular attributes of health claims on the food label make them inherently misleading" (Dunkelberger & Taylor, 1993, p. 634). It also holds that, under its regulations, "the presence of an unapproved health claim on a food label or labeling renders the product adulterated, and exposes the company and its officials to criminal prosecution" (Dunkelberger & Taylor, 1993, p. 634).

Many new products contain engineered ingredients, however, such as artificial sweeteners or processed vegetable protein. Identity standards are less applicable to these products, and the FDA must adjust its nutrition labeling and monitoring efforts, particularly if these ingredients have a long-term health impact. Study will continue in several areas, including organic foods, biotech labeling, and health claims. Indeed, one industry group has filed a health-claim petition with the FDA, seeking permission to make claims that sugarless chewing gums (which use "sugar alcohols") do not promote tooth decay.

The food industry believes that the FDA has underestimated NLEA compliance costs substantially. Sensing a more receptive political environment, the industry wants to roll back some of the FDA's regulatory safeguards and positions. The industry wants a more permissive health-claims framework, to encourage health claims and promote nutritious diets and consumer health. To reduce the cost of compliance with federal, state, and local regulations, it also wants legislation that creates national uniformity for all labeling and safety requirements.

Despite this pressure, the FDA continues to insist on strict regulations, particularly in regard to significant health risks associated with dietary supplements. In early 1995, for instance, the FDA found, after receiving numerous complaints, that a dietary supplement containing the Chinese herb "ma huang," when ingested as a dietary supplement along with kola nuts, caused serious illnesses, from heart attacks and hepatitis to death.

Consequently, the FDA has not backed off from regulating certain dietary supplements. Although the agency has granted the supplement industry until the end of 1996 to complete DSHEA nutrition labeling, it has moved in other ways to assert control. Three months after Congress passed the DSHEA, the FDA proposed new iron supplements packaging-and-labeling guidelines, maintaining that, although the DSHEA removed the FDA's authority to regulate the packaging under its food-additive authority, the FDA still can govern them under other regulations.

Although far from perfect, U.S. food law effectively protects people on several levels. First, the law ensures that foods are wholesome and safe to eat. Second, the law establishes assistance programs to underserved populations. Finally, the law mandates truthful and informative food labeling. As a result food law plays an enduring and critical role in society's health and nutrition.

NOTES

1. Pub. L. No. 59–384, 34 Stat. 768 (repealed).
2. Pub. L. No. 75–717, 52 Stat. 1040 (1938), as amended 21 USC §§ 301–394 (1988).

3. Pursuant to the Federal Meat Inspection Act, 21 U.S.C. §§ 601–695; the Poultry Products Inspection Act, 21 U.S.C. §§ 451–470; and the Egg Products Inspection Act, 21 U.S.C. §§ 1031–1056 (1988).
4. Pursuant to the Federal Trade Commission Act, 15 USC §§ 41–77 (1988).
5. This case is officially known as *U.S. v. Mytinger and Casselberry, Inc.* (S.D. Calif. 1951).
6. Pub. L. No. 85–929, 72 Stat. 1784, codified at 21 USC § 348 (1988).
7. Pub. L. No. 89–755, 80 Stat. 1296 (1966), codified at 15 USC §§ 1451–1461 (1988).
8. CONN. GEN. STAT. § 21a–29 (1995).
9. CONN. GEN. STAT. § 21a–118 (1995).
10. Pub. L. No. 94–317, 90 Stat. 695 (1976), codified at 42 USC § 300u (1988).
11. Pub. L. No. 94–278, 90 Stat. 401 (1976), codified at 21 USC § 350 (1988).
12. Pub. L. No. 101–445, 104 Stat. 1034, codified at 7 USC §§ 5301–5342 (1988 & Supp. IV 1992).
13. Pub. L. No. 101–535, 104 Stat. 2353, codified at 21 USC §§ 343(q), 343(r), and 343–1 (1988 & Supp. IV 1992).
14. Pub. L. No. 102–571, 106 Stat. 4491, amending 21 USC §§ 343(q), 343(r) (Supp. IV 1992).
15. Pub. L. No. 103–417, 108 Stat. 4325, amending various statutes.
16. Pub. L. No. 103–417, 108 Stat. at 4325 § 2(3)(A).

REFERENCES

Arent v. Shalala, 886 F.Supp. 6 (D.C.D.C. 1994).

Back Seat for Food Safety? (1995). *Los Angeles Times*, June 7, p. B6.

Bessonette, C. (1995). Q & A On The News, *Atlanta Journal and Constitution*, June 4, p. A2.

Center, J. (1995). Why punish poor children? *San Francisco Chronicle,* June 6, p. A19.

Christoffel, T. (1982). *Health and the law: A handbook for health professionals.* New York: Free Press.

Cooper, R. M., Frank, R. L., & O'Flaherty, M. J. (1990). History of health claims regulation. *Food Drug Cosmetic Law Journal, 45,* 655–691.

Dunkelberger, E., & Taylor, S. E. (1993). The NLEA, health claims, and the first amendment. *Food Drug Law Journal, 48,* 631–664.

FDA to issue supplement rules this month. (1993, December 20). *Food Chemical News, 35.*

FDA's Scarbrough came to NLEA implementation with the right stuff. (1995, January 26). *Food Labeling News, 3.*

Federation of Homemakers v. Schmidt, 539 F.2d 740 (D.C. Cir. 1976).

Greenberg, E. F. (1990). The changing food label: The Nutrition Labeling and Education Act of 1990. *Loyola Consumer Law Reporter, 3,* 10–15.

Health claims petition on sugarless products accepted for filing. (1995, January 19). *Food Labeling News.*

Hutt, P. B. (1986). Government regulation of health claims in food labeling and advertising. *Food Drug Cosmetic Law Journal, 41,* 3–73.

Hutt, P. B., & Hutt, P. B., II (1984). A history of government regulation of adulteration and misbranding of food. *Food Drug Cosmetic Law Journal, 39,* 2–73.

Hutt, P. B., & Merrill, R. A. (1991). *Food and drug law: Cases and materials* (2nd ed.). Mineola, NY: Foundation Press.

Iannarone, A. J. (1992). Scientific basis for health claims for dietary supplements. *Food Drug Law Journal, 47,* 665–676.

Janssen, W. F. (1975). America's first food and drug laws. *Food Drug Cosmetic Law Journal, 30,* 665–672.

Janssen, W. F. (1980). The U.S. food and drug law: How it came; How it works. *Food Drug Cosmetic Law Journal, 35,* 132–142.

Kassel, M. A. (1994). From a history of near misses: The future of dietary supplement regulation. *Food Drug Law Journal, 49,* 237–269.

Kirschbaum, N. E. (1983). Role of state government in the regulation of food and drugs. *Food Drug Cosmetic Law Journal, 38,* 199–204.

Lev, L. L. (1952). The nutrilite consent decree. *Food Drug Cosmetic Law Journal, 7,* 56–69.

Levitt, G. M. (1993). FDA enforcement under the Nutrition Labeling and Education Act. *Food Drug Law Journal, 48,* 119–124.

Line between food and drug claims seen as blurred. (1992, December 10). *Food Labeling News,* 1.

Lyons, J., & Rumore, M. (1993). Food labeling—Then and now. *Journal of Pharmacy & Law, 2,* 171–183.

"The MacNeil/Lehrer NewsHour." (1995, March 28). Transcript #5193.

McCutcheon, J. (1994). Nutrition labeling initiative. *Food Drug Law Journal, 49,* 409–414.

McVicar, J. (1995, April 17). Getting the glitches out of WIC. *San Diego Union-Tribune,* p. B7.

Nestle, M. (1994). The law and nutrition. *New York State Bar Journal, 66,* 38–41.

NFPA urges Congress to pass food safety legislation. (1995, June 7). *PR Newswire.*

Peterman, P. (1995, April 16). WIC: A good program fares badly in Congress. *St. Petersburg Times,* p. 6D.

Shank, F. R. (1990). The Nutrition Labeling and Education Act of 1990. *Food Drug Law Journal, 47,* 247–252.

Sidak, M. L. (1993). Dietary supplements and commercial speech. *Food Drug Law Journal, 48,* 441–461.

Sinclair, U. (1906). *The jungle.* New York: New American Library.

Taylor, S. E. (1988). Health claims for foods: Present law, future policy. *Food Drug Cosmetic Law Journal, 43,* 603–621.

U.S. v. Mytinger and Casselberry, Inc. (S.D. Calif. 1951).

Wax, P. M. (1995). Elixirs, diluents, and the passage of the 1938 Federal Food, Drug and Cosmetic Act. *Annals of Internal Medicine, 122,* 456–461.

Wodicka, V. O. (1990). The 1970's: The decade of regulations. *Food Drug Cosmetic Law Journal, 45,* 59–67.

CHAPTER 5

Food: Production, Processing, Distribution, and Consumption

Paul A. Lachance

T he occupants of 92 million or so households in America search for their "at home" food supplies from nearly 140,000 supermarkets and spend 11.5% of their disposable income on food. On average, supermarkets contain 30,000 items and with mergers creating larger one-stop shopping markets, the number of items is increasing. The annual retail sales by food stores approaches $385 billion (Manchester, 1994). On average, 40% of the household food dollar is spent in purchasing food that is eaten outside the home. The amount of money spent on "off premise" food exceeds $235 billion.

Whereas personal consumption expenditures for food at home increased 3.1% between 1992 and 1993, expenditures for food away from home increased 8.9%. There is a startling empirical correlation between the rate of increase in away- from-home eating and the increase in the prevalence of obesity. The propensity to select foods of lower nutrient density when eating away from home may be related to a psychological phenomenon described as "disinhibition" of a more careful "restraint," concerning food selections (Klesges, Isbell, & Klesges, 1992). "Restraint" eating is believed to correlate with the degree of consumer "nutrition or health" knowledge. Eating donuts, for example, becomes OK any time of day (i.e., "disinhibition" occurs) if eaten away from home. Allred (1995) has documented an inverse relationship between the increase in obesity from 27% of adults to 34% of adults in only 10 years, but with a concomitant decrease in the intake of fat expressed as percentage of calories from fat from 42% to 34%. Decreasing fat calories evidently does not decrease the prevalence of obesity. The total of calories ingested away from home is higher than that consumed at home; therefore, the suggestion of a positive correlation with eating away from home has merit.

FOOD COMMODITIES

The entire food supply is provided by U.S. farmers and from imported raw agricultural commodities. Imported food either cannot be grown in the United States (e.g., bananas) or is grown in insufficient amounts to meet demand (e.g., orange-juice concentrate), or needed to meet demand out of season (e.g., fruits and vegetables). An increasing number of ethnic foods are imported to meet the increased cultural diversity of Americans. American agriculture is estimated to approach $1 trillion in value. The United States exports $42 billion of raw agricultural commodities and imports food valued at $24 billion.

The United States had estimated wheat stocks in 1995 of 968 million bushels (down 6% from the prior year) and corn stocks of 5,591 million bushels (up from 3,996 million the previous year, low because of the effects of extensive flooding in the Midwest).

The world production (1994–1995) of cereal grains (wheat, rice, and coarse grains like corn) was 1,750 billion metric tons; for major oil seeds (soy, cotton, peanut, sunflower, rape, copra) production is 251 million metric tons, of which one quarter becomes edible oil. The world produces 160 million metric tons of meat and has a fish catch of 98 billion metric tons. In 1992 the United States produced 41 million metric tons of meat, and the United States fish catch was 5.6 billion metric tons. It is evident that the majority of the world's population gets most of its energy, and the major portion of its protein needs, from cereal grain products. Those who reside near the sea eat fish for protein.

PRODUCTION VARIABLES ON NUTRITIVE VALUE

Of the several variables in the production of commodities, namely, variety and strain (genetic makeup); agronomic practices (e.g., till, no-till);

fertilization practices (types, quantities and frequencies); pesticide practices, and abiotic factors (sunlight, rainfall, etc.); there is consensus that genetics has the greatest impact on yield, resistance to disease, and macronutrient composition. The quality of protein; lipid (type of fatty acid, degree of unsaturation, etc.); type and quantity of starch; and vitamin content can be genetically manipulated, but genetic engineering for these attributes is rarely practiced, because yield or disease resistance take economic precedence. The farmer is paid by the bushel or pound and nutritive value is not a factor. The mineral composition of plant foods is highly variable because it reflects the composition of the soil as well as the mineral composition of fertilizers and of the water applied (Karmas & Harris, 1988)

PREHARVEST AND PREMORTEM NUTRITIVE LOSSES

Many factors can cause loss of food commodities prior to harvest or slaughter. Even with sophisticated technology, food commodity losses approach 20%. Without pesticides, herbicides, and animal drugs, which keep preharvest/slaughter losses low, field losses, particularly in developing countries, approach 50%. Quality losses after harvesting, but before preservation or cooking, are due to decay and senescence (overripening) and decreased resistance to microbial spoilage, as well as contamination with food-poisoning microorganisms.

GARDEN versus MARKET FRESH

Harvesting and handling can obviously affect nutritive values. Practically all fruits and vegetables continue a metabolism of respiration after harvesting. The blanching and/or cooking steps arrest metabolism and inactivate enzymatic activity. Therefore one can distinguish acceptance qualities when fruits and vegetables are freshly harvested (i.e., "garden" fresh), in contrast to "market"-fresh produce, grown and harvested in another state or country and shipped to a wholesaler who redistributes fruits and vegetables to retail outlets; or harvested in one season and held under controlled storage (e.g., potatoes, apples) for sale in other seasons of the year.

Major processors of fruits and vegetables contract with farmers, with specifications not only for a given crop, but also for the specific varieties of seed to be used. Specifications also often include the agronomic practices (types, quantity, and frequency of fertilizers, pesticides, etc.) to be carried out and a scheduled " window" of expected date of harvest. Thus, with major packers, the time between harvesting and processing is measured in hours and the goal is to process "garden"-fresh produce in order to optimize for and assure quality products. This approach does not apply to cereal grains and legumes, for which the farmer's goal is high yield and choosing the proper time when to sell grain to be stored in grain elevators (Breene, 1994).

The concept of freshness is not applicable to animal products. Animal products are processed post mortem. Further, research on twin animals has demonstrated no advantage in nutritive value whether the animal is luxus fed throughout life, or range fed and then fattened a few weeks before slaughter.

INTACT FOOD in Contrast to PARTITIONED FOOD

Intact foods are recognizable as products of plant or animal agriculture. The consumer readily identifies with the product at the retail level and in the cooked state, for example, a pea or diced carrot particle in a soup or stew.

Partitioned foods are food ingredients separated in a pure or almost complete state from an intact commodity that itself may or may not be edible. For example, corn bran, corn oil, and corn starch are partitioned from corn, whereas cottonseed flour and cottonseed oil are partitioned from cottonseeds. The latter is a commercial commodity associated with textiles and the history of slavery, but rarely classified as edible. Usually the consumer cannot identify the source of the oil or flour without reading the label.

A refined food is an intact or partitioned food whose principal component (sugar, oil, protein) is further processed primarily to enhance wholesomeness, shelf life, and cost. It is typically used as an ingredient in formulated or fabricated food. Examples are table sugar (sucrose), wheat flour, and most edible oils.

Partitioning or refining a food commodity places emphasis on obtaining a value-added product/ingredient; invariably this is a macronutrient (protein, fat, starch, or bran). The micronutrient constituents are sacrificed in the process. Therefore the formulation and especially the fabrication of a new food requires that attention be paid to including those micronutrients that are likely to be contained in the product being emulated. For example, vitamins A and D should be added to margarine because it emulates butter. Sadly, emulation fortification is not a routine practice unless dictated by law. Consequently, our food intake becomes increasingly impoverished as more and more products that are poor in or devoid of micronutrients become a part of the diet.

FORMULATED in Contrast to FABRICATED FOODS

A formulated food product is one whose ingredients are for the most part intact and/or can be prepared from a recipe in a kitchen. Bread/cake, ice cream, home-canned vegetables, and even sausages are formulated foods. These products are often offered as "convenience" foods, for example, condensed soup, stew, pot pie, TV dinners. These products are readily prepared in fast-food operations, or purchased ready to cook or reheat. Because of its rapid action, the microwave oven has become the major appliance for this practice.

A fabricated food product is one whose ingredients are for the most part derived from partitioning technology and require manufacturing technology to prepare. These products tend to emulate a known intact or formulated food but are in fact quite unrelated in chemical and nutrient composition. Examples are margarine that emulates butter, Bacos®, which emulate chips of cooked bacon, Cool Whip® as a substitute for whipped cream, Hamburger Helper®, which extends ground beef, and Tang® for fruit drinks.

FOOD PROCESSING/FOOD SERVICE

In the United States there are 17,000 food processing companies with 1.6 million employees; and an additional 5.5 million individuals are employed in the food-service industry. Historically, a basic objective of food processing has been to increase the shelf life of food and to provide foods all year round. Today the emphasis of food processing and preparation is to make the food safe, that is, to eliminate potential microbiological harm to the consumer. In addition, since World War II, providing "convenience" food has been a major processing activity. The advent of the double-income household leaves little time to prepare food from classic ingredients. "Convenience" foods have become part of practically every American household and food-service establishment. Moreover, microwave ovens with their rapid reheating capability add to the "convenience." Ready-to-eat food is available through fast-food outlets, and ready-to-reheat food is available at the modern supermarket. Table 5.1 gives a synopsis of major food categories by their degree of perishability, deterioration factors, critical preservation factors, and thus estimated shelf life.

Table 5.1 Food Perishability: Type, Deterioration Factors, and Shelf Life

Food product	Deterioration (assuming an intact package)	Critical effect factors	Shelf life (average)
Perishables			
Fluid milk and fluid milk products	bacterial growth, oxidized flavor, hydrolytic rancidity	oxygen, temperature	7–14 days at refrigerated temperature
Fresh bakery products	staling, microbial growth, moisture loss causing hardening, oxidative rancidity	oxygen, temperature	2 days (bread) 7 days (cake)
Fresh red meat	bacterial activity, oxidation	oxygen, temperature, light	3–4 days at refrigerated temperature
Fresh poultry	pathogen growth, microbial decay	oxygen, temperature, light	2–7 days at refrigerated temperature
Fresh fish	bacterial growth	temperature	14 days when sorted on ice (marine fish)

continued

Table 5.1 *(continued)*

Food product	Deterioration (assuming an intact package)	Critical effect factors	Shelf life (average)
Fresh fruits and vegetables	microbial decay, nutrient loss, wilting, bruising	temperature, light, oxygen, relative humidity, soil & water physical handling	

Semiperishables and perishables

Fried snack foods	rancidity, loss of crispness	oxygen, light, temperature, moisture	4–6 weeks
Cheese	rancidity, browning, lactose crystallization	temperature	processed cheese 4–24 months, natural cheese 4–12 months
Ice cream	graininess caused by ice and lactose crystallization, loss of solubilization (caking), lysine loss	fluctuating temperature (below freezing)	1–4 months

Long shelf-life foods

Dehydrated foods	browning, rancidity, loss of pigment, loss of texture, loss of nutrients	moisture, temperature, light, oxygen	dehydrated vegetables 3–15 months, dehydrated meat 1–6 months, dried fruit 1–24 months
Nonfat dry milk	flavor deterioration, loss of solubilization, (caking), lysine loss	moisture, temperature	12 months

Table 5.1   *(continued)*

Breakfast cereals	rancidity, loss of crispness, vitamin loss, particle breakage	moisture, temperature, rough handling	6–18 months
Pasta	texture changes, staling, vitamin and protein loss	moisture too high or too low, temperature	pasta with egg solid 9–36 months, macaroni and spaghetti 24–48 months
Frozen concentrated juices	loss of turbidity or cloudiness, yeast growth, loss of vitamins, loss of color or flavor	temperature	8–30 months
Frozen fruits and vegetables	loss of nutrients, loss of texture, flavor, color, and formation of package ice	temperature	6–24 months
Frozen meats, poultry, and fish	rancidity, protein denaturation, color change, desiccation	temperature	beef 6–12 months, veal 4–14 months, pork 4–12 months, fish 2-8 months, lamb 6–16 months
Frozen convenience foods	rancidity in meat portions, weeping and curdling of sauces, loss of flavor, loss of color	oxygen, temperature	6–12 months
Canned fruits and vegetables	loss of flavor, texture, color, nutrients	temperature	12–36 months
Coffee	rancidity, loss of flavor and color	oxygen	ground, roasted, vacuum-packed, 9 months; instant coffee 18–36 months

(continued)

Table 5.1 *(continued)*

Food product	Deterioration (assuming an intact package)	Critical effect factors	Shelf life (average)
Tea	loss of flavor, absorption of foreign colors	moisture	18 months

Adapted from T. P. Labuza & J.W. Erdman (1984). *Food science and nutritional health: An introduction* (pp. 235-236). St. Paul, MN: West Publishing Co.

CAUSES OF SPOILAGE

Benefits of Food Preservation

The three major causes of food spoilage are: microbes, enzymes, and physical deterioration (Nickerson & Ronsivalli, 1980). Food spoilage leads to decreased acceptance and, eventually, complete decay. Controlling the microbiological causes of food spoilage decreases food spoilage per se and the risk of food-borne disease.

Physical damage to food is caused by poor handling and packaging. Fruit that is bruised, even though the skin may be intact, undergoes enzymatic browning under or at the bruise. Hardier commodities, such as walnuts and corn have outer protective "shells" and thus can be handled by machine. Improper packaging of meats permits "freezer burn" and the destruction of tissue. Modern harvesting technology can be sophisticated. Tomatoes intended for the production of tomato paste, sauce, or ketchup are genetically bred species selected for hardier skins that resist bruising and can be machine harvested at a rate of tons per hour; and, with the help of on-board electronic scanners, the unripe culls are left in the field as organic matter; thus only tomatoes suitable for processing enter the manufacturing stream. The harvesting step triggers a natural increase in respiration of produce of up to 15-fold. Much of this activity is hydrolytic and the slow deterioration of complex macromolecules begins. The rate of ripening and or eventual spoilage is accelerated and shelf-life is shortened.

Microbiological spoilage may be caused by bacteria, yeast, or fungus (mold). No food-commodity surface is microbiologically sterile, although the interior usually is. Thus any break in the surface, caused by harvesting and handling, introduces the opportunity for microbial spoilage. Conditions during plant growth (e.g., high humidity favors mold growth), or during storage or delays before final processing increase the opportunity for microbiological growth and the risk of spoilage, as well as growth of food-borne pathogens.

Both enzymatic and microbiological spoilage are affected by factors in the product environment, namely, moisture, temperature (if more than-25°C to less than 90°C), oxygen, pH, and the nature of the substrate. Therefore, to control spoilage, that is, to preserve foods, means controlling these factors.

Controlling Moisture

Primitive man learned that drying food in the sun or over a fire preserved some foods, but dramatically altered their appearance and taste. Because drying changes the relative humidity, that is, the activity of water in the food, enzymatic activity is slowed. By controlling water activity in a food, microorganisms fail to grow at a water activity less than 0.6. In addition to drying one can control the amount of available water by adding sugar or salt. Strawberry preserve is 55% sugar by weight and this requirement for jams and jellies is codified in the standard of identity regulations. For many years supersaturated solutions of salt brine were used to preserve slabs of salt pork and some other meats. Today salt (sodium chloride) is used less widely, but is a component (2.5–3%) in "cured" foods, such as sausage, ham, and bacon.

For most commodities there is an applicable drying technology. Cereal blends, as well as molasses, can be dried, and often "instantized," that is, they are precooked, very economically, on a drum dryer. Spray drying is very effective for drying milk-based products and for incorporating nutrients in powdered products, such as infant formula and instant-breakfast beverage powders. Fruit and vegetable pieces or small vegetables (e.g., peas) can be dried in a tunnel dryer or countercurrent air dryer. A better but more expensive process is to freeze food and vacuum dry it at the same time, that is, "freeze drying." Foods for backpacking, some space foods, and higher cost ingredients in selected foods justify the use of this more expensive technology.

Thermal Processing

Napoleon realized that to wage effective war and occupation over several countries, one needed more than the ability to scavenge the land en route;

therefore, he offered a substantial prize to anyone who could devise a method that preserved an array of different foods. Nicholas Appert (Nickerson & Ronsivalli, 1980), a pharmacist, won this prize in 1809 by demonstrating that several selected foods could be individually stuffed in champagne bottles, heated to boiling temperatures for substantial times, and sealed while still hot. With the advent of cans just a few years later, the process became known as "canning." Another Frenchman, Louis Pasteur (Nickerson & Ronsivalli, 1980), began to explain the science of this technology in 1853. A temperature greater than 90°C will denature enzymes, and therefore control enzymatic spoilage; however, food spoilage and hazardous microorganisms, especially spores, are more resistant. Today effective heat (thermal) processing is based on thermal death time–temperature curves, which assure that the spores of *Clostridium botulinum* are killed. Food-borne pathogens are killed by pasteurization (e.g., 1 second at 88.3°C in the case of fluid milk), which represents less heat than that needed to kill spores and to preserve the food.

Referigeration and Freezing

Early man and Eskimos discovered that food could be preserved in ice. Commercial preservation with ice (1875) and later (1895) mechanical refrigeration made frozen food storage of meat and fish suitable. Between 1932–1934 Clarence Birdseye (Nickerson & Ronsivalli, 1980) developed over 100 different quick-frozen food items. Although the quality of frozen foods is superior to that of thermally processed foods, the shelf life is considerably shorter because chemical spoilage can occur in micro pockets of unfrozen water. Refrigerated and frozen foods are often uncooked and therefore are at greater risk for microbial spoilage.

Oxygen

Oxygen content is best controlled by packaging, especially vacuum packaging; however, one must be certain that no anaerobic microorganism such as *Clostridia* are present. One can control enzymatic browning by excluding oxygen. Polyphenols in food are readily converted to melanins in the presence of the enzyme polyphenol oxidase and oxygen. Thus excluding air retards the reaction, as for example, by covering peeled potatoes with water. Prolonging the shelf life of fruit by controlled-atmosphere storage in environments high in carbon dioxide and low in oxygen works well for apples, but for few other fruits or vegetables.

pH

The optimum pH for bacteria is 4–7; 2.5–8.5 for yeast, and 1.5-11 for molds, however, pathogenic bacteria will *not* grow at a pH below 4.5. This principle accounts for the greater safety when high acid foods, such as those that contain tomatoes, are preserved. The degree of thermal processing required is therefore less for high acid foods. Certain fermented foods, such as sauerkraut, pepperoni, and similar sausages, benefit from this concept. The conversion of milk lactose into lactic acid contributes to the preservation of yogurt and permits an increased tolerance to lactose. The pH of other foods can be altered through the use of acidulants, such as citric acid. Microbial food safety relies on the combination of defensive technologies described as "hurdles." By taking advantage of naturally occurring antibiotics (e.g., bacteriocins) in the food, lowering the pH (acidulants), and controlling water activity one can achieve "triple-hurdle preservation."

Microbiological Safety

Today, with no food shortages, processing is critical to the control of food-borne diseases. Although improper processing does on occasion lead to outbreaks of disease, the major incidence of food-borne disease is the result of improper handling procedures in the home and in food-service establishments. The cost of food-borne disease includes the cost of the illness or death, including medical costs and productivity losses. The costs do not include the expense expended to prevent food-borne illness. The pathogen *Salmonella sp.*, particularly prevalent in undercooked chicken and eggs, beef, and pork, exacts an annual disease cost of $1.2–1.6 billion; *Campylobacter sp.*, in raw poultry and raw milk, exacts an annual cost of $1.0 billion; and the coliform 0157:H7 exacts a cost of $200–$600 million. Other pathogens are *Staphylococcus aureus*, *Clostridium perfringens*, *Bacillus cereus*, *Listeria monocytogenes*, *Shigella sp.*, *Clostridium botulinum*, *Vibrio sp.*, and *Norwalk* virus (cf. Chapter 3).

The factors that contribute to food-borne outbreaks are one or a combination of the following (a) improper cooling (46%) such as previously cooked food left on the counter rather than refrigerated; (b) time lapse between preparation and serving (21%), as with home parties; caterers, and so on; (c) infected persons touching food (20%); (d) inadequate cooking (16%); (e) inadequate reheating (12%); (f) contaminated raw food (11%); (g) improper cleaning and cross contamination (each 7%).

Shellfish, fish, and meat stews are involved in 35.5% of outbreaks. Fruits, vegetables, salads are involved in 12.2 % of outbreaks; milk and dairy products in 5.4%; poultry in 5.2%; Mexican foods in 3.3%; baked products and beverages each account for 2.2%; and mushrooms account for 1.5% of outbreaks.

In the preceding section, the key mechanisms to controlling microbiological problems were briefly reviewed. A process of food preservation that has not been mentioned but that has undergone considerable research with favorable results is food irradiation. Its use in Europe and Japan is substantial in comparison to use in the United States. Only one commercial food irradiation facility is available in the United States; it is used to pasteurize poultry. Fear of radiation in U.S. consumers evidently far exceeds their general concern with food cleanliness and safety.

FOOD PREPARATION

A major reaction in baking, cooking, and food preparation is chemical (nonenzymatic) browning. The crust of bread, cookies, the toasting of bread, bagels, English muffins, and the browning of meat are all examples of browning caused by chemical changes. The principal reaction is Maillard browning, which is the result of the reaction between an amino group (often of the amino acid lysine) and a reducing sugar, such as glucose. The nutritive value of these products in terms of protein (e.g., the crust of bread) is essentially nil because humans do not have a digestive enzyme that can cleave the Maillard reaction product, even in the colorless stage that precedes the appearance of browning. Browning does provide sensory (flavor and texture) properties that are frequently considered desirable. However, the production and distribution of high-protein cookies in an effort to combat protein malnutrition has overlooked that these products provide no effective protein nutrition. Another, but different, example of chemical browning is the caramelization of sugars.

CHANGES IN NUTRITIVE VALUE

The greatest losses in the overall nutritive value of common foods occur in the home and in food-service establishments (Clydesdale, Ho, Mandy,

& Shewfelt, 1991; Karmas & Harris, 1988). Together with an increasing array of partitioned and fabricated processed foods to which micronutrients have *not* been restored, the cooking losses are believed to contribute to states of subclinical malnutrition and to fail in mitigating the incidence of chronic diseases. The vast array of food choices, food fortification, and the use of vitamin and mineral supplements, minimizes the occurrence of specific vitamin/mineral deficiency diseases, but does little to overcome or mitigate the major causes of the morbidity and mortality encountered in developed countries.

TYPICAL NUTRITIVE LOSSES

Figure 5.1 illustrates the percentage of nutrient retention for typical vegetable products. In comparison with the ideal retention for a "garden-fresh" product brought to serving temperature, an individually quick-frozen version of the same product would exhibit no greater losses even though consumed out of season. A boil-in-the-bag version of the produce would give ideal retention because no water would come in direct contact during the reheating of the food. The thermally processed (i.e., canned) equivalent food would have less retention because the process is harsher, but it does provide a 2-year shelf life. Losses became even greater if the liquid of the reheated product is decanted prior to serving. In years gone by this nutrient-rich liquor was added to the daily-modified soup. Dried foods have the poorest retention, with freeze-dried and spray-dried products being superior to tunnel dried products.

Given a choice of cooking methods, the best retention (least leaching) of nutrients occurs when cooking is done with microwaves, by steam basket, or the wok method. Braising (frying) in nonstick or lecithin-coated cookware or the minimal use of oil is superior to broiling and baking. One-pot slow cooking is superior to multi-pot cooking of several foods. Properly cleaned raw foods can be recommended even though the bioavailability of some nutrients is poorer than with the cooked version (e.g., carrots).

FOOD-INTAKE COMBINATIONS

It might be a "tempest in a teapot" to fret about nutrient changes with pro-

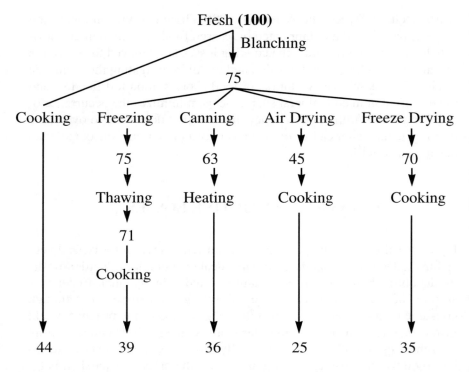

Figure 5.1 Nutrient retention varies with type of commodity; however, nutrients in vegetables are good indicators of the "worst" case. In general, water-soluble nutrients and fat-soluble antioxidant nutrients are more labile than other vitamins.

Based on: Mapson, L.W. (1956). *Br. Med. Bull.*, *12*:73-77.

cessing and preparation in view of the fact that national surveys have repeatedly reported that Americans do not make daily food combinations as recommended by various educational schemes and public and private education programs. No more that 20% of Americans on a given day select and consume at least five servings of fruits and vegetables (Kant, Schatzin, Harris, Zegler, & Block, 1993). Five servings have been recommended as minimal by the National Cancer Institute, and the new food-guide pyramid recommends the *daily* ingestion of no fewer than 2 servings of fruits, and no fewer than 3 servings of vegetables. Lachance (1989) reported that every major national survey demonstrates that Americans continue to consume a 60:40 ratio of animal to plant foods, whereas the recommended

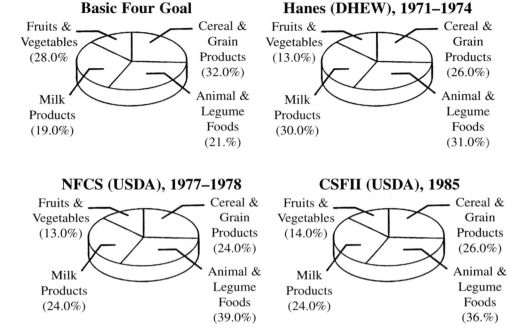

Figure 5.2 Comparison of the Basic Four recommendation to actual eating patterns. The Basic Four recommendation approximates the recommended 4:4:2:2 servings per day of key food groups. What Americans have been eating is reflected in the 1971–1974 Health and Nutrition Examination Survey data, the 1977–1978 National Food Consumption Survey data, and the 1985 Continuing Survey Food Individual Intakes data. Rather than consuming two servings of plant-derived food for each serving of animal-derived food, as recommended by the Basic Four food-guide concept, the consumer is doing the opposite.

From LaChance (1989).

pattern for about 50 years has been 40:60. One only needs to observe the food combinations ordered at fast-foods outlets and the food proportions served in restaurants to confirm that the emphasis is on the most expensive nutrient we purchase: protein, preferably of animal origin. Repeated national surveys (see Figure 5.2) demonstrate this phenomenon. From the first National Health and Nutrition Examination Survey (NHANES) follow-up study of 4,160 men and 6,264 women, Gladys Block (Kant et al., 1993) has compiled impressive data on dietary diversity and its significance on mortality. The abstract on page 434 of the article states:

> Although less than 5% of respondents reported omitting foods from the
> meat and grain groups on the survey day, 46% reported no fruit, 25% no
> dairy, and 17% reported no vegetable. Among those consuming two or
> fewer food groups more than 90% did not report fruit and more than
> 80% omitted foods from the dairy and vegetables groups. . . . Diets that
> omitted several food groups were associated with an increased risk
> (RR=1.4–1.5) of mortality.

PUBLIC HEALTH FORTIFICATION

Deaths directly attributable to beriberi, ariboflavinosis, and pellegra,
prevalent prior to and at the onset of World War II, became rare within 10
years after the vitamins thiamin, riboflavin, and niacin were added by
Presidential Executive Order to all wheat, corn, and rice flour and their
cereal products. The public health nutrition community (and the then
newly established Food and Nutrition Board of the National Academy of
Science), without placebo-controlled, double-blind clinical trials, convinced Franklin Delano Roosevelt to issue an Executive Order for the
duration of World War II. By 1945 when the Executive Order expired, several states had already moved to mandate the "enrichment" process. In
1941, the Food and Nutrition Board of the National Research Council of
the National Academy of Sciences (US) was formed and the first recommended dietary allowances were issued in 1943. Beginning in 1938 the
Standards of Identity for major classes of foods were promulgated by the
Food and Drug Administration. The "standard" incorporated the "enrichment" nutrients; however, no changes in the permitted nutritive ingredients
of these "standards" have been possible in over 50 years, even though the
Food and Nutrition Board (FNB) made concrete suggestions in 1974 to
expand "enrichment" to six vitamins and four mineral micronutrients,
rather than three vitamins and only one mineral (iron). A petition to the
FDA 4 years ago to make mandatory the 1943 optional addition of calcium
in the enrichment of flours, on the grounds that the extent and incidence
of four major chronic diseases (osteoporosis, colon cancer, hypertension,
and lead poisoning) can be reduced, has been pigeonholed. Table 5.2
reveals the best estimates of what micronutrient fortification contributes to

Table 5.2 Percentage of Nutrient Contribution of Enrichment and Forti
fication to Foods in the United States

Nutrient	Nutrient contribution (%)	
	1970	1985
Vitamin A	10	13
Vitamin C	10	8
Thiamin (B-1)	40	24
Riboflavin (B-2)	15	20
Niacin (B-3)	20	18
Vitamin B-6	4	6
Folacin	—	6
Vitamin B-12	2	4
Iron	25	24

From Lachance (1989).

the American diet (Lachance, 1989). Noteworthy is the fact that iron fortification has *not* altered the incidence of iron-deficiency anemia over the
last 50 years. This is true, even after the type of iron used as a fortificant
was changed from the poorly soluble ferric orhophosphate to highly
bioavailable forms, such as ferrous sulfate. This change was a result of
pressure at the 1969 White House Conference on Food Nutrition and
Health. The lack of effect probably indicates that one or more other
micronutrients are more limiting in iron-deficiency anemia than iron.
These may include vitamin B-6, folic acid, magnesium, and zinc, nutrients
that the 1974 FNB recommended to include in the "enrichment" flour
standards. In the face of clinical evidence for the need to enrich flour with
folic acid, and of the specific recommendation of the Centers for Disease
Control, a sister agency, the FDA, has recently promulgated a regulation
permitting folic acid enrichment of grain products to become mandatory
in January 1998. The addition of folate, even if only to restoration levels
(compensating for loses due to milling) would enhance daily intakes of all
Americans by 125 mcg. The impact on the incidence of spina bifida,
ancephaly, and the increased resistance to several cancers, because of the

role of folate in DNA synthesis and repair, seem logical grounds for an intervention to benefit the American public. Fortification technology makes possible complete meal-replacement products, and selected restorations and public health enrichments. Technology is no longer limiting further advances in the improvement in nutrient delivery via food systems (Bauernfeind & Lachance, 1991).

CONCLUSIONS

The worldwide supply of agricultural commodities is currently sufficient to meet the dietary needs of the world population, but the lack of food preservation and poor or hampered infrastructures for distribution promote areas of starvation, hunger, and malnutrition. An array of advanced preservation and fortification technologies is available, but these are seriously lacking in developing countries.

Americans (and some individuals in other developed countries) are consuming an increasing proportion of their diet away from home. The away-from-home diet has a higher energy and poorer nutrient density than the typical diet consumed at home. A phenomenon of "disinhibition" (of learned restraint) may contribute, along with a more sedentary lifestyle, to the increase in the prevalence of obesity (34% in the United States).

Nutrient fortification practices account for as much as 25% of the intake of selected nutrients (e.g., thiamin, iron) in the United States. Without fortification, pockets of micronutrient deficiency diseases would possibly be more prevalent. Food-fortification technology directed to remedying specific micronutrient deficiencies, vitamin A, iodine, and iron, in particular, is being adopted increasingly in developing countries.

REFERENCES

Allred, J. B. (1995). Too much of a good thing? An overemphasis on eating low-fat foods may be contributing to the alarming increase in overweight among US adults. *Journal of the American Dietetic Association, 95,* 417–418.

Bauernfeind, J., & Lachance, P. A. (Eds.). (1991). *Nutrient additions to food: Nutritional, technological and regulatory aspects.* Trumbull, CT: Food and Nutrition Press.

Breene, W.M. (1994). Healthfulness and nutritional quality of fresh versus processed fruits and vegetables: A review. *Journal of Foodservice Systems, 8,* 1–45.

Clydesdale, F. M., Ho, C. T., Lee, C. Y., Mondy, N. I., & Shewfelt, R. L. (1991). The effects of postharvest treatment and chemical interactions on the bioavailability of ascorbic acid, thiamine, vitamin A, carotenoids and minerals. *Critical Reviews in Food Science and Nutrition, 30,* 599–638.

Kant, A. K., Schatzin, A., Harris, T. B., Ziegler, R., & Block, G. (1993). Dietary diversity and subsequent mortality in the First HANES epidemiological follow-up study. *American Journal of Clinical Nutrition, 57,* 434–440.

Karmas,E., & Harris, R. S. (Ed.). (1988). *Nutritional evaluation of food processing* (3rd ed.). New York: Van Nostrand Reinhold.

Klesges, R. C., Isbell, T. R., & Klesges, L. M. (1992). Relationship between dietary restraint, energy intake, physical activity, and body weight: A prospective analysis. *Journal of Abnormal Psychology, 98,* 499–503.

Lachance, P. A. (1989). Nutritional responsibilities of food companies in the next century. *Food Technology, 43*(4),144.

Manchester, A. (1994). 1993 food spending picked-up. *Food Review* (USDA/ERS), *17*(3), 33–42.

Nickerson, J. T. R., & Ronsivalli, L. J. (1980). *Elementary food science* (2nd ed.). Westport, CT: AVI Publishing.

PART 2

Nutrition-Related Conditions and Diseases: Policies and Approaches

CHAPTER 6

Intervention Strategies for Undernutrition

Eileen T. Kennedy

D espite considerable progress in understanding the nature and causes of malnutrition, it continues to be a problem of staggering proportions in developing countries throughout the world. The Sixth World Food Survey (Food and Agricultural Organization of the United Nations [FAO], 1992) estimates that 20% of the world's population is energy deficient. In addition, the United Nations' Subcommitte on Nutrition (UN/SCN, 1992) report entitled, *The World Nutrition Situation,* indicates that 36% of preschool-aged children are moderately to severely malnourished, based on weight for age.

In the United States the nutrition situation is different. Problems of underconsumption and nutrient deficiencies that were common in the early part of the 20th century have been replaced, on average, by problems of excesses and imbalances. Food insecurity and inadequate nutritional status still affect portions of the U.S. population, however, primarily low-income groups.

A variety of nutrition interventions has been implemented in both developing and developed countries to deal with problems of undernutrition. This chapter provides a conceptual framework for identifying the factors influencing nutritional status at the individual, household, community, national, and international level. This chapter presents and critiques methods for assessing nutritional status, reviewing the most common interventions for mitigating undernutrition both at the individual and household level, as well as assessing their effectiveness. The chapter ends with a summary of "lessons learned" about the cost-effectiveness of nutrition interventions in developing countries and the United States.

CONCEPTUAL FRAMEWORK AND TOPOLOGY OF NUTRITION INTERVENTIONS

Policymakers have used a variety of approaches over the years to tackle the problem of undernutrition. Strategies have ranged from broad-based economic development policies intended to increase the incomes of the poor to more targeted food/nutrition interventions, aimed specifically at the most vulnerable members of society. Not all interventions have worked equally well in achieving their stated objectives. The imperative need to implement effective policies and programs that reduce the number of people suffering from undernutrition forces a reexamination of past interventions in an effort to learn from experience.

Although poor nutritional status (undernutrition and overnutrition) and malnutrition manifest themselves at the individual level, the causes typically reflect a combination of individual, household, community, national, and even international factors. The schema presented in Table 6.1 illustrates the range of causes of malnutrition and potential program and policy-intervention options, both for the United States and developing countries.

CAUSES OF MALNUTRITION

Food availability at the national, regional, or local level is one factor that can affect household-level food availability, but is generally not the most important. Until recently, emphasis was placed by many developing country policymakers on food production self-sufficiency as a means of achieving food security for the population. Many believed that national food self-sufficiency would alleviate malnutrition.

There are two major flaws with this argument. First, food insecurity and malnutrition are primarily problems of distribution, not production (World bank, 1986). It is common to have 20% to 30% of a country's population consuming less than 80% of the necessary caloric requirements, even though

Table 6.1 Schematic Overview of Factors Influencing Status and Policy Options

Issues influencing principal factors	Principal factors determining nutritional status	Programs and policies influencing the principal factors
Food production Food distribution (place, time) International trade and aid Processing and nonfood demands	Food availability, (national, regional, and local)	Research and technological changes in food and nonfood production Rural development schemes Input and output price policies Resource-ownership policies Changes in rural institutions Foreign trade and aid policies Other policies affecting area utilization and yields
Money income Prices Income in kind Own production	Ability to obtain available food (household)	Income-generating policies Income-transfer programs and policies Food-transfer programs and policies Food-price policies with or without explicit subsidies Food supply and demand policies with price effects Programs and policies affecting production for home consumption

continued

Table 6.1 *continued*

Issues influencing principal factors	Principal factors determining nutritional status	Programs and policies influencing the principal factors
		Policies and programs affecting the cost of nonfoods that complete for the household budget
Intrahousehold income distribution Outside influences Perceived food needs Perceived nutrition needs		
Past consumption, traditions, and social, cultural, and religious factors	Desire to obtain available food (household)	Policies and programs affecting intrahousehold distribution of control over incomes and spending Promotion and advertising Policies and programs affecting the range of spending opportunities perceived by the household
Intrahousehold food distribution Child care Weaning/feeding patterns Intrahousehold food processing	Utilization of obtained food to meet nutritional needs (household and individual)	Nutrition education

Table 6.1 *continued*

Food characteristics and composition Time constraints		
Water/sanitation	Health of the individual	Programs to supply macro- and micronutrients Child care and breast-feeding programs Food fortification Programs and policies regulating formulated foods
Prior nutritional status Diarrhea Infectious diseases Parasites Maternal nutritional status Activity patterns/work load	Nutritional status (individual)	Public health programs Integrated nutrition and health programs Water improvement and sanitary programs Disease prevention and cure Growth monitoring/growth promotion

Source: From Kennedy and Pinstrup-Andersen (1983).

national-level food availability is at or greater than 100% (World Bank, 1986). Clearly in the United States the overall nutrient and calorie content of the food supply is well above national needs (U.S. Department of Agriculture [USDA], 1995). It is the household's ability to obtain food that is critical in ensuring household food security. As the purchasing power of households increases, access to food increases.

The second flaw in the food self-sufficiency argument relates to the links between hunger and malnutrition. Hunger and malnutrition are not synonymous. Food is only one of a series of inputs into the production of health and nutritional status. Factors such as the health/sanitation environment, including hygienic practices within the household, availability of health services, food distribution within the household, cultural practices related to weaning, and child feeding practices can have a greater influence on nutrition than simply the amount of food available at the household level.

This is not to argue that macroeconomic policies (including those affecting food production) are not important. Clearly, national-level development policies have a direct effect on market prices, household income, and availability of publicly provided health and social services. These community- and household-level factors, then, have an impact on the health and nutritional status of individual family members.

IMPORTANCE OF APPROPRIATE INTERVENTIONS

The implementation of appropriate interventions depends on the ability to identify relationships between principal factors and the health and nutritional status of households and individuals. The type of interventions that will be most effective depends on which factor or combination of factors constitute the most limiting constraint in achieving good nutrition. The lack of empirical nutrition information in a context-specific setting has resulted in the implementation of interventions that have not addressed the underlying causes of the malnutrition problem. For example, on a macro level, the assumption has been that by focusing on income alone, the problem of malnutrition would be resolved. Clearly, this is not the case (Kennedy, Bouis, & von Blaun, 1992). Alternatively, on a more micro or targeted level, the supplementary schemes for preschoolers in developing countries, as typically implemented, have had only limited effects (Kennedy & Alderman, 1987).

The choice of the most appropriate intervention will depend on who is malnourished and why. This sounds obvious; yet, over and over again, an effective nutrition program or project has failed when transplanted to a new setting. The interventions may not be ineffective per se, but, more likely, are inappropriate given the nature and causes of the specific malnutrition problem in the new setting.

The list of nutrition interventions outlined in Table 6.1 covers the range of approaches that have typically been used to alleviate malnutrition and/ or improve nutritional status. Each of the interventions is based on different assumptions about who is malnourished and what are the causes of malnutrition. Are the malnourished simply those with a lower calorie diet, or are there other micro-nutrient needs? Are the causes of malnutrition primarily a result of food shortages, or are they due to a combination of factors, including exposure to infection and parasites, and lack of access to adequate sanitation and potable water supplies? Is malnutrition a national problem, a household problem, or a preschooler problem? Part of the continuing controversy as to which type of nutrition intervention is most effective results from the fact that policymakers are identifying different factors as the most limiting constraint in causing malnutrition.

Summary of Nutrition Interventions

There continues to be tension among policymakers in the use of broad-based economic policies as a means of dealing with undernutrition and more targeted food/nutrition interventions. This section summarizes the range of policies and programs that have been used to address problems of undernutrition in developing countries and the United States.

INTRODUCTION TO BROAD STRATEGIES

The direct relationship between increasing household income, poverty alleviation, and improved food consumption has been well documented (Alderman, 1986; Kennedy & Bouis, 1993). Strategies that increase the incomes of the poor will result in significant decreases in hunger. In developing countries, where the majority of people live in rural areas, an emphasis on agricultural policies and programs is a starting point for income-generating strategies to alleviate hunger and improve nutritional status. The main policy vehicles have been modernization and technological change and the commercialization of agriculture.

Modernization and Technological Change in Agriculture

New Seed Varieties

Investments in agricultural research have resulted in technologies that rely heavily on modern seed varieties and have had dramatic effects on food production, most notably in Asia and Latin America (Pinstrup-Andersen & Hazell, 1985). The increases in agricultural production have resulted in lower food prices, which directly benefit the urban consumer, the rural landless, and the smallholder producer who is a net purchaser of food. In rural areas, the production increases resulting from use of the new technologies have raised household incomes. For example, in North Arcot, India, households that adopted the new rice varieties more than doubled the real value of consumption of food and other consumer goods between 1973 and 1983/84 (Hazell, 1987); there was also a shift toward more varied diets within these households.

Technological change in agriculture has also generated increased demand for hired labor and has thus provided a means of increasing the income of the rural landless. Recent evidence suggests that labor intensity in crop production has diminished somewhat in the second phase of the green revolution (Binswanger & von Braun, 1991). New technologies have been estimated initially to have increased labor demand by about 25%. However, the labor requirements for rice production have declined somewhat since 1973/1974 because of the increased mechanization of irrigation pumping and paddy threshing. Although the global output of food supplies has increased because of high-yielding cereals, the pattern of growth across regions of the world has been uneven and variable (Anderson, 1985). The unirrigated areas of Asia are suffering energy deficiencies at least as severe as 10–15 years ago, and most of Africa is without modern varieties and is poorer than in the 1970s (Anderson, 1985). In some instances households have migrated from less favorable to more favorable growing environments, where modern varieties have substantially increased productivity. This is not to argue that the green revolution has been ineffective; rather, that additional approaches need to be pursued for regions that have been missed by these technological advances.

In Africa the main staples include millet, sorghum, cassava, and maize. With the exception of high-yielding varieties of maize in eastern and southern Africa, few advances have occurred in the production of millet and sorghum in Africa (Matlon & Adesina, 1991). As a result, the area devoted to millet and sorghum cultivation has expanded by about 1.0% per year in response to rapid population growth and fallow periods have declined. This may have negative implications for the sustainability of yields in the future because often there is no replacement in the soil.

The modernization of agriculture that has taken place over the past 25 years has involved heavy reliance on purchased inputs. Increased use of fertilizer and pesticides in combination with the new seed varieties has contributed to the production increases that have been observed. Notwithstanding higher input costs, the increase in agricultural output that has resulted from technological change has led to a decrease in production costs per unit of output.

Development and dissemination of modern cereal varieties over the past 25 years have dramatically increased food production. Successes in wheat and rice breeding are estimated to have increased global production of these commodities by about 40 million metric tons (Herdt & Capule, 1983). The resulting supply expansion has resulted in decreased food prices that have benefited the poor. In addition, there have been income and employment benefits for many of the households via multiplier effects for the rest of the economy, resulting in strong income/food consumption links. The links appear less strong for the relationship between income and individual nutritional status, however.

Commercialization of Agriculture

The deteriorating economic situation in the 1980s forced many developing countries to adopt a series of policy reforms. A common element of these economic adjustment programs has been emphasis on the commercialization of agriculture. Policymakers view export/cash crops as a means to generate foreign exchange, provide income-earning possibilities for the poor, and improve food security and nutrition.

Critics of the commercialization of agriculture have argued that national-level food security will deteriorate as farmers shift land from staple food crops into cash crops. National-level data suggest that this deterioration has not occurred, however. An analysis of data from 78 countries has indicated that countries that did well in the growth of export agriculture also had positive rates of growth in staple food production (von Braun & Kennedy, 1986). Appropriate policies for input supply, output marketing, and rural infrastructure have benefited both food-crop and cash-crop production. Expansion of export agriculture therefore need not be at the expense of staple-food production.

The most contentious issues in the cash-crop/food-crop debate have revolved around the impact of commercial agriculture on household food security and the nutritional status of individuals. Proponents of commercial agriculture contend that the transition from semisubsistence to a more commercialized agriculture will increase household income and, in turn, improve food intake and therefore health and nutritional status. Critics of cash-crop policies have argued that, in many cases, household income does not increase, and even in situations where household income improves, food security can deteriorate because income control has shifted from women to men.

A series of case studies recently conducted by the International Food Policy Research Institute (IFPRI) in The Gambia, Guatemala, Kenya, the Philippines, and Rwanda looked at the links between entry into commercial agriculture and the health and nutritional status of women and children (von Braun & Kennedy, 1994). The five case studies used a similar protocol, emphasizing the links between commercialization of agriculture and individual nutritional status.

A key assumption is that a primary positive effect of agricultural commercialization is to increase household incomes. These in turn could lead to increased food consumption, as well as increased expenditures on health and health maintenance. In addition, as a result of hiring labor for farm work and less need to seek employment outside the home, more time could be made available for nurturing behavior.

In all five case studies, The Gambia, Guatemala, Kenya, the Philippines, and Rwanda, the incomes of the more commercialized households increased; at least a portion of this increase was due to cultivation of the new cash crop. There was also a conscious effort on the part of smallholder farmers to maintain subsistence production along with the commercial crop, even though the returns to land and labor in most cases are higher for the cash crop than the staple crop. This appears to be the response of households to high transaction costs and market, employment, and production risks.

Similar to the findings on introduction of modern cereal varieties, entry into commercial agriculture tends to occur earlier and more often for richer farmers. A longitudinal study from Kenya found that it was the wealthier, larger landholding farmers who began sugarcane production soonest (Kennedy, 1989). Once it was established that sugarcane production could be profitable, the poorer farmers entered the scheme. These new entrants had returns to land and labor that were as good as, or in some cases better than, those of the earlier participants. This is a general theme in the literature: the risk-averse, poorer farmers are late adopters but, having adopted, can profit from the innovations.

Earlier entry of farmers with smaller than normal farms could be facilitated by easier access to services. Credit is often difficult for poor farmers to obtain, and agricultural extension services are typically biased against smallholders, particularly women farmers (Staudt, 1978). Government policies can relieve these and other constraints for the poor (Binswanger & von Braun, 1991).

Commercialized agriculture has also resulted in increased employment (von Braun & Kennedy, 1994); however, the employment effects are very crop and location specific and are a function of the technologies introduced. Choice of crop and technology, therefore, has a major influence on the actual employment; when the commercial crop involves more processing, the demand for hired labor is likely to increase substantially.

The generally positive income effect of cash cropping has resulted in an increase in food expenditures and household calorie consumption. The impact of commercialization on food expenditures was greater than on calories, because households tended to purchase more varied, higher priced sources of calories, such as meats and fruits. Higher household calorie intakes were associated with increases in the energy consumption of preschoolers. The increases, although statistically significant, were modest, however. A doubling of household income in Kenya and the Philippines resulted in an increase in preschooler energy intake of only 4% and 7%, respectively, whereas the average calorie intake was 20 to 30% below recommended levels. Because the food-consumption analysis was limited primarily to calories, however, the income/micronutrient impact of cash-cropping schemes may have been underestimated.

In the IFPRI commercialization studies, increases in household income were not usually found to be associated with a significant decrease in the morbidity of preschool-aged children (Kennedy et al., 1992). This is because the poor health/sanitation environment in the study areas overshadowed any potential positive effect of increasing household income on child health. The one exception was in Guatemala, where participation in an export vegetable scheme was associated with a decrease in the incidence of illness in preschool-age children. Interestingly, the export cooperative had a health/social welfare component financed out of profits generated from the smallholders' scheme. The positive health effect was related to this rather than the increment in household income.

Interventions Targeted to the Individual or Household

Critics of broad agricultural and economic policies have argued that there is a long lead time for these approaches to improve significantly overall health and nutritional status of low-income populations. Therefore, the argument is made that in the short to medium term, interventions targeted to vulnerable individuals and/or households also need to be implemented.

Supplementary Feeding Programs

Supplementary feeding programs are a common type of nutrition intervention in developing countries. Typically, these schemes provide supplementary food, either on-site or for taking home. Generally, the food supplement is made available to preschool-age children and, to a lesser extent, to pregnant women and school-age children. Supplementation programs are based on the premise that food given directly to nutritionally vulnerable groups, such as women and children, will do more to improve their energy and nutrient intake than interventions directed to the household.

However, a review of over 200 supplemental feeding programs in developing countries concluded that such programs, as normally operated, have not been very effective in alleviating malnutrition (Beaton & Ghassemi, 1982). Often, these programs tended to have erratic participation and large leakage of the supplement to nontarget individuals, thereby significantly increasing cost. In contrast, supplementation programs that were effective in improving nutritional status tend to have certain characteristics in common: provision of a high level of calories (often close to 100% of requirements); targeting to moderately and severely malnourished individuals; and regular participation over a 3- to 12-month period (Kennedy & Alderman, 1987).

The modest impact of many supplemental feeding programs led to a rethinking of these schemes, with an emphasis on selective use of food combined with growth monitoring/promotion activities. The Tamil Nadu Nutrition Program in India is an example of the successful application of this approach (Berg & Austin, 1984). All children are weighed monthly, but only one-third of the most vulnerable (those who failed to gain weight or those children who lost weight) are given supplemental food. Food is given only for a 3-month period; those children who fail to improve during this 90-day period are then referred for more intensive care.

Although most supplementation programs are targeted to preschoolers, it is supplementation of pregnant women that is often most cost-effective. Energy supplementation of high-risk pregnant women is associated with significant decreases in neonatal and infant mortality.

Special Supplemental Food Program for Women, Infants and Children

Despite the somewhat lackluster success, on average, of many supplemental feeding programs in developing countries, the experience in the United States has been different. The Special Supplemental Feeding Program for Women, Infants and Children (WIC), was created, in part, as a response to the recommendation of the 1969 White House Conference on Food, Nutrition and Health that pregnant women and preschool-age children be given a top priority for nutrition programs (cf. Chapters 13 and 14).

WIC began as a 2-year pilot project in 1972. The program provides supplemental food, nutrition education, and serves as an adjunct to health care. As of 1994, WIC was serving 6.5 million participants operating through 85 state agencies and 8,000 local agencies. Currently, WIC serves 40% of all infants born in the U.S. and one out of four pregnant women in the country. Why is WIC so popular?

One reason is the accumulating body of research evidence that WIC has been successful in improving nutritional status. A series of studies conducted from 1974 to the mid-1980s, using a variety of research designs, each with different strengths, has documented a consistent pattern of positive, significant health/nutrition benefits associated with participation in the WIC program (Kennedy & Summer, 1989). A number of studies have also been done to analyze the cost-effectiveness of WIC's prenatal component. Participation in WIC prenatally results in $1.77 to $3.90 in health care savings per individual per dollar spent (Devaney & Schirm, 1993). Data from five U.S. states, Florida, North Carolina, South Carolina, Minnesota, and Texas, indicate that infant mortality had significantly decreased with WIC participation in all states but Minnesota. Most of the decline has been due to a decrease in neonatal mortality.

Several factors account for WIC success in improving nutritional status; the high level of energy supplementation; targeting of program benefits to high-risk individuals; and an integrated approach to providing food, health care, and nutrition education (Kennedy & Summer, 1989).

Weaning Foods/Formulated Foods

Formulated or blended foods were originally conceived of as a low-cost, commercially available processed food used during weaning. A formulated food is a nutrient-dense dietary supplement based primarily on a mixture of a local staple and vegetable proteins. Commercial weaning foods come in a variety of forms, including beverages, pastas, and biscuits. Examples include Incaparina, a beverage available in Guatemala; Superamine, an Algerian pasta; and Wheat Soy Blend Flour, which is sometimes provided as part of Food Aid.

Commercial weaning foods have had limited success. First, cost has been the principal barrier to widespread use. On a nutrient-per-dollar basis, commercial weaning foods are between 8 and 40 times more expensive than homemade traditional foods (Kennedy, 1983). Even with substantial government subsidies, the cost of these foods is prohibitive for many poor households. Second, the acceptability of commercial weaning foods has been low. Third, there is an urban bias in distribution because marketing channels and commercial vendors are not as readily available in rural areas.

As a result of the limited success in formulated or blended weaning foods, most governments are now stressing the use of home-produced weaning foods. This type of weaning food can be produced at lower cost, with better acceptability, and is made up of indigenous household foods (Kennedy, 1983).

The most successful weaning-food interventions have been combined with nutrition education, using social marketing techniques. There are instances, however, in which nutrition education regarding the needs of the child being weaned is not the limiting factor in providing adequate food for the child. Financial constraints within the household may preclude sufficient calories for the preschooler. In this case, a weaning food could be provided as part of an integrated health/nutrition intervention and distributed free to vulnerable households. If possible, such a weaning food should be one that is prepared locally in villages and not manufactured on a large-scale commercial basis.

Fortification

Diets of low-income households and young children in developing countries are often characterized by a lack of diversity. Staple grains, such as rice, wheat, and corn, are only occasionally supplemented with vegetables and small bits of meat or fish. These cereal-based diets are the major source of calories and micronutrients. Countries in which a single grain supplies a disproportionate share of the total dietary intake consistently show a higher prevalence of micronutrient deficiencies (Kennedy, el Lozy, & Gershoff, 1979).

Vitamin A, iodine, and iron-folate are the three most common micronutrient deficiencies in developing countries. As a result, fortification programs have typically focused on one or a combination of these nutrients. The most dramatic results have been obtained by the addition of iodine to salt. Iodination of salt has almost completely eliminated goiter and cretinism in the United States and some parts of Latin America and Asia (Austin et al., 1981).

The results of vitamin A fortification programs are less clear-cut. Vitamin A deficiency is associated with night blindness, xerophthalmia, and, if left untreated, eventual blindness. An accumulating body of evidence now suggests that vitamin A supplementation decreases mortality and certain types of morbidity. Vitamin A fortification of sugar in Guatemala and of monosodium glutamate (MSG) in the Philippines has had some success in increasing serum vitamin A levels. The MSG fortification program also showed a reduction in the clinical signs of vitamin A deficiency.

The success of fortification with any nutrient depends on identifying a food that is consumed regularly by the target population. Where this is not feasible, a mass-dose program is a possible alternative. A recent randomized clinical trial in India, involving 15,419 preschool-age children, delivered low doses of vitamin A weekly to children with the aid of community health volunteers (Rahmathullah et al., 1990). There was a significant decrease (54%) in mortality among children receiving the vitamin A supplement.

Mass dose distribution programs have been less successful in other countries, particularly in Africa, where coverage of the target population is poor. Some of the principal reasons for the poor coverage include irregular or short supply of the vitamin, lack of supervision by program personnel, and lack of preparedness of the community. A weekly distribution of vitamin A, as done in India, would be much more difficult to implement in parts of rural Africa, where infrastructure is poorly developed. The difficulty in accessing convenient distribution points is compounded by the long distances that people must travel in rural Africa.

Iron-folate supplementation programs have proved successful in some areas in improving the hematological status of pregnant women (Sood et al., 1975). Programs for preschoolers have had less success, primarily because of sporadic coverage and infrequent participation by the intended beneficiary.

Success in improving preschooler growth in some programs without the distribution of food strengthened the inference that a lack of nutrition knowledge or awareness limited improvement of nutritional status in, at least, some households (Rohde, Ismail, & Sutrinso, 1975). Interventions under the general label of "nutrition education" have been used to address this knowledge or attitudes gap. However, the freestanding nutrition education interventions that were common in the 1960s and 1970s have been replaced by programs in which nutrition education is provided in conjunction with other activities. Thus, a weaning-foods intervention integrates nutrition-education skills as part of the program.

Given the checkered success rate of nutrition interventions targeted to specific individuals, many policymakers believe that interventions aimed at households may be a more cost-effective way of improving the nutritional status of vulnerable individuals. Berg (1981) has concluded that even if policymakers were interested in reaching only preschoolers, it would often be more cost-effective to reach them through programs that would affect households as a whole. Many of the intervention strategies outlined in Table 6.1 have a household orientation.

Targeted Consumer-Price Subsidies

Targeted food-price subsidies are a popular and common type of intervention aimed at increasing food consumption of poor households. Subsidized food items are provided to consumers at below market prices. Lower food prices increase the real incomes of the poor; this approach generally results in higher expenditures on food. Subsidy programs are attractive policy instruments because they are highly visible and allow governments to reach a large number of poor people easily. Food price subsidies have been criticized as being expensive, however, even when part of well-targeted schemes.

Most subsidy programs are intended to achieve broad social and political goals. Better nutrition may be a stated or unstated objective of these programs. A recent multicountry study of the nutrition impacts of subsidy schemes (Kumar & Alderman, 1989) found that such schemes can have a significant impact on household food consumption. The nutritional effectiveness of a specific subsidy program will increase if it is aimed at those households with the greatest caloric deficits and, in turn, at those individuals within the household who are most nutritionally vulnerable (Pinstrup-Andersen, 1989). The potential nutrition effect of any food subsidy will be enhanced if the subsidy can be applied to a food normally consumed in large amounts by the malnourished population, but that is not eaten by other income groups. This type of "self-targeting" food was used successfully in Pakistan and Bangladesh (Rogers et al., 1981).

Food Stamps

Food-stamp programs are potentially a less costly alternative to food-subsidy schemes. Sri Lanka switched from a ration system to food stamps in 1979 and reduced total government expenditures from 14% to 7% (Edirisinghe, 1984). Jamaica also garnered a substantial saving in government expenditures by replacing a general food-subsidy system with a food-stamp program.

U.S. Food Stamp Program

The U.S. Food Stamp Program (FSP) was established in the mid-1960s to provide adequate food-purchasing power for low-income households. The basic premise underlying the FSP is that use of food stamps will increase food expenditures, which in turn will improve food consumption/ nutrient intake and ultimately improve health. A number of studies have documented that food expenditures increase with participation in the FSP (Basiotis, Johnson, Morgan, & Chen, 1987; Fraker, 1990; West, 1984).

In addition, data from the USDA show that diets of the poor have improved dramatically between the period 1965/1966 and 1977/1978, a period that marked the nationwide expansion of the Food Stamp Program (Kennedy, 1995); the lower intake of a range of nutrients noted in 1965/ 1966 in low-income groups was not apparent in 1977/1978. Between 1965 and 1977, the average group nutrient intake levels for households in the lowest income group improved more than those in other income groups. A part of this improvement was due to participation in the Food Stamp Program.

Food-Stamp Summary

Empirical evidence suggests that the food consumption of low-income households increases as a result of participation in both food-subsidy and food-stamp programs. There is little documentation of the effect on nutrition of individual family members when a household participates in these programs, however. This failure to demonstrate an observable effect on individual nutrition status is related in part to the complex linkage between household food expenditures, household caloric intake, individual member caloric intake, and, ultimately, growth.

Table 6.2 Summary of Nutrition Interventions

Program	Effectiveness	Constraints
Consumer food-price subsidies	There is some evidence that subsidies improve family caloric consumption, but little evidence to suggest that subsidies can alleviate preschooler or maternal malnutrition. They are most effective as preventive strategy for improving nutrition.	Subsidies are difficult to implement on a small scale and expensive to implement on a large scale. They are administratively difficult to implement in rural areas. They are most cost-effective when combined with some type of targeting— either to lowest income groups or by use of self-targeting food.
Food stamps	Like subsidies, there is some evidence that food stamps can increase family nutrient intake, but no evidence to date that food stamps are effective in improving maternal or preschooler nutritional status. Focus is preventive rather than therapeutic.	Food stamps are feasible only where households rely on the marketplace for food purchases; in this sense they are subject to urban bias.
	U.S. program has consistent evidence that the Food Stamp Program increases food expenditures and nutrient intake.	Urban bias is less apparent in the U.S.
Food-for-work	Information on nutritional effectiveness is	Most programs rely heavily on food aid.

Table 6.2 Summary of Nutrition Interventions

	limited. Given the focus of most programs (1 to 3 months of participation), it is most effective in alleviating seasonal fluctuations in consumption.	
Supplementary feeding	As these programs have been typically operated, they are not very effective in improving preschooler malnutrition. They are most effective when targeted to high-risk individuals. Programs that offer a small ration (200-300 calories) to a large number of people are unlikely to show a measurable impact on growth.	The level of supplementation provided has not taken into account leakage to nontarget group individuals. As a result, net calories consumed by a child are not enough to cover the energy gap and/or improve growth. Also, programs are administratively intensive, requiring moderate amounts of infrastructure and logistical support.
	WIC program is an exception; strong evidence from a series of studies that WIC participation improves neonatal outcome, including decreasing low birth weight and infant mortality. Studies also document improvements in children's growth and/ or hematological status.	WIC program capitalizes on strong health infrastructure. Longer participation in WIC is equated with more positive impact. Some programs are more effective than others in encouraging early and frequent participation.

continued

Table 6.2 *continued*

Program	Effectiveness	Constraints
Integrated health/nutrition	An appropriate mix of health/nutrition services is effective in improving maternal and child health. Successful projects have targeted services to high-risk persons, have used supplementary feeding selectively, and tailored program components to individual needs.	Program usually requires some health infrastructure and is very labor intensive.
Formulated foods	Only limited success in improving nutritional status of preschoolers has been observed.	Cost is a primary barrier for commercially available weaning foods. Low consumer acceptability has also limited use of these foods.
Home gardens	Some evidence suggests an impact on increasing micronutrient intake, but the effect on increasing macronutrient consumption appears limited.	Land and labor is insufficient for cultivation of home garden by the most nutritionally needy families.

CONCLUSIONS ON INDIVIDUAL OR HOUSEHOLD INTERVENTIONS

The preceding review illustrates that nutritional effectiveness of various interventions has been mixed. Table 6.2 summarizes what is known about the effectiveness of and constraints to successful implementation of the programs just reviewed.

Part of the discrepancy in nutritional effectiveness across programs is related to the differences in objectives of the interventions. Most family-oriented programs—food subsidies and food stamps—emphasize obtaining food. By providing food or purchasing power, these programs concentrate on making it possible to provide an adequate household diet. It is not the stated objective of these family interventions to alleviate malnutrition; rather the focus of these programs is to prevent dietary insufficiency and hunger.

Programs directed toward specific individuals within a household often have a therapeutic focus. For example, many of the supplemental feeding programs reviewed target benefits only to children who are already malnourished.

Given the range of objectives for the different programs, it is not surprising that success in achieving the various objectives has varied. A food-subsidy program that is effective in maintaining family calorie consumption is probably an inappropriate vehicle for treating severely malnourished children.

SUMMARY

Consumption and nutritional status can be improved in a variety of ways. The choice of a particular policy instrument should be dictated in large part by the nature of the malnutrition problem and the goals of the intervention. Planners are frequently ambivalent about what a program should do. This, of course, affects evaluation.

Broad-based agricultural and macroeconomic policies often need implementation of complementary health/nutrition interventions in order to protect the vulnerable population in the short to medium term.

For interventions aimed at either an individual or a household, some form of targeting almost always improves the cost-effectiveness of the approach. The most appropriate targeting strategy will depend on the local environment. Geographical targeting as a means of reaching households with malnourished members can work if it is possible to identify an area with a high proportion of energy-deficient households and/or a high proportion of malnutrition.

Nutrition programs typically have a variety of goals that the government is trying to achieve, however. Because of the need of governments for political support, interventions often cover a group larger than those that would be defined as nutritionally needy. Although this broad approach might be attractive, it can be expensive.

Policy decisions about whether and how to invest in nutrition are made at the country and/or donor level, whereas implementation typically occurs at the local level. Nutrition officers or nutrition workers need to be able to identify the nature of the malnutrition problem and to point to feasible solutions within the local environment.

In the United States, over the past 30 years, an effective nutrition safety net has developed that involves a variety of programs. Low-income households at risk of hunger have access to food purchases via the Food Stamp Program. The nutrition worker at the local level, by encouraging and facilitating participation, can be the link between vulnerable households and the Food Stamp Program. At-risk households members—children, women, the elderly—often require special nutrition interventions targeted to the individual. For low-income women and children, the WIC program complements the household-oriented Food Stamp Program, by providing supplemental foods, health care, and nutrition education to high-risk individuals. Inasmuch as the program is currently serving only approximately 60% of eligible individuals, the local nutrition worker can serve as the link between the program and the at-risk individual. For the nutritionally vulnerable elderly person, a combination of congregate feeding programs and/or home-delivered meals would complement the Food Stamp Program. Some of the proposals put forward in 1996 by the United States Congress could have changed the basic structure of the U.S. nutrition programs by providing block grants that would have allowed states to determine a state-specific level of benefits and in some cases, even eliminate programs. In the final analysis, the welfare reform proposals did not block grant the nutrition programs and thus the U.S. nutrition safety net has been maintained.

In developing countries the task is more complicated for the nutrition worker because the level of nutrition need is usually greater than in the United States, but the resources are fewer. Nonetheless the hunger/undernutrition problem typically requires a multifaceted approach of interventions that are focused on both household and the individual. Targeted food subsidies and/or food-for-work programs can be an effective way of increasing the food purchases of vulnerable households. In addition, interventions aimed specifically at malnourished pregnant women and children, in which supplementary foods combined with health care are provided, enhance the nutrition effectiveness of family-oriented interventions. Here also, the nutrition worker can be the lynchpin, linking the household and the individual to available interventions within the community.

Where nutrition interventions have been successful in alleviating malnutrition and/or improving nutritional status, it has almost always involved a combination of appropriate macroeconomic policies in conjunction with appropriately implemented community programs. Research suggests that this national/community focus will continue to be important. The nutrition officer can play a significant role in translating economic policy at the community level and in calling attention to specific problems at the local level.

REFERENCES

Alderman, H. (1986). *The effect of food price and income changes on the acquisition of food and income changes on the acquisition of food by low-income households.* An IFPRI Occasional Paper. Washington, DC: International Food Policy Research Institute.

Anderson, J. (1985). *International agricultural research centers: Achievements and potential.* Washington, DC: The Consultative Group on International Agricultural Research (CGIAR) Secretariat.

Austin, J. E., Belding, T. K., Pyle, D., Solon, F. S., Fernandez, L., Latham, M., & Popkin, B. M. (1981). *Nutrition intervention in developing countries, study III: Fortification.* Cambridge, MA: Oelgeschlager, Gunn and Hain.

Basiotis, P., Johnson, S. R., Morgan, K. J., & Chen, J. S. (1987). Food stamps, food costs, nutrient availability and nutrient intake. *Journal of Policy Modeling, 9,* 383.

Beaton, G., & Ghassemi, H. (1982). Supplementary feeding programs for young children in developing countries. *American Journal of Clinical Nutrition, 34,* (Suppl.) 864–916.

Berg, A. (1981). Malnourished people: A policy view. *Poverty and Basic Needs Series.* Washington, DC: World Bank.

Berg, A., & Austin, J. (1984). Nutrition policies and programs: A decade of redirection. *Food Policy,* (November), 304–312.

Binswanger, H., & von Braun, J. (1991). Technological change commercialization of agriculture: The effect on the poor. *Bank Research Observer, 6,* 57–80.

Devaney, B., & Schirm, A. (1993) *Infant mortality among medicaid newborns in 5 states: The effects of prenatal WIC participation.* Princeton, NJ: Mathematica Policy Research.

Edirisinghe, N. (1984, May). *The implications of the change from ration shops to food stamps in Sri Lanka for fiscal costs, income distribution, and nutrition.* Paper prepared for Workshop on Consumer-Oriented Food Subsidies held by International Food Policy Research Institute, Washington, DC.

Food and Agricultural Organization. (1995). *Sixth world food survey*—Rome.

Fraker, T. (1990). *The effects of food stamps on food consumption: A review of the literature.* Washington DC: Mathematica Policy Research.

Hazell, P. B. R. (1987). Changing patterns of variability in cereal prices and production. In Mellor, J. W., & Anned, R. (Ed.), *Agricultural price policy for developing countries*, (pp. 27–52). Baltimore, MD: Johns Hopkins University Press.

Herdt, R. W., & Capule, C. (1983). *Adoption spread and production impact of modern rice varieties in Asia.* Los Banos, Laguna, Philippines: International Rice Research Institute.

Kennedy, E. (1983). Determinants of family and preschooler food consumption. *Food and Nutrition Bulletin, 5,* 22–29.

Kennedy, E. (1989). *The effects of sugarcane production on food security, health, and nutrition in Kenya: A longitudinal analysis.* Research Report 78. Washington, DC: International Food Policy Research Institute.

Kennedy, E. (1995). *Public policy implications of emerging legislation's for USDA food assistance and nutrition programs.* Paper presented at Experimental Biology meetings, April, Atlanta, GA.

Kennedy, E., & Alderman, H. (1987). *Comparative analyses of nutritional effectiveness of food subsidies and other food-related interventions.* Joint WHO–UNICEF Nutrition Support Program. An IFPRI occasional paper. Washington, DC: International Food Policy Research Institute.

Kennedy, E., & Bouis, H. (1993). *Linkages between agriculture and nutrition: Implications for public policy.* Washington, DC: International Food Policy Research Institute.

Kennedy, E., Bouis, H. E., & von Braun, J. (1992). Health and nutrition effects of cash crop production in developing countries: A comparative analysis. *Social Science and Medicine, 35,* 689–697.

Kennedy, E., el Lozy, M., & Gershoff, S. N. (1979). Nutritional need. In J. E. Austin (Ed.), *Global malnutrition and cereal fortification* (pp. 15–34). Cambridge, MA: Ballinger.

Kennedy, E., & Summer, L. (1989). The U.S. WIC program: Elements of success. In *Successful nutrition programs: What makes them work?* Rome, Italy: United Nations, subcommittee on Nutrition.

Kumar, S., & Alderman, H. (1989). Food consumption and nutritional effects of consumer-oriented food subsidies. In P. Pinstrup-Andersen (Ed.), *Food subsidies in developing countries: Costs, benefits, and policy options*, (pp. 36–48). Baltimore, MD: Johns Hopkins University Press.

Malton, P., & Adesina, A. (1991, September). Prospects for sustainable growth in sorghum and millet productivity in West Africa. In S. Vosti, T. Reardon, & W.

von Urff (Eds.), *Agricultural sustainability, growth, and poverty alleviation: Issues and policies*, (pp. 363–387). Proceedings of an international conference, Feldafing, Germany.

Pinstrup-Andersen, P. (1989). *Cash cropping, food security, and nutrition: Conceptual relationships and assessment approaches.* World Bank Staff Working Paper No. 456. Washington, DC: World Bank.

Pinstrup-Andersen, P., & Hazell, P. B. R. (1985). The impact of the green revolution and prospects for the future. *Food Review International, 1,* 1–25.

Rahmathullah, L., Underwood, B. A., Thulasiraj, R. D., Milton, D., Ramaswarny, K., Rahmathullah, R., & Babu, G. (1990). Reduced mortality among children in southern India receiving a small weekly dose of vitamin A. *New England Journal of Medicine, 323,* 929–935.

Rohde, J. E., Ismail, D., & Sutrinso, R. (1975). Mothers as weight watchers: The road to child health in the village. *Journal of Tropical Pediatrics, 21,* 2295–297.

Rogers, B. L., Overholt, C. A., Kennedy, E. T., Sanchez, F., Chavez, A., Belding, T. K., Timmer, C. P., & Austin, J. E. (1981). *Nutrition intervention in developing countries, Study V: Consumer food price subsidies.* Cambridge, MA: Oelges-chlager, Gunn & Hain.

Sood, S. K., Ramachandran, K., Mathur, M., Gupta, K., Ramalingaswamy, V., Swarnabai, C., Ponnial, J., Mathan, V. I., & Baker, S. J. (1975). WHO sponsored collaborative studies on nutritional anemia in India, I. The effects of supplemental oral iron administration to pregnant women. *Quarterly Journal of Medicine, 44,* 241–258.

Staudt, K. (1978). Agricultural productivity gaps: A case study of male preference in government policy implementation. *Development and Change, 9,* 439–457.

United Nations Administrative Committee on Coordination, Subcommittee on Nutrition. (1992). *World nutrition situation report.* Geneva: ACC/SCN.

U.S. Department of Agriculture. (1995). *Nutrient content of the U.S. food supply.* Washington, DC: Center for Nutrition Policy and Promotion.

von Braun, J. J., & Kennedy, E. (1994). *Agricultural commercialization, economic development and nutrition.* Baltimore, MD: Johns Hopkins University Press.

von Braun, J. J., & Kennedy, E. (1986). *Commercialization of subsistence agriculture: Income and nutritional effects in developing countries.* Working Papers on Commercialization of Agriculture and Nutrition No. 1. Washington, DC: International Food Policy Research Institute.

World Bank. (1986). *Poverty and hunger: Issues and options for food security in developing countries.* A World Bank Policy Study. Washington, DC: World Bank.

West, D. A. (1984). *Effects of the Food Stamp Program on food expenditures.* Agricultural Research Center. Research Bulletin XB 0922. Pullman, WA: Washington State University.

CHAPTER 7

The Obesity Epidemic: Nutrition Policy and Public Health Imperatives

Barbara J. Moore, C. Everett Koop, and Judith S. Stern

THE PROBLEM OF OBESITY

Obesity is the leading form of malnutrition in the United States, affecting nearly 60 million adults (U.S. Dept. Health and Human Services, 1995). Even more alarming are the results from the National Health and Nutrition Examination Survey III (NHANES III), which reveal that one out of five children aged 7 to 19 years is overweight (Troiano, Flegal, Kuczmarski, Campbell, & Johnson, 1995). These figures represent approximately a 30% increase in obesity prevalence since the late 1970s (NHANES II). In an analysis of deaths in the United States during 1990, McGinnis and Foege (1993) concluded that diet and inactivity—known to be major contributors to obesity—are the "actual causes" of more than 300,000 preventable deaths. Subsequent analysis of the relationship between body mass index (BMI) and premature mortality by Manson et al. (1995) has corroborated that number.

Because obesity is linked to 5 of the 10 leading causes of death and health disability in the United States, it represents a multibillion dollar drain on the U.S. economy. Obesity is linked to heart disease, adult-onset diabetes, hypertension, atherosclerosis, stroke, and certain types of cancer. Its costs have been estimated at more than $100 billion annually (Colditz, 1992; Institute of Medicine [IOM], 1995). This includes $46 billion in direct costs, such as hospital care and physician services—or 6.8% of all health care costs, $33 billion on weight-reduction products and services; $19 billion in the indirect costs of lost output, and $4 billion in work days lost to illness attributable to obesity. In addition, researchers calculate that the number of work days lost to weight-related health problems amounts to about 53 million.

THE CONTEXT OF OBESITY: THE BALANCE OF INTAKE AND EXPENDITURE

Until recently, most humans engaged in high levels of activity in the form of physical labor. Since the dawn of the industrial revolution, large segments of the population have been freed of the necessity for heavy physical labor on a daily basis. In the past, a large appetite was prized and, indeed, there was a need to maintain a robust appetite so that one might consume the quantities of food necessary to balance the large daily expenditure of energy in the form of physical labor. A large appetite was seen as both healthful and desirable; hence, an entire course in a multicourse dinner was devoted to whetting the appetite—the appetizer course. Socially, the challenge was to make enough food available to laboring classes so that they might continue to sustain their daily levels of caloric expenditure.

Today, the daily energy expenditure on the part of the majority of men and women living in industrialized nations like the United States is considerably lower than it was at the beginning of the 20th century, when the majority of people worked in the agricultural sector. Whereas an agricultural laborer might have to expend 3500 to 4000 calories a day during the planting or harvesting of crops, today's office laborers typically need to expend only half that amount of energy. In order to avoid weight gain, modern men and women must struggle to contain their robust appetites within the bounds needed to match their much more modest daily energy expenditures. This state of affairs faces all countries that have sizable segments of the population in more sedentary job categories. In short, modern men and women are faced with a mismatch of appetite and required expenditure.

Certainly there are some individuals who have no difficulty consuming small amounts of food, that is, they have appetites that are appropriate for the more modest energy demands of the modern, more sedentary society. For others, the mismatch of appetite and energy expenditure is a source of constant struggle and consternation.

Why do some people have no difficulty eating less food to match contemporary society's reduced demands on individual energy expenditure, whereas for others it is a constant struggle? Genetic factors seem to modulate the mechanisms that control appetite. Thus, the recent discovery of leptin, a protein that functions as a putative satiety signal in appetite regulation in rodents, is a promising development that may one day lead to therapeutic interventions that influence appetite.

The list of single-gene mutations that cause obesity in rodents includes: diabetes (*db*), fat (*fat*), obese (*ob*), tubby (*tub*), adipose (*Ad*) and Yellow (*A*^{y}) in the mouse, and fatty (*fa*) in the rat (Friedman, Leibel, & Bahary, 1991). Several of these genes have been cloned (Warden & Fisler, 1996). Investigations of these animals continue, with db/db and ob/ob mouse models yielding important research into the generation and reception of satiety signals that appear fundamental to the regulation of food intake and energy balance. Bray (1996) has summarized recent discoveries in the ob/ob mouse, calling attention to the startling discovery that the genetic defect was expressed only in adipose tissue. As a consequence, abnormally low levels of leptin are produced and secreted into the blood. When the obese animals are injected with the protein, food intake is reduced and body fat content normalizes (Bray, 1996). By powerfully implicating the genetic basis for energy intake and a sense of satiety, these findings may ultimately find application in the treatment of obesity. The path to such interventions will likely not be straightforward because it is known that in obese humans, leptin is elevated.

Considering the problem from the expenditure side of the equation, it might also be asked why some individuals willingly increase their energy expenditure through physical activity during leisure or discretionary time so that their daily energy expenditure is elevated through physical activities, such as walking, jogging, biking, and so on. The effort made by these individuals may or may not be described as a struggle. For some, physical activity is pleasurable and may not require the prodigious application of discipline; for others, it may require daily discussion and self-examination as one weighs how one allocates one's time between the couch and the treadmill. Exercisers address the mismatch between appetite and the reduced physical demands of contemporary society not by struggling to decrease their appetite and intake of food, but by increasing daily energy expenditures in an attempt to balance appetite and expenditure. Still, others may choose to combine the two strategies of curbing the appetite and increasing physical activity.

Genetic and metabolic factors that characterize voluntarily active individuals have been less well studied and there is, as yet, no discovery or breakthrough on the expenditure side of the energy-balance equation that corresponds to the discovery of leptin on the intake/appetite side of the equation. There may well be subtle metabolic factors that influence energy expenditure by influencing thermoregulatory mechanisms or other components of the resting energy expenditure. For example, leptin, when injected into mice, increases metabolic rate, body temperature, and activity levels (Pelleymounter et al., 1995). Further research may yet yield information that one day could lead to helpful therapeutic interventions.

In the absence of a detailed understanding of the mechanisms of appetite and satiety that control food intake and energy expenditure, and because of the conspicuous lack of long-term therapeutic interventions that permit maintenance of weight loss, modern societies are faced with a number of difficulties. First, is the struggle to increase voluntary activity. This is an imperative even in individuals of normal weight because there is clear evidence that a sedentary lifestyle compromises health. Second, because increased physical activity may not be sufficient to bring about energy balance, food intake may have to be moderated as well. Third, those who refuse to or cannot increase activity are left with the sole (and difficult) strategy of moderating food intake.

To remain in energy balance, because of today's sedentary lifestyles, most people can afford to eat only 1800 to 2400 kilocalories each day. This raises the challenge to make each calorie count, that is, for the diet to deliver the most nutritional value in terms of long-term health benefits. This chapter aims to discuss these issues, with a particular focus on the policy and environmental factors that can and must serve to promote increased activity and healthy eating. There is a genuine need to achieve healthier eating and a more active lifestyle in order to stem the growing epidemic of obesity and reduce the suffering and expense associated with it. Obesity is a threat to the public health. Therefore, resources need to be allocated or reallocated to combat this insidious disease condition.

KEY ISSUES RELATED TO OBESITY AND THE ACHIEVEMENT OF A HEALTHY WEIGHT

Eating Disorders: Anorexia and Bulimia

Eating disorders (anorexia and bulimia) occur most often among teenage girls and young women, and represent a growing concern in industrialized societies. Whereas eating disorders are killing fewer than 5,000 people annually, poor diet and sedentary lifestyles that lead to obesity have been linked to more than 300,000 premature deaths in the United States annually (McGinnis & Foege, 1993). To the uninformed, eating disorders may appear to be nothing more than a dieting strategy that has run amok, but the prevalence of these eating disorders should not constitute a rationalization for ignoring obesity. Indeed, many young people suffering from eating disorders were never overweight or obese to begin with. Although some report that the onset of their disease was associated with dieting, adoption of a diet in the absence of overweight is a hallmark of compulsion and of the distorted self-image characteristic of eating disorders. The assertion that dieting *causes* eating disorders lacks scientific support.

Self-Perception in Females

The distorted self image of anorexic individuals—who see themselves as fat, even when painfully thin to the point of emaciation—is an extreme case of the unfortunate social phenomenon that is part of our time and our society: women are less content with, and even contemptuous of, the shape of their bodies. They express contempt for their bodies by calling themselves fat when, by any reasonable standard, they are not. This distortion in body image and an inappropriate standard for fatness are obscuring the need for a campaign to combat true obesity. An appropriate standard for overweight is a body mass index over 27.8 in males and 27.3 in females (IOM, 1995), with obesity defined as a BMI in excess of 30.[1] It should be pointed out that in adults in the United States, most of the overweight is attributable to excess fat that represents a threat to health. Only in certain athletes, laborers, and body builders, are elevations in BMI sometimes seen in the absence of excess fat.

Concern about body weight among individuals whose BMI falls between

---

1. Body mass index = Body weight (in kilograms) divided by height (in meters) squared.

25 and 27 may or may not be appropriate. But excessive concern among individuals whose BMI is less than 25 may signal the presence of a distorted body image that needs to be sensitively addressed by a health professional specifically trained to identify and treat eating disorders.

Ethnic Differences

NHANES III data clearly indicate that obesity disproportionately affects certain minority populations: obesity prevails in adult female African Americans, Hispanics, Pacific Islanders, and certain American Indian populations, to a degree that greatly exceeds the ratio of one in three adults who are overweight or obese in the general population. It should be pointed out that the above definitions of overweight and obesity, based on BMI, are those used by the National Center for Health Statistics to measure the prevalence of overweight and obesity in these populations.

Self-perception of females in the above ethnic populations can differ in important ways from that of their white counterparts. For example, the female preoccupation with slimness so prevalent among whites is often absent among African American females. In the Hispanic and other cultures, a rounder female form is widely appreciated as more attractive than the slim counterpart coveted in white culture. Public health measures targeted to these communities for reducing the prevalence of obesity can and must respect and take into account these differences in standards for beauty.

Major studies relating body weight to premature mortality, such as the recent study by Manson et al. (1995) have focused primarily on mortality experience among white female Americans. Comparable data need to be obtained for other ethnic populations. Data are also lacking that evaluate how weight loss contributes to reducing risk for chronic disease and premature mortality in ethnic populations. For these reasons, obesity prevention and treatment efforts among these ethnic populations may be hampered by different aesthetic standards and cultural values that must be taken into account. Adapting and tailoring public health prevention and treatment efforts to suit these different ethnic communities is a particular challenge to those concerned with public health.

Relationship to Income

It has long been known that in the United States and other developed countries, obesity is more common among individuals of lower socioeconomic status. Exactly how such status translates into the imbalance between energy intake and energy expenditure is not well known. *Shape Up America!*— a nonprofit public health initiative to combat obesity—recently conducted a survey to examine some factors related to income that they hypothesized played a role as barriers to healthy eating and increased physical activity in urban residents. From September 27 through October 5, 1995, Moore, Glick, Romanowski, and Quinley (1996) conducted a telephone survey of 1,599 individuals living in urban centers throughout the United States. By design, half the respondents were male, half female; half earned less than $25,000 annually, half earned more; all were at least 18 years of age or older. Of those responding to the survey, 31.3% were nonwhite (see Figure 7.1).

As shown in Figure 7.1, the lack of safety is an impediment to some individuals who are interested in walking or jogging in their neighborhoods, and safety is cited as an impediment twice as often by individuals earning less than $15,000 per year as it is by individuals who earn more than $25,000 per year. Figure 7.2 shows that lack of affordable recreational facilities is also a barrier with 50% of the low-income individuals unable to afford membership in a gym. With respect to the issue of healthier eating habits, especially the consumption of high-fiber low-fat foods, individuals earning more than $25,000 are relatively unlikely to report that the cost of fruits and vegetables is an impediment to healthy eating, but the percentage jumps from 7.9% in this group to 25.2% among people earning less than $15,000 (Figure 7.3). It has long been known that income is inversely related to the prevalence of obesity. If the growing obesity epidemic is to be stemmed the need for safe neighborhoods, sidewalks, and parks for recreation and exercise is even more critical for low-income individuals than for persons with greater income. Furthermore, for low-income individuals, strategies to promote fruit and vegetable consumption are very important, both as a weight-management and disease-prevention strategy.

Safe neighborhoods, parks and sidewalks, and affordable supplies of fruits and vegetables should not be viewed as luxuries; they are essential components of a health-promoting community and play a vital role in supporting the public health. The individuals who need them most are often at the margins of society by virtue of their limited financial reserves. When disease conditions develop as a consequence of obesity in these individuals, they quickly lose their financial resources and wind up being picked up by the health care system that all taxpayers support. Treating disease

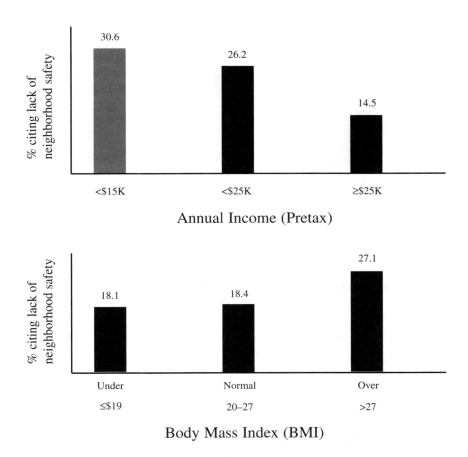

Figure 7.1 (Top) The effect of income on the percentage of adults living in urban areas who report that lack of neighborhood safety is a barrier to walking or jogging. Half the population (*n*=757) earned less than $25,000 annually and half (*n*=738) earned more (dark bars). Those earning less than $15,000 (shaded bar, *n*=333) are included in the group earning less than $25,000 (6% of those surveyed refused to provide income information). (Below) The relationship between lack of neighborhood safety and overweight or obesity. The percentage of individuals with body mass index (BMI) > 27 (*n*=387) reporting that neighborhood safety is a barrier to walking or jogging is significantly greater than the percentage with normal (*n*=1079) or low BMI (*n*=83). BMI was based on self-reported height and weight.

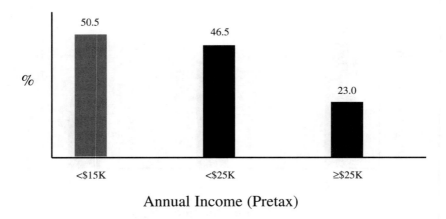

Annual Income (Pretax)

Figure 7.2 The effect of income on the percentage of adults in urban areas who report that lack of affordable recreational facilities is a barrier to increased physical activity. Number of subjects is the same as for Figure 7.1.

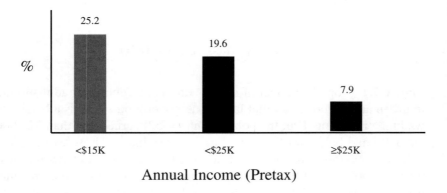

Annual Income (Pretax)

Figure 7.3 The effect of income on the percentage of adults in urban areas who report that affordability is a barrier to increased consumption of fruits and vegetables. The population and number of subjects are as described in the legend for Figure 7.1.

conditions that are known to be linked to obesity represents an ongoing financial drain because they are chronic diseases, including diabetes, atherosclerosis, hypertension, stroke, and certain types of cancer. From a financial standpoint, an investment in measures to improve the safety of neighborhoods and the availability of parks, gyms, and sidewalks is a prudent and wise investment in health.

Obesity and Smoking

There is evidence that some people—particularly teenage girls and women —use smoking as a strategy to manage their weight. Smoking is currently the number one cause of preventable death (McGinnis & Foege, 1993). It has been suggested that the rising prevalence of obesity, in some measure, reflects the success of efforts to promote smoking cessation. Yet, according to recent statistics released by the National Center for Health Statistics, the prevalence of obesity among children and teens has doubled over the past 20 years. Surely this trend cannot be explained as a sole consequence of quitting smoking. Furthermore, although smoking cessation has contributed to weight gain amounting to 9.4 lbs (4.4 kg) for men and 12.1 lb. (5.0 kg) for women (Flegal, Troiano, Pamuk, Kuczmarski, & Campbell, 1995), it cannot fully account for the 8 pounds that all Americans have gained, on average, over the past decade. In any case, the pounds of weight gain that many people experience when they quit smoking are avoidable and may not represent a significant threat to their health, whereas continuing to smoke assuredly does.

Available Remedies

The Institute of Medicine has recently described the various resources available to individuals who are overweight and obese and who are interested in losing weight (IOM, 1995). The IOM has also listed considerations that might guide an individual's choice. Figure 7.4 highlights the lifelong process of weight management, including criteria for matching the consumer and program, treatment options, and outcomes.

Key considerations to guide selection of a weight-loss strategy should be as follows:

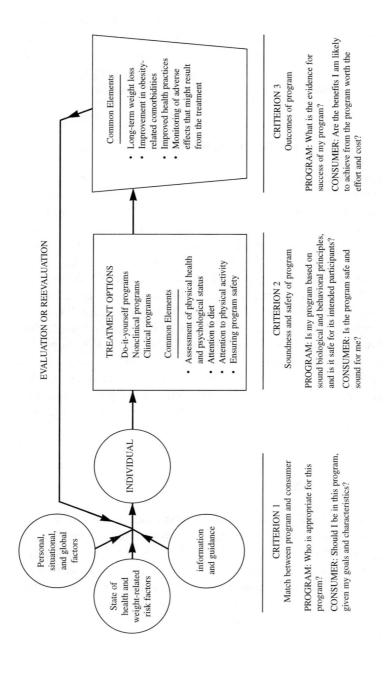

Figure 7.4 For an individual, weight management includes obtaining information from a variety of sources, considering treatment options, evaluating treatment outcomes, and reevaluating outcomes periodically. An individual's history, including demographic variables, will influence the decision-making process. From: *Weighing the Options*, Institute of Medicine, National Academy of Sciences Press, 1995, reprinted with permission.

1. Does the strategy include physical activity?
2. Does the strategy clearly teach how to construct a healthy diet based on the Dietary Guidelines and the Food Guide Pyramid published by the U.S. Departments of Agriculture and Health and Human Services?
3. Does the strategy clearly teach portion control?
4. Does the strategy advocate targeting the loss of only 5–10 pounds (or 5%–10% of body weight) at a time?
5. Does the strategy address psychological, social and environmental factors that may erode commitment to the strategy?
6. Does the strategy include a weight-maintenance strategy?
7. Does the strategy advocate a slow rate of weight loss of no more than one pound per week?

A "no" to any of the above questions signals a serious deficit in the strategy under consideration.

Table 7.1 outlines considerations the IOM recommends individuals should weigh when choosing a particular weight-management program. The IOM has recommended that the various weight-management programs collect and make available data to potential clients of such programs. The IOM recommendations for data collection are outlined in Table 7.2.

Weight Cycling and Recidivism

Studies have shown that 95% of individuals who successfully lose weight regain it within 2 years (IOM, 1995). This observation has given rise to two major concerns. First, that current weight-loss strategies are ineffective and second, that repeated cycles of weight loss and regain lead to physiological, metabolic, and/or psychological damage. The National Task Force on the Prevention and Treatment of Obesity (1994) conducted an exhaustive review of the literature on weight cycling in humans, and concluded that convincing evidence of metabolic or physiological damage was lacking. From a psychological standpoint, there is greater agreement that repeated cycles of weight loss and regain are associated with damage to self-esteem and a poor self-image, but which comes first still appears controversial.

The fact that recidivism is common is not necessarily proof that weight-loss strategies are ineffective. Rather, it is more accurate to state that either

Table 7.1 Program Disclosure of Information

All potential clients of weight-management programs should receive information, such as the following:

- A truthful, unambiguous, and nonmisleading statement of the approach and goals of the program. Part of such a statement might read, for example, "We are a program that emphasizes changes in lifestyle, with group instruction in diet and physical activity."
- A brief description of the credentials of staff, with more detailed information available on request. For example, "Our staff is composed of one physician (M.D.), two registered nurses (R.N.s), three registered dietitians (R.D.s), one master's-level exercise physiologist, and one Ph.D-level psychologist. At your first visit, you will be seen by the physician. At each visit, you will be seen by a dietitian and exercise physiologist and after five visits by the psychologist. Resumes of our staff are available on request."
- A statement of the client population and experiences over a period of 9 months or more. For example, "To date, we have seen 823 clients for at least three visits each. Although only 26 clients have participated in this program for more than 1 year, they have maintained an average weight loss of 12 pounds."
- A full disclosure of costs. For example, "If you avail yourself of all our facilities with one weekly visit for a period of 1 year, the total cost to you will be between $2,000 and $2,500." Costs should include the initial cost; ongoing costs and additional costs of extra products, services, supplements, and laboratory tests, and costs paid by the average client. Programs may also wish to provide information on the experiences clients have had in recovering their costs from third-party payers.
- A statement of procedures recommended for clients. For example, "We urge that each of our clients see a physician before joining our program. If you have high blood pressure or diabetes, you should see your physician at intervals of his or her choosing while with our program."

Table 7.2 Collection of Data by Weight-Management Programs

1. The number of people who attend the first treatment session. (This is the group of potential clients and those who will become actual clients.)
2. Number of clients attending their first two treatment sessions (a gauge of those who have really begun a program) and the percentage that continue to participate in the program at 1, 3, 6, and 12 months. (These time points seem reasonable but are selected somewhat arbitrarily, for although there is no set of ideal time points, it is important to have a set for standardization and comparison among programs. Programs may, of course, use additional time points.)
3. The average weight, height, BMI, and waist to hip ratio (WHR) of clients attending the first two sessions and appropriate measures of change in these variables at 1, 3, 6, and 12 months in the program. (These data should be assembled by gender and, if possible, by race, age, and starting weight or BMI.)
4. The percentage of actual clients who complete each of the stages of the treatment program. This means either the number of clients who complete the program's prescribed number of sessions (e.g., 8 weeks for an 8-week program) or the number of clients in treatment at 3 months.
5. The percentage of actual clients who reenroll in the same program for further treatment. (This figure should not necessarily be interpreted as a measure of clients failure in a program; it may indicate satisfaction with the program.)

Reprinted with permission from The Institute of Medicine, National Academy of Sciences, IOM, 1995, p. 150.

there have been no weight *maintenance* strategies or that most have been ineffective. Retrospective studies of weight maintenance indicate that increased physical activity is a key component of successful weight maintenance (IOM, 1995; Kayman, Bruvold, & Stern, 1990). Hence, public health strategies that help prevent obesity must also include measures that lead to the successful maintenance of weight loss over the long term. These strategies should emphasize increased physical activity.

The National Task Force on the Prevention and Treatment of Obesity (1994) concluded that weight loss and regain is not dangerous although it may be psychologically damaging. Failure to maintain weight loss should not deter efforts to lose weight. Furthermore, it has been shown that even very modest weight losses are clearly associated with such benefits as improvements in blood pressure, lipid profiles, and glucose disposal and handling. Weight loss in small (5–10 lb) incremental steps with periods of weight maintenance between permits the individual to develop both realistic, achievable goals, as well as vital weight-maintenance skills and strategies that will reduce the likelihood of recidivism.

PUBLIC POLICY RECOMMENDATIONS

Make public education about the prevention and treatment of obesity a national priority. As a first step, new education efforts must "redefine" the overweight issue for Americans. Healthy weight is both achievable and maintainable and, in an overweight individual, any loss of body fat is a measure of success and is beneficial for those who have too much. Further, educators must communicate messages that are positive and enabling, culturally sensitive, and relevant to the specific lifestyles and concerns of targeted populations. These include, in particular, minority and low-income population groups who are at greatest risk for developing obesity. Equally necessary to the success of public education efforts is the need to expand beyond the current activities of the federal government and national health-related organizations to include American industry, the mass media, the education community, youth groups and community-service organizations to make the public aware that healthy weight and physical activity must be a priority.

Create new economic and workplace incentives for weight-reduction efforts. Based on 1988 data, about a third (32.4%) of work sites with 250 to 749 employees and more than half (53.7%) of workplaces with over 750 employees have health-promotion programs. Employers should be encouraged to include in these programs added emphasis on weight-reduction activities. Likewise, companies can promote physical activity and weight control by allowing time for their employees to exercise, installing showers, paying for weight-loss programs, and providing health information to their workers. Further, employees can be motivated to enter weight-loss programs if health insurance companies build in economic incentives to their insurance plans, such as reduced premiums or rebates for individuals who are not overweight.

Generate public support for the increased funding and availability of school and community-based physical-fitness and nutrition programs. The evidence showing the link between physical activity and weight control notwithstanding, there has been a disturbing decline in participation in physical education and community recreation programs. Currently, almost half of all high-school students (48%) are not enrolled in physical-education classes, only one in five attends these classes on a daily basis; and only 37% of high-school students get 20 minutes or more of vigorous exercise three or more times a week. What these statistics make clear is that every youth-serving agency, educational institution, the public-health community, and parents must devote new energies to expand school- and community-based programs that promote physical fitness. Such programs should include sound information about diet and food and about healthy weight.

Mobilize the nation's physicians and other health care workers to combat obesity. Because the average American has 5.4 contacts with physicians a year, the opportunities for physician intervention in obesity prevention and weight management are plentiful. In practice, because of the demands of the changing health care environment, physicians have less time to spend with individual patients. In addition, many physicians still do not recognize obesity as a serious chronic disease. For this reason, a major education effort is required to make physicians aware of the nature of obesity, the difficulties inherent in treating the disease, and the importance of counseling patients about realistic goals for weight reduction. At the same time, physicians should be encouraged to identify at-risk individuals and to educate them about lifestyle changes that will promote a healthier weight.

Put development and approval of drugs to treat obesity on a fast track. Until 1996 no drugs to treat obesity had been approved in the United States since 1973. This is not the case in other nations. In November 1995, the Food and Drug Administration (FDA) Endocrinologic and Metabolic Drug Advisory Committee voted six-to-five to recommend approval of a drug, dexfenfluramine, which has been used to treat over 10 million obese patients in 65 countries outside the United States. Based on this recommendation, the FDA approved this drug in 1996. This action will help stimulate the development of other effective drugs to treat obesity, one of which is under FDA review at this time.

Expand research efforts into the prevention, causes, and treatment of obesity. Compared with cancer research, which receives $1.4 billion per year in federal funding, and research in heart disease/stroke ($930 million per year), funds spent on obesity research by the National Institutes of Health (NIH) are only $34 million a year—this is less than 50 cents per overweight person. Little research has been conducted with NIH support on obesity prevention or intervention. It is imperative that the public health community unite behind the recent call for a significant increase in federal funding for obesity research (National Science & Technology Council on Health Safety & Food). This will enable scientists to uncover molecular, genetic, environmental, and behavioral causes of obesity, as well as develop effective intervention strategies at the individual, workplace, and community level.

WHAT CAN THE PUBLIC HEALTH/ NUTRITION OFFICER DO?

The public health/nutrition officer should be prepared to implement policies that promote *both* physical activity and healthy eating. The 1995 Dietary Guidelines, released jointly by the United States Departments of Agriculture and Health and Human Services, advocate balancing the food eaten with physical activity. This is the first time that physical activity has become part of the dietary guidelines and sets the stage for taking a view that integrates physical activity with healthy eating.

The following action list represents activities that nutrition officers in a public health setting should encourage or adopt:

1. Promote collaborative planning among school personnel, students, families, community agencies, and businesses to develop, implement, and evaluate nutrition and physical activity education and programs for youth and adults.
2. Include appetizing and appealing selections of vegetables, fruits, grains, and legumes wherever and whenever foods are offered at school and community functions. Provide recipes and preparation instructions whenever possible.
3. Encourage the employment of professionally prepared teachers of physical education, health education, and nutrition.
4. Make parents and the public aware of the need *not* to use food as a tool to punish or reward. Similarly, discourage the use of physical activity as punishment; rather, encourage its use as a reward.

5. Reward educators who excel in the promotion of physical activity and healthy eating.
6. Commit adequate resources including time, budget, training, and facilities for physical education, health education, and nutrition education.
7. Encourage school officials and parents to assure that youngsters have adequate time to eat meals in a pleasant and safe environment and to be physically active for at least 30–45 minutes every day.
8. Encourage students and parents to provide input in-school food-service programs.
9. Ensure that school and community facilities for physical activity are safe, affordable, and available to all members of the community before and after the school day.

REFERENCES

Bray, G. A. (1996). Hereditary adiposity in mice: Human lessons from the yellow and obese (ob/ob) mice. *Obesity Research, 4,* 91–95.

Colditz, G. A. (1992). Economic costs of obesity. *American Journal of Clinical Nutrition, 55,* 5035–5075.

Flegal, K. M., Troiano, R. P., Pamuk, E. R., Kuczmarski, R. J., & Campbell, S. M. (1995). The influence of smoking cessation on the prevalence of overweight in the United States. *New England Journal of Medicine, 333,* 1165–70.

Friedman, J. M., Leibel, R. L., & Bahary N. (1991). Molecular mapping of obesity genes. *Mammaliam Genome, 1,* 130–144.

Institute of Medicine, & Thomas, P. R. (1995). *Weighing the options: Criteria for evaluating weight-management programs* (p. 282). Washington, DC: National Academy Press.

Kayman S., Bruvold W., & Stern J.S. (1990). Maintenance and relapse after weight loss in women: Behavioral aspects. *American Journal of Clinical Nutrition, 52,* 800–807.

Manson J. E., Willett, W. C., Stampfer, M. J., Colditz, G. Z., Hunter D. J., Hankinson, S. E., Hennekens, C. H. & Speizer, F. E. (1995). Body weight and mortality among women. *New England Journal of Medicine, 333,* 677–85.

McGinnis, J. M., & Foege, W. H. (1993). Actual causes of death in the United States. *Journal of the American Medical Association, 270,* 2207–2212.

Moore, B. J., Glick N. L., Romanowski, B., & Quinley, H. (1996). Neighborhood safety, child care and high cost of fruits and vegetables identified as barriers to increased activity and healthy eating and linked to overweight and income. *FASEB Journal, 10,* A562.

National Science and Technology Council Committee on Health, Safety, and Food. (1996). *A research agenda for America's health, safety, and food.* Executive Office of the President, Office of Science and Technology Policy (OSTP). Washington, DC: U.S. Government Printing Office.

National Task Force on the Prevention and Treatment of Obesity. (1994). Weight cycling. *Journal of the American Medical Association, 272,* 1196–1202.

Pelleymounter, M. A., Cullen, M. J., Baker, M. B., Hecht, R., Winters, D., Boone, T., & Collin, F. (1995). Effects of the gene product on body weight regulation in ob/ob mice. *Science, 269,* 540–543.

Troiano, R. P., Flegal, K. M. Kuczmarski, R. J., Campbell, S. K., & Johnson, C. L. (1995). Overweight prevalence and trends for children and adolescents. *Archives of Pediatrics and Adolescent Medicine, 149,* 1085–1091.

U.S. Department of Health and Human Services. Public Health Service. (1995). *Health, United States, 1995* (p. 183). DHHS Publ. No (PHS) 96–1232. Washington, DC: U.S. Government Printing Office.

Warden C., & Fisler, J. (1996). Molecular genetics of obesity. In C. Bouchard and G. A. Bray (Eds.), *Handbook of obesity.* New York: Marcel Dekker.

CHAPTER 8

Coronary Heart Disease and Public Health Nutrition

Aryeh D. Stein

T his chapter is concerned with the relationship between dietary habits and coronary heart disease, particularly the latter's manifestations as angina pectoris and myocardial infarction. It is not intended to be a comprehensive review—a task that would far exceed the available space and has been performed extensively elsewhere (National Research Council, 1989)—but rather to illustrate some key points of increased relevance to public health nutritionists. Following a brief description of the clinical and epidemiologic characteristics of this disease, the chapter provides a framework for determining the potential benefits of population-based dietary modification programs, focusing on reduction of total fat intake. Because it is unlikely that major changes in the dietary habits of Americans will occur, the particular focus is the examination of benefits to be expected from modest dietary changes.

CORONARY HEART DISEASE

The heart consists of four chambers. On the right side, the atrium accepts venous blood from the body while the ventricle pumps this blood to the lungs for oxygenation. The left atrium receives the oxygenated blood from the lungs, while contractions of the left ventricle provide the force that circulates blood through the body. Blood leaves the ventricle through the aorta, which then branches to form the arteries. One of these, the coronary artery and its further branchings, supplies the coronary muscles with oxygen and nutrients. For further details, readers are referred to any standard medical textbook.

The generally accepted model of atherosclerosis suggests that over time, the arterial endothelium is infiltrated by fatty deposits, which may eventually become calcified and cause substantial narrowing of the lumen, thus restricting blood flow. Coronary artery disease consists of a range of clinical entities that result from this progressive damage to the coronary arteries. Angina, a symptom of temporary insufficiency of the blood supply during physical effort (increasing the heart rate and thus the heart's own requirement for oxygen), which is relieved once effort ceases and requirements decline, is caused by partial blocking of the arterial lumen. Myocardial infarction represents the result of complete blockage of a coronary artery due to thrombosis, resulting in permanent damage to myocardial muscle. Three pathological processes appear to be of primary influence on the risk of experiencing disease: narrowing of the arterial diameter through progressive accumulation of atherosclerotic plaque, reduction in the contractility of the arteries, and changes in the tendency to clotting. Of these, accumulation of atherosclerotic plaque appears to be the most affected by modifiable lifestyle characteristics, and thus the most amenable to influence through public health activities.

TRENDS IN MORTALITY FROM CORONARY HEART DISEASE

Coronary artery disease remains the most common cause of death of both men and women in most developed countries. In the United States, age-adjusted mortality rates increased steadily from early in the century to 1968, and have been declining every year since then. In 1990 mortality rates were below those observed in 1950, and had dropped 50% compared to the peak years of the epidemic (Thom & Maurer, 1988). Trends in western Europe have followed the U.S. pattern, but with some delay, whereas central and eastern Europe, and the industrializing sectors of countries elsewhere, have been reporting dramatic increases in mortality rates over the past 20 years (Uemura & Pisa, 1988).

In the United States and elsewhere, there has also been substantial changes in the age, gender and social class distribution of death rates from coronary heart disease (Marmot, Adelstein, Robinson, & Rose, 1978). The early years of the epidemic were marked by an excess of premature deaths of middle- and upper-class males in their economically active ages. This group has also experienced the most dramatic reversal of this excess. Among the elderly, there is much less difference in the death rates of men and women, and the rate of decline in death rates has not been as dramatic. As a result, the decline in overall death rates has been accompanied by an increase in the median age at death from coronary heart disease, an increase in the proportion of women among coronary-heart-disease deaths, and a relative increase in the proportion of deaths occurring among people of lower social class, including members of ethnic minority groups.

The impact of improvements in medical treatment of acute myocardial infarction (MI) on the overall mortality rate is not clear. All states in the United States and most countries maintain registries of vital events, and all deaths are recorded, although low autopsy rates and lack of standardization of diagnosis may reduce cross-population comparability. Incidence data are much more sparse, as few population-based coronary-heart-disease registries exist. More common are hospital-based registries, developed primarily to investigate the outcome of treatment rather than etiology; these, moreover, exclude outpatient diagnoses and out-of-hospital deaths. One notable effort to establish a coronary-heart-disease registry is the MONICA project, sponsored by the World Health Organization (WHO), which monitors disease incidence in 38 communities in 26 countries (WHO MONICA Project Principal Investigators, 1987). This project has shown that the variation in mortality rates between communities is paralleled by variation in incidence rates; this suggests that both prevention and treatment continue to be important components of the fight against this disease. A conference in 1986 concluded that the initial decline in mortality rates could not be adequately explained by the introduction of improved treatments, and therefore had to be caused by reduced incidence, reflecting the impact of prevention activities, primarily management of hypertension and smoking cessation, with perhaps some changes in dietary habits and physical activity responsible for a small proportion of the decline (Higgins & Luepker, 1988). Since the early 1980s, however, advances in medical technology, particularly thrombolytic therapy, coronary artery bypass grafts, and balloon angioplasty, have markedly improved the prospects for survival and full recovery among patients who have access to these services. Thus mortality rates provide only a surrogate measure for estimating the impact of coronary heart disease in a population.

EARLY PRECURSORS OF
CORONARY HEART DISEASE

Evidence for the chronic, cumulative course of coronary heart disease (CHD) comes from several sources. Early clinical observation had noted fatty deposits in the arteries of persons (generally elderly) dying of acute MI. These deposits were subsequently determined to contain high concentrations of cholesterol. An early autopsy series of children and young adults in Louisiana showed that fatty streaks could be observed in the arteries of very young children, with the prevalence and intensity of infiltration increasing with age (Holman, McGill, Strong, & Gea, 1958; Strong & McGill, 1962). During the Korean and Vietnamese conflicts, autopsies performed on U.S. casualties revealed the same fatty streaks (Enos, Holmes, & Beyer, 1953; McNamara, Molot, Stremple, & Cutting, 1971). It was not known if these were predictive of future disease, however, and it was not known whether the development of fatty streaks and atherosclerosis was in any way affected by diet and other lifestyle factors. It was hypothesized that dietary cholesterol is related to the development of atherosclerosis, but it was impossible to assess development of these deposits except by necropsy, as no noninvasive technology existed. Experimental studies were therefore limited to work with animals. Studies of the etiology of coronary heart disease in humans were limited to the noninvasive assessment of putative risk factors (anthropometric measures, behavior, diet, markers found in serum and urine) and of clinically relevant events. Recent developments in imaging technologies, although still too expensive and invasive to be used routinely as screening instruments in asymptomatic people, have made it possible to verify findings seen in animal studies as occuring in people. Nevertheless, the majority of epidemiologic research continues to focus on noninvasive technologies.

THE DIET–HEART DISEASE HYPOTHESIS

Most nutrition policy as it relates to coronary artery disease results from the acceptance of the classic diet–heart disease model. This model suggests that there is a sequence of events, starting with changes in the quantity and composition of dietary fat, which affect circulating serum cholesterol levels. Increased serum cholesterol results in an intensification of atherosclerosis. This in turn ultimately leads to clinical symptoms. This basic model has undergone refinements and modifications as techniques have developed to differentiate between serum cholesterol fractions and as the role of thrombosis in acute myocardial infarction has become clear. Nevertheless, the underlying model still remains at the core of public health policy.

Serum Cholesterol and Coronary Heart Disease

The role of total serum cholesterol concentration in influencing coronary artery disease risk has been clearly and consistently demonstrated. The Framingham study, a long-term observational study of middle-aged residents of the town of Framingham, Massachusetts, was among the first to establish that the incidence of coronary heart disease increases with increased level of serum cholesterol (Kannel, 1992). This relationship held for both men and women, and at all age groups studied. Later studies have consistently replicated this finding—one of the largest of these, the Multiple Risk Factor Intervention Study (MRFIT), in which over 350,000 men were screened for coronary disease risk, found that risk of coronary events was related to total serum cholesterol level measured at the initial screening (Stamler, Wentworth, & Neaton, 1986). There was no evidence of a threshold below which lower cholesterol levels had no additional benefit. Trials among hypercholesterolemic individuals, in which serum cholesterol levels were lowered using dietary manipulation or pharmaceutical agents, have consistently demonstrated reduced disease risk in proportion to the reduction in serum cholesterol. In general, every reduction of 1% in serum cholesterol resulted in approximately 2% reduction in risk of coronary disease (National Research Council, 1989).

More recent work has led to the identification of low-density lipoprotein (LDL) cholesterol as the fraction most sensitive to changes in dietary fat composition. The cardioprotective high-density lipoprotein (HDL) fraction, conversely, appears to be more sensitive to physical activity and smoking than to dietary changes. A recently identified key stage in the development of atherosclerosis appears to be the peroxidation of the LDL cholesterol, which renders it more likely to adhere to the endothelium. This work has led to the hypothesis that antioxidant vitamins may have a role in the prevention of plaque formation (Steinberg, Pathasarathy, Carew, Khoo, & Witzum, 1989). The role of antioxidants is examined later in this chapter.

Evidence for Influences of Dietary Habits on CHD

Total Energy

Over time, energy expenditure by persons has to equal their energy intake from food. Otherwise a change in weight will occur. People who gain weight are consuming calories in excess of their requirements. It cannot be assumed, however, that overweight individuals are eating more calories than individuals who do not gain weight, because energy intake is a function of metabolic rates and individuals with high intake may also have high rates of energy expenditure. The net effect of energy intake on coronary-heart-disease risk is unpredictable. On the one hand, excess relative weight (an indirect measure of obesity) and weight gain (including the periodic weight gain associated with weight cycling) are consistently and strongly associated with increased risk of coronary heart disease. On the other hand, regular physical activity shows a clear benefit in terms of reducing risk. Willett (1990) concludes that the expected finding from well-conducted studies is that energy intake should be inversely associated with coronary-heart-disease risk, due primarily to the beneficial effects of exercise, and that failure to account for the effects of energy intake may seriously confound estimates of the effect of individual nutrients.

Even small imbalances between energy intake and expenditure, if sustained, will result in substantial weight gain over adult life. If we take a weight gain of 20 kg (44 lb) over 30 years, for example, which would result in a healthy 25-year-old becoming a fairly overweight 55-year-old, this represents an increase of 0.67 kg per year, or approximately 2 g per day. This 2 g is composed primarily of fat in adipose tissue, with an energy content of 9 kcal/g or approximately 18 kcal. If we assume metabolic efficiency of 33%, then it is apparent that considerable weight gain over the life span is a result of a seemingly trivial imbalance of approximately 50 kcal per day. This is the energy content of 1 teaspoon of margarine or butter, of 1/2 bottle of beer, of one thin slice of bread, or of the fat in one glass of whole milk. These examples show that only very small dietary restrictions would be required to reinitiate energy balance in most people. (Weight loss will require more stringent dietary restriction.) Similarly, small increases in routine physical exercise, such as using stairs or walking short distances instead of driving, would compensate for the excessive energy intake by increasing energy expenditure. Although these small increases in energy expenditure may be adequate to control weight gain, they will not enhance cardiovascular fitness, which requires a more intensive exercise regimen.

Fat Density and Fat Composition

In ecologic studies (in which mean dietary intakes in several populations are related to population disease or mortality rates), such as the Seven Countries Study (Keys, 1980), there is a consistent relationship between the mean total fat density of the food eaten and incidence rates of coronary heart disease. It has been extremely difficult to establish the direct link between dietary fat intakes and clinical coronary heart disease in studies within populations, however (Willett, 1990).

Ornish and colleagues have been promoting a very-low-fat diet as part of a program to induce regression of coronary disease (Gould et al., 1992; Ornish, 1993). In this program, which is prescribed to individuals with diagnosed coronary artery disease, dietary fat is reduced to approximately 10% of calories, whereas total energy intake is unrestricted. The diet requires the complete elimination of animal products, except for a small amount of egg whites and skim-milk or nonfat yogurt. The diet may appear extreme to most North Americans, but is sustainable within the context of foods available in U.S. supermarkets and is comparable to vegetarian diets that are commonly consumed in several parts of the world, notably India. Recent developments in imaging techniques make it possible to assess the impact of this risk-factor modification on the extent of atherosclerosis, even before clinical events occur. The results to date have been encouraging—atherosclerosis regresses in patients who successfully adhere to the diet and stress-management program, but progresses in those who are less successful. It should be remembered that this program was designed to be therapeutic, and may be more restrictive than is required to prevent the development of atherosclerosis in the first place. Furthermore, the degree to which such a program would be acceptable to the general population has not been evaluated. Nevertheless, the results suggest that there is little to be lost, and potentially much to be gained, from a radical dietary change.

Partially Hydrogenated Oils

Saturated fats are characterized by the absence of double bonds between the carbon atoms of the fatty acids in the triglyceride molecule. They are usually solid at room temperature, giving them characteristics of importance in food preparation. In contrast, oils with a high unsaturated fatty-acid content are generally liquid at room temperature. Hydrogenation, the process of replacing double bonds with hydrogen bonds, gives these unsaturated oils the characteristics of saturated fats. By manipulating the conditions under which hydrogenation occurs, the desired proportions of saturated, monounsaturated, and polyunsaturated fatty acids, and hence the degree of hardness of the resulting fat, can be achieved. Such industrially hydrogenated oils are quite similar to their naturally occurring corresponding fatty acids, except for their stereo-specificity. Industrial hydrogenation results in both cis- and trans-isomers of the resulting monounsaturated fatty acids, whereas naturally occurring monounsaturated fatty acids are all cis-isomers. Willett and colleagues have suggested that the industrial hydrogenation of unsaturated fats may be atherogenic (Ascherio et al., 1994; Willett and Ascherio 1994; Willett et al., 1993). This is an evolving area of research, particularly as the food industry is highly responsive to felt or expressed consumer concerns and is continuously modifying the transfatty-acid content of foods. It remains to be clarified whether, in fact, guidelines for transfatty acids are required, or whether a general guideline to reduce fat intake overall is sufficient.

Antioxidants

Oxidized LDL cholesterol may be more atherogenic than LDL in its native state (Steinberg et al., 1989). If this is so, then differences in antioxidant intakes should be associated with differences in the risk of coronary heart disease. Among the antioxidants, vitamin E and A (as carotene) are lipophilic, whereas vitamin C is hydrophilic. The hypothesis that vitamins A (particularly the precursor provitamin beta-carotene) and vitamin E (alpha-tocopherol) play a role in the prevention of LDL peroxidation has been widely tested. Nevertheless, published studies although suggestive, (Kardinaal et al., 1993; Rimm et al., 1993; Stampfer et al., 1993), do not provide conclusive evidence of the benefit of encouraging all individuals to use antioxidant supplements.

QUANTIFYING THE POSSIBLE IMPACT
OF DIETARY CHANGE ON CVD

Public health practitioners are charged with developing and implementing policy based on the best scientific evidence available. This includes not

only firm evidence about the presence (and strength) or absence of a relationship, but also information concerning the prevalence of the risk-factor,
and the expected reduction in prevalence that might be induced by public
health activities. If little change in risk factor levels is likely, then little
benefit is to be expected.

The epidemiologic concept of attributable risk provides a useful tool for
integrating these three factors. For a risk factor that can be either present
or absent, the potential reduction in disease incidence (the population
attributable risk fraction) is a function of the prevalence of the risk factor
and the relative risk associated with that risk factor. Thus it may be as
important to intervene on a risk factor that is very common but does not
increase risk dramatically, as on a stronger but less common risk factor.

For risk factors such as dietary intakes there is no true unexposed group,
as all tend to consume some quantity of each nutrient. The potential benefit of dietary modification depends on the degree to which the individual's
diet can be modified to conform to an ideal. This approach may be illustrated through a hypothetical example.

Let us consider the results of a large prospective study, in which dietary
fat intake and other variables of interest were measured and the participants followed for disease onset. The observed elevation in risk associated
with increased fat intake is provided in Table 8.1. There is a threshold.
When total fat provides less than 30% of energy, there is no relationship
between total fat density and risk of disease. Once total fat density exceeds
30% of calories, however, the risk of disease increases with increasing fat
density. For example, individuals consuming 40% of energy as fat have 3.0
times the risk of disease than do individuals consuming less than 20% of
energy from fat.

Let us now apply these results to a hypothetical population of 1 million
people, whose dietary fat intake is distributed as described in Table 8.1

Over 50% of the population eats a diet with 35% or more of energy
from fat, and only 2.5% have "ideal" diets. Twenty percent of the population are currently meeting the dietary guidelines for total fat intake. For
individuals in each category of intake, we can estimate the potential benefit of reducing fat intake to that of the group with the lowest risk, by cal-
culating the number of disease events to be expected if that group had the
risk of disease observed in the group with the lowest risk (here assumed to
be 100 events per 25,000 people), and subtracting that from the number
expected if no dietary change were made. Obviously, the group with the
lowest risk cannot reduce their risk of disease by further modifying their

Table 8.1 Expected Change in Coronary Heart Disease Event Rates Following Dietary Fat Reduction in a Community

Fat intake		Population distribution		Baseline expected events	Model 1: Change to optimal diet		Model 2: Change to <30 of energy from fat		Model 3: Change by one exposure category	
Percentage of energy	Relative risk	Number	Percentage		Expected events	Prevented events	Expected events	Prevented events	Expected events	Prevented events
<20	1.00	25,000	2.5	100	100	—	100	—	100	—
20–24.99	1.05	75,000	7.5	315	300	15	315	—	315	—
25–29.99	1.10	100,000	10.0	440	400	40	440	—	440	—
30–34.99	2.00	250,000	25.0	2,000	1,000	1,000	1,100	900	1,100	900
35–39.99	2.50	500,000	50.0	5,000	2,000	3,000	2,200	2,800	4,000	1,000
40+	3.00	50,000	5.0	600	200	400	220	380	500	100
Total reduction		**1,000,000**		**8,455**	**4,000**	**4,455** **52.7%**	**4,375**	**4,080** **48.3%**	**6,455**	**2,000** **23.7%**

dietary fat intake, so their potential benefit is zero. Conversely, if those in the highest fat group (over 40% of energy as fat) were to reduce their fat intake to below 20% of calories, only 200 events would be expected, compared to 800 if no dietary changes were made, a dramatic reduction of 75%. To estimate the overall potential benefit of a complete, population-wide change to an ideal diet, we perform this calculation for all fat intake categories, and sum them. In this hypothetical case, a total of 4,455 cases of heart disease could have been prevented, or 53% of those expected in the absence of dietary change. Although the risk of heart disease was highest in the group with extremely high fat intakes, and the reduction in disease risk was 75% in this group, this constitutes only 5% of the total population, so that these individuals do not contribute overwhelmingly to the total benefit of fat reduction. Most events (3,000) were prevented among those individuals who derived 35%–39.99% of energy from fat, largely because these individuals were the most numerous. This example illustrates the difference between a high-risk approach, in which individuals with extremely high fat intakes are identified and their diets modified, and a population-based approach, in which it is recommended that all individuals modify their diet.

It is, of course, highly unlikely that all will reduce their diet to the optimal level of fat intake. Two alternative scenarios are provided in Table 8.1. In the first, individuals with intakes above 30% of energy as fat reduce their fat intake to just below 30%, whereas those in the below 30% groups make no change to their diet. This scenario corresponds to comprehensive adoption of the dietary guidelines, which recommend that total fat intake be reduced to below 30% of energy intake. Those in the very-high-fat-intake groups are called on to make more radical dietary changes than those whose diets are currently close to the guidelines. Under this scenario, the expected benefits (a reduction of 48% in cardiovascular events) would be almost as large as in the "ideal" scenario, as most of the population, and most of the risk, is concentrated in the categories with higher fat intake (>35% of energy from fat). It is these individuals who would be making comprehensive dietary modifications, whereas little additional benefit will be gained from further reductions in fat intake below the 30% threshold.

As a third scenario, all individuals consuming over 30% of energy from fat reduce their fat intake a consistent amount, so that they shift to one lower exposure category. This corresponds to an overall shift in dietary habits of a uniform nature in the higher-risk population, without a more dramatic behavior change in the extremely high-risk population. Under this scenario, not all people would attain the dietary guidelines recommendation, although mean intakes would approach 30% of energy from fat. If this degree of change were made, a total of 2,000 events (24% of baseline) would be prevented. Although still substantial, this represents only about one half of the potential benefit of full adherence to the dietary guidelines.

All three scenarios assume that everyone in each fat-intake category makes similar dietary modifications. A more complex scenario, not illustrated in Table 8.1, is one in which a proportion of people in each fat-intake category make changes in their fat intake, whereas the remainder do not. This is the situation most commonly encountered in public health education, as not everyone in the population is receptive to the campaign message. Indeed, the proportion affected may well vary across fat-intake categories. Obviously, if not everyone adopts the program, the expected effect in the overall population will be smaller. The magnitude of the expected benefits is therefore subject to the distribution of fat intake in the population, to the increased risk associated with varying levels of fat intake, and to the extent to which a dietary modification campaign affects all members of the population.[1] As new research is published, the expected benefits of dietary change may need to be modified.

So what is the public health nutrition officer to do? It goes without saying that the national campaigns (such as the 5-a-day campaign to encourage fruit and vegetable consumption) should be publicized. It is not clear that individuals are adopting the campaign message, however, even though they are aware of the message content. It is possible that short-term economic considerations play a role, as fruits and vegetables are, calorie for calorie, more expensive than high-fat, high-sugar processed foods. This economic disincentive to a healthy diet needs to be addressed at a policy level. Although not within the scope of the individual local nutrition officer, one might start to envisage (and mobilize support for) cost-shifting programs that penalize fat consumption and reward low-fat foods. One such route might be through a "fat-excise" levied at the point of production (and therefore, presumably passed on to the consumer) in relation to the number of grams of fat per standard serving size. This would make

---

1. The reader is encouraged to examine the effects of varying the underlying assumptions. This can be performed easily using a spreadsheet. For an example, implemented in Microsoft Excel™, please send a diskette to the chapter author.

high-fat foods more expensive, without affecting the price of low-fat foods, which would then become more competitive. Although such a plan has appeal, it still requires much formulation and concerted, national action. Local initiatives are unlikely to be acceptable, as food manufacturers would be unhappy with a myriad of pricing structures required to conform to local ordinances. Nevertheless, the success of initiatives to discourage tobacco use among youth by raising the excise tax levied on cigarettes shows that such initiatives can be instituted and have an impact. Further research needs to be undertaken to examine the price elasticity of fat, in order to determine a level of excise that would result in behavior change. Until such time as the political mood swings in favor of improving public health through personal financial incentives, education, at points of food purchase and consumption (supermarkets, restaurants, etc.) and at other times when the individual may be receptive (such as in a medical encounter) provides the most likely method of encouraging reduction in dietary fat intakes.

CONCLUSIONS

Premature coronary heart disease (i.e., the appearance of clinical symptoms in persons under 70 years of age) is overwhelmingly a disease of social and environmental origin, including the increased mechanization of daily activities, and cigarette smoking. Evidence that nutritional and dietary factors affect the risk of premature coronary artery disease comes from cross-cultural comparisons, observational and experimental studies among human populations, and a wealth of supporting evidence from animal and in vitro investigations. Physical activity reduces coronary-heart-disease risk through its impact on weight balance and cardiovascular fitness, whereas caloric restriction alone is rarely effective as a means of weight loss. Isocaloric replacement of saturated fat by monounsaturated fats and unhydrogenated polyunsaturated fats can be moderately beneficial, as such replacement affects serum profiles, but few well-conducted trials with clinical endpoints have been reported. Major reductions in the incidence of CHD events should occur if total fat intake is substantially reduced, but even moderate changes in fat intake are likely to benefit those whose fat intake is currently high. The guideline that all Americans consume less than 30% of energy as fat is a useful target, but is unlikely to be reached without major changes in food production and consumption patterns. The role of antioxidants appears to be minor in the quantities usually present in the diet, but may be more influential in pharmacological doses, and particularly so among smokers.

There continues to be a role for dietary change in the fight against premature coronary artery disease in the United States and elsewhere. Population-based programs aimed at encouraging a low-fat diet should be implemented, but planners need to have realistic and modest expectations of benefits at a population level, as message adoption is not likely to be widespread.

REFERENCES

Ascherio, A., Hennekens, C. H., Buring, J. E., Master, C, Stampfer, M. J., & Willett, W. C. (1994). Trans-fatty acids intake and risk of myocardial infarction. *Circulation, 89,* 94–101

Enos, W. F., Holmes, R. H., & Beyer, J. (1995). Coronary disease among United States soldiers killed in action in Korea: Preliminary report. *Journal of the American Medical Association, 152,* 1090–1093.

Higgins, M. W., & Luepker, R. V. (Eds.), (1988). *Trends in coronary heart disease mortality: The influence of medical care.* New York: Oxford University Press.

Holman, R. L., McGill, H. C. Jr, Strong, J. P., & Geer, J. C. (1958). The natural history of atherosclerosis: The early aortic lesions as seen in New Orleans in the middle of the 20th century. *American Journal of Pathology, 34,* 209–235.

Gould, K. L., Ornish, D., Kirkeeide, R., Brown, S., Stuart, Y., Buchi, M., Billings, J., Armstrong, W., Ports, T., & Scherwitz, L. (1992). Improved stenosis geometry by quantitative coronary arteriography after vigorous risk factor modification. *American Journal of Cardiology, 69,* 845–853.

Kannel, W. B. (1992). The Framingham experience. In G. Marmot & P. Elliott (Eds.), *Coronary heart disease epidemiology: From aetiology to public health.* Oxford, UK: Oxford University Press.

Kardinaal, A. F. M., Kok, F. J., Ringstad, J., Gomez-Aracena, J., Mazaev, V. P., Kohlmeier, L., Marin, B. C., Aro, A., Kark, J. D., Delgado-Rodriguez, M., Riemersma, R. A., van 't Veer, P., Huutunen, J. K., & Martin-Moreno, J. M. (1993). Antioxidants in adipose tissue and risk of myocardial infarction: The EURAMIC study. *Lancet, 342,* 1379–1384.

Keys, A. (1980). *Seven countries: A multivariate analysis of death and coronary heart disease.* Cambridge MA: Harvard University Press.

Marmot, M. G., Adelstein, A. M., Robinson, N., & Rose, G. (1978). Changing social class distribution of heart disease. *British Medical Journal, 2,* 1109–1112.

Marmot, M. G. (1992). Coronary heart disease: the rise and fall of a modern epidemic. In G. Marmot & P. Elliott (Eds.), *Coronary heart disease epidemiology: From aetiology to public health.* Oxford, UK: Oxford University Press.

McNamara, J. J., Molot, M. A., Stremple, J. F., & Cutting, R. T. (1971). Coronary artery disease in combat casualties in Vietnam. *Journal of the American Medical Association, 216,* 1185–1187.

National Research Council. (1989) *Diet and health: Implications for reducing chronic disease risk.* Washington DC: National Academy Press.

Ornish, D. (1993). Can lifestyle changes reverse coronary heart disease? *World Review of Nutrition and Dietetics, 72,* 38–48.

Rimm, E. B., Stampfer, M. J., Ascherio, A., Giovanucci, E., Colditz, G. A., & Willett, W. C. (1993). Vitamin E consumption and the risk of coronary heart disease in men. *New England Journal of Medicine, 328,* 145–1456.

Stamler, J., Wentworth, D., & Neaton, J. D. (1986). Is the relationship between serum cholesterol and risk of premature death from coronary heart disease continuous or graded? Findings in 356,222 primary screenees of the Multiple Risk Factor Intervention Trial (MRFIT). *Journal of the American Medical Association, 256,* 2823–2828.

Stampfer, M. J., Hennekens, C. H., Manson, J. E., Colditz, G. A., Rosner, B., & Willett, W. C. (1993). Vitamin E consumption and risk of coronary disease in women. *New England Journal of Medicine, 328,* 1444–1449.

Steinberg, D., Pathasarathy, S., Carew, T. E., Khoo, J. C., & Witzum, J. L. (1989). Beyond cholesterol: modification of low-density lipoprotein that increases its atherogenicity. *New England Journal of Medicine, 320,* 915–924.

Strong, J. P., & McGill, H. C. Jr. (1962). The natural history of coronary atherosclerosis. *American Journal of Pathology, 40,* 37–49

Thom, T. J., & Maurer, J. Time trends for coronary heart disease mortality and morbidity. In M. W. Higgins & R. V. Luepker (Eds.), *Trends in coronary heart disease mortality: The influence of medical care.* New York: Oxford University Press.

Uemura, K., & Pisa, Z. (1988). Trends in cardiovascular mortality in industrialised countries since 1950. *World Health Statistics Quarterly, 41,* 155–178

WHO MONICA Project Principal Investigators. (1987). WHO MONICA Project: Geographic variation in mortality from cardiovascular diseases. *World Health Statistics Quarterly, 40,* 171–184.

Willett, W. (1990). *Nutritional epidemiology.* New York: Oxford University Press.

Willett, W. C., Stampfer, M. J., Manson, J. E., Colditz, G. A., Speizer, F. E.,

Rosner, B. A., Sampson, L. A., & Hennekens, C. H. (1993). Intake of trans fatty acids and risk of coronary heart disease among women. *Lancet, 341,* 581–585

Willett, W. C., & Ascherio, A. (1994). Trans fatty acids: Are the effects only marginal? *American Journal of Public Health, 84,* 722–724.

CHAPTER 9

Nutrition in the Etiology, Prevention, Control, and Treatment of Cancer

Carole A. Palmer and Johanna T. Dwyer

INTRODUCTION: INTERRELATIONSHIPS
BETWEEN NUTRITION AND CANCER

Nutritional factors may play a role in the prevention, initiation, promotion, progression, and treatment of cancer. Primary prevention involves identifying food-related factors which contribute to cancer incidence and prevalence, controlling risks by regulations, and effective communication to the population resulting in altered eating behaviors and improved food supply. Secondary prevention focuses on early diagnosis and anticancer and dietary treatment. Both cancer itself and its treatment can have profound and deleterious effects on the nutritional status of the cancer patient. Nutrition support can play a major role by promoting the cancer patient's ability to respond successfully during treatment, and by preventing the development of secondary malnutrition. Tertiary prevention involves providing nutritional therapy and support to the cancer patient after treatment to maximize function, provide palliation, and enhance quality of life. This chapter provides an overview of the many relationships between diet, nutrition, and cancer.

Prevalence of Cancers in the U.S. Population

More than 1 million Americans develop cancer each year. Of these, 18% are prostate; 15% breast; 14% lung; 11% colon or rectal; 5% hematopoetic (lymphomas); 4% (each) bladder or uterus; 3% (each) skin or oral/laryngeal; 2% (each) pancreatic, leukemia, kidney, ovarian, and 1% stomach (American Cancer Society, 1996). Breast cancer, one common diet-related cancer, is the most common site of new cancers in women and lags behind only lung cancer as the leading cause of cancer deaths in women. In 1993 approximately 182,000 new cases of invasive breast cancer were diagnosed and 46,000 deaths expected (Advance Data, 1994). There has been a steady rise in cancer mortality in the United States in the last 50 years as the population has grown older. Lifestyle factors, including nutrition, may be involved in the pathogenesis of up to 60% of cancers in women and 40% in men. Dietary modifications may be associated with as much as a 35% reduction in overall cancer mortality, according to some experts, with the actual risk-reduction estimates ranging from 10%–70% depending on the type of cancer (Doll, 1994). Because of the complexity of food and cancer relationships and the many determinants of carcinogenesis, however, it is almost impossible to separate the effects of specific dietary factors from the many other environmental and genetic determinants of cancer in specific individuals. Current research focuses on determining both nutrient and nonnutrient dietary factors that initiate or promote cancer development and those that reduce cancer risks and act as inhibitors of carcinogenesis.

Proposed Mechanisms for Relationships Between Nutrition and Cancer

The exact mechanisms by which dietary factors influence carcinogenesis are unknown but may operate on several levels. Preventive factors help prevent carcinogenesis, often via free-radical quenching. Initiators of carcinogenesis probably directly affect cellular deoxyribonucleic acid (DNA). Only a few dietary constituents (such as saffrole and aflatoxin) have been identified as possible initiators. Food components usually operate at the cancer promotion or progression stages. Promotion refers to the time it takes for cells to progress or the numbers of cells that progress from initiated to fully developed neoplastic cells. Promoters or cocarcinogens help accelerate the process, whereas inhibitors slow it down. Dietary factors may also act in later stages (after the cancer cell develops) to speed or slow metastasis; this stage is known as cancer progression. Diet appears to modify risk, rather than being the only factor involved in causing or preventing the myriad diseases called cancer.

Research Approaches

Many research approaches are used to study diet–cancer relationships. These include population studies, retrospective and prospective case control studies, and prospective clinical trials. Animal models are often used to test hypotheses of relationships between specified substances and cancer initiation, promotion, and prevention. Compounds that cause mutations in bacteria and experimental animals are often also mutagens in humans. There are relatively high ($r^2 = .8–.9$) correlations between findings of carcinogenity in animal models and humans for most common cancers involving diet. Because of the ethical considerations involved in human investigations, only interventions thought to decrease (rather than increase) human cancers are tested in clinical trials. Problems in research design of experimental human diet–cancer studies include the inherent difficulty of estimating dietary intakes, the effects of confounding and interacting variables in the diet, the low cancer risks associated with specific food constituents or nutrients, long latency, and the large populations needed to study rare diseases (Lee, 1993).

Epidemiological studies are either retrospective or prospective with respect to their time frames. They analyze population groups to determine factors most significantly associated with cancer risk. For example, migrants are often studied. When Japanese women (who have a low breast cancer incidence) migrate to Hawaii, their breast cancer rates increase to the level of the native Hawaiians or Caucasians by the third generation in the United States; this indicates an association between dietary change and cancer risk (Henderson, 1995a). Diet is also associated with colon cancer risk (Steele, 1995; Weisburger & Williams, 1995). For example, Seventh Day Adventists who have a low risk of colon cancer also have different diets in some respects than do other Americans (Mills, Beeson, Phillips, & Fraser, 1994). Nurses who have high-fat, low-fiber diets have a higher incidence of colon cancer than those with other dietary patterns (Willett et al., 1987).

Epidemiological research observes associations between factors and cancer without intervening, and cannot be used to demonstrate causation. It is helpful, however, in identifying potential factors for further study.

Intervention studies are prospective in nature and manipulate variables, including diet, to observe their effects on cancer outcomes. Likely factors thought to be related are generated by the epidemiologic and animal research previously described. Many cancer risk-reduction studies are now in progress and will be described in the Section entitled "Nutrition Factors that May *Reduce* Cancer Risks" (p. 180).

PRIMARY PREVENTION: NUTRITION IN CANCER INITIATION AND/OR PROMOTION

A variety of food-related compounds have been implicated in cancer development (Bal, Nixon, Foerster, & Brownson, 1995; Weisburger & Williams, 1995).

Intentional Additives

The carcinogenic risk to humans from the 3,000 intentional food additives appears to be minimal, as the Food, Drug and Cosmetic Act requires that food additives be tested for carcinogenicity before they are approved for use (cf. Chapter 3). In the early 1970s the Food and Drug Administration (FDA) established a committee to evaluate all Generally Recognized as Safe (GRAS) substances, and the Select Committee on GRAS Substances (SCOGS) developed evaluations of safety for a large number of substances (U.S. Department of Health and Human Services, 1989). The Delaney Amendment to the Food, Drug and Cosmetic Act requires that any additive or food found to be carcinogenic in animals at any level will not be permitted on the market. Of additives tested to date, and found to be carcinogenic in animals, only one weak carcinogen, saccharin, is permitted in the food supply, because of special legislative dispensation granted by Congress before other alternative sweeteners were available. Some intentional food additives may actually decrease cancer risks, such as BHA (butylated hydroxyanisole), BHT (butylated hydroxy toluene), vitamins C and E, and carotenoids. Other food additives retard spoilage and may also have a positive role. Indeed, one of the explanations for decreases in stomach cancer incidence is that the quality of food preservation has improved (Hwang, Dwyer, & Russell, 1994)

Environmental Contaminants and Naturally Occurring Carcinogens

Environmental contaminants also add to cancer burdens. About 12,000 unintentional food additives and environmental contaminants may be present in food. They pose different problems because they are not deliberately added. In the future, food technology and bioengineering may make it possible to modify food crop composition and contaminants to minimize the levels of these carcinogens in the food supply. In the meantime, levels of these substances are monitored by the Food and Drug Administration, the Environmental Protection Agency, and other government agencies.

A variety of food constituents influence cancer development and are considered naturally occurring carcinogens. Among the more common factors are dietary fat and alcohol. Aflatoxin, produced by fungi on plants, has been linked to increasing risks of some forms of liver cancer. Others include benzo(a)pyrene and other polynuclear aromatic hydrocarbons (formed when high-protein foods are cooked at high temperatures), the heterocyclic amines that are formed on foods cooked over charcoal, and compounds in salted, smoked and pickled foods. Salt, nitrite-preserved foods, and pickled vegetables appear to increase stomach cancer risk in some studies (Tominaga & Kato, 1992), but chronic *H. pylori* infection may be even more important in causing stomach cancer than dietary factors (Hwang et al., 1994). High consumption of chili powder and foods cooked over wood has been linked to increased risk of oral cancers (Winn, 1995). Some constituents of coffee, tea, spices, and certain alcoholic beverages may also be carcinogenic.

Dietary Fat

The traditional high-fat (e.g. 35%–40% of kilocalories from fat) Western diet may be associated with five of the six most common cancers: breast, colorectal, pancreatic, prostate, and uterine (Schapira, 1992; Weisburger & Wynder, 1991). Ovarian cancers may aso be associated with high-saturated-fat, low-fiber diets (Risch, Jain, Marrett, & Howe, 1994). The mechanisms thought to implicate fat in the development of cancers are several. The metabolism of sex hormones, especially estrogen, may be altered; prostaglandins that promote carcinogenesis may be involved; or other factors may be operative. These other factors are difficult to study because high-fat diets are often also diets high in calories (Weisburger &

Wynder, 1991). The evidence associating high-fat diets with cancers is strongest when comparing populations between countries whose usual intakes of dietary fat differ by 20% or more. In some studies, animal sources of calories, protein, and fat are linked to increased risks of colon and pancreatic cancers, but it is difficult to distinguish between levels and sources of the nutrients, as the two are highly correlated (Ghadirian, Ekove, & Thovez, 1992).

Only about half the differences in breast cancer risk can be explained by known risk factors (Henderson, 1995b). Even the new work on genetic markers for breast cancer provides only partial explanations for remaining differences in risks. Studies in experimental animals and correlation studies in humans across countries implicate both the total amount and the type of fat consumed as risk factors. In Japan, for example, the age-adjusted risk of breast cancer has been increasing for the past 20 years as diets have increased in fat, energy, and protein (Kodama, Miura, & Yoshida, 1991). A recent study showed a 50% increase in relative risk for breast cancer in women consuming high saturated fat (Hankin, 1993). In other human studies, however, only weak and inconsistent associations with dietary fat intake have been found for both breast and prostate cancers; small but positive effects are seen in some cohort studies but not in others (Weisberger & Williams 1995). Conflicting results may reflect methodological limitations, such as the inherent difficulty in collecting the dietary data.

In addition to dietary fat, other factors involving diet may influence breast cancer risk. Physical activity may be protective. Breastfeeding in early childhood has also been hypothesized to reduce subsequent risk of breast cancer incidence in adulthood (Freudenheim et al., 1994). Nutrition in adolescence may also be important because it affects the age at which menarche occurs and possibly differentiation of the ducts in the breast.

Body Weight and Obesity

Increased incidence of and mortality from many cancers has been associated with increased body weight. Two thirds of the case-controlled studies in one recent review found positive associations between body weight and cancers of the breast, endometrium, kidney, ovary, prostate, and colorectum (Albanese & Taylor, 1990). Body fat distribution may also be important. Women with upper body fat localization are at significantly higher risk for developing breast cancer and endometrial cancer than women with other phenotypes (Schapira, 1992). Obesity may be associated with breast cancer for several reasons. Fat tissue can convert androgens to estrogens. In obese postmenopausal women this may be sufficient to alter endocrine status in a way that favors breast-tumor production. Or, obesity may merely make it more difficult to locate tumors already present or be a marker for some other process or agent responsible for increased risk. Finally, obesity may cause alterations in immune status.

Alcohol and Oral Irritants

The incidence rate of head and neck cancers is increasing worldwide, especially among males, primarily because of smoking, but other factors may also be involved. A high intake of alcohol is a major risk factor for cancers of the mouth, larynx, esophagus, and respiratory tract, especially when accompanied by heavy smoking (Boffetta, Mashberg, Winkelmann, & Garfinkel, 1992). Populations with relatively raised oral cancer incidence also have diets low in fruits and vegetables, or high intakes of oral irritants, such as very hot beverages. Cancer of the esophagus has a more varied geographical incidence and distribution than other common cancers of the head and neck. This suggests that environmental effects are present and that factors in addition to alcohol may be involved.

In a region of northern Iran where esophageal cancer is higher in women than in men, a favorite food during pregnancy contains strong black pepper and sharp crushed pomegranate seeds, both of which irritate the esophagus (Ghadirian, 1992).

Other Dietary Factors

Dietary factors may affect cancer indirectly through their effects on immune function. Factors that depress immunocompetence are thought to enhance the risk for some infectious diseases and for cancer. Dietary deficiencies that contribute to reduced immune function include those of ascorbic acid, selenium, and vitamin E, and protein-calorie malnutrition. In animal studies both obesity and consumption of high-fat diets, particularly of saturated fat, depress immunocompetence (Maki & Newberne, 1992). Therefore dietary deficiencies and excesses may both play a role in compromised immunity.

NUTRITIONAL FACTORS THAT MAY *REDUCE* CANCER RISKS

Dietary Fiber and Fat

Low consumption of dietary fiber, particularly of insoluble fiber, is associated with increased risk of colon cancer. Insoluble fiber is found in the support structures of plants and is not metabolized by humans, passing through the digestive tract undigested. It is thought to reduce colon cancer risk by decreasing the type and timing of contact of carcinogens with the colon wall. According to another hypothesis, increased peristalsis or the greater bulk or consistency of materials left after digestion prevents debris from becoming lodged in the diverticular pouches of the intestinal wall where bacterial toxins that can promote carcinogenesis accumulate. Low-fiber diets are also associated with an increased risk of breast cancer (Ganz & Schag, 1993).

Conversely, high-fiber diets are associated with hormonal changes that may decrease cancer risks (Goldin et al., 1994). Some data suggest that high-fiber/low-fat combinations may also modulate estrogen metabolism, thereby resulting in a decreased cancer risk. A diet of less than 10% of calories from fat and 40 g of fiber daily, including fruits and vegetables, has been proposed to decrease the risk of breast and colon cancer, but there is no evidence to support this contention. A more moderate fat-restricted diet high in fiber is being tested in the National Polyps Trial and in the Women's Health Initiative studies approved by the National Institutes of Health (Greenwald, 1993).

Constituents of Fruits and Vegetables

Many epidemiological studies have shown a strong positive association between the consumption of fruits and vegetables and a decreased risk for various cancers. Whether these associations are caused by cancer-protective nutrients, such as vitamins C or E, beta-carotene, selenium, dietary fiber, or phytochemicals such as xanthines or isoflavonoids, or other food components, is currently under study. Epidemiological studies have consistently shown that a diet high in fruit intake is associated with a 20%–80% reduction in oral cancer risk (Winn, 1995).

Vegetarian lifestyles that have lasted 20 years or more are also associated with a decreased mortality from some cancers. Such a lifestyle often includes high consumption of fiber and fruits and vegetables, as well as abstinence from alcohol and tobacco, and a physically active lifestyle (Frentzel-Beyme & Chang-Claude 1994). Whether high quantities of protective substances or low quantities of toxins are responsible factors in vegetarian diets requires further study.

Vitamin A, Carotenoids, and Lycopenes

Evidence from many epidemiological studies shows that populations with the highest serum levels of beta-carotene and the highest consumption of carotenoid-rich diets have lower risks of lung, oral cavity, esophagus, stomach, larynx, and bladder cancers, among others (Bendich, 1993). Carotenoids are pigments that give fruits and vegetables their yellow, orange, and red colors. Of the more than 600 carotenoids found in nature, the most plentiful is beta-carotene, whose primary function is conversion to vitamin A in the body. Other functions of carotenoids, unrelated to vitamin A activity, may also play a role in cancer prevention. These include singlet oxygen quenching, antioxidant activity, and the activation of gene expression. Beta-carotene prevents singlet oxygen (high-energy oxygen) from producing free radicals in cells by quenching it. Free radicals, produced by single oxygen action, can attack cell components, leading to cell destruction. Other carotenoids, such as lycopene, lutein, and zeaxanthin also have singlet oxygen-quenching ability. Beta-carotene itself can also serve as an antioxidant, by scavenging free radicals directly, and functioning in the cell like vitamin C and vitamin E, although the latter may operate at different cell sites (Bendich, 1993).

In 89% of studies reviewed in the period 1975–1992, there was a twofold reduction in lung cancer risk in individuals with the highest dietary or serum levels of beta-carotene. A significant protective effect of carotenoids in food and/or serum was also found for the risk of cancers of the head, neck, and stomach (Block, Patterson, & Subar, 1992; Byers, 1991; Gaby & Singh 1991). Interactions with other risk factors are apparent as well. Smokers with the highest consumption of beta-carotene-rich foods have lower risks of head, neck, esophagus, and stomach cancers than do their peers with lower intakes (Block et al., 1992; Byers, 1991; Gaby & Singh 1991).

Associations between carotenoids and cervical, ovarian, and breast cancer risks are weaker. The association with reproductive-tract cancers is strong when the intake of fruits and vegetables rather than of carotenoids is analyzed, however. This suggests that there may be food components such as lycopenes or other biologically active substances responsible for the protective effects (Block et al., 1992; Byers, 1991; Gaby & Singh 1991).

Of three large prospective intervention trials of beta-carotene in lung cancer risk reduction so far, one study is incomplete, one, in Finland, was negative, and one, in China, showed conflicting positive results (Taylor et al., 1994). The apparent conflict between the conclusions of the Chinese and Finnish studies has prompted much analysis. The Chinese population had very low levels of many nutrients and responded positively to the supplements. On the other hand, the Finnish men were well nourished, their long-time smoking may have overwhelmed any protective effect of the carotene, and the high doses of beta-carotene used (20 mg/day as compared to the recommended 5–6 mg) may actually have had a harmful prooxidant effect at those levels (Meister,1994).

In a study of patients who had skin cancer, no beneficial effect of beta-carotene supplementation was seen on the rate of development of subsequent skin cancers (Greenberg et al., 1990). Thus, the benefit of carotenoids for the prevention of these cancers is as yet unproven.

Not only is high carotenoid status associated with reduced risk of oral cancer, but recent studies have shown that supplementation with beta-carotene can actually reverse and prevent the progression of premalignant oral lesions (leukoplakia) (Garewal, 1992; Kaugers, Brandt, Carcaise-Edinboro, Strauss, & Kilpatrick, 1990; Stich, Rosin, Hornby, Mathews, & Sankaranarayanan, 1988; Toma, Benso, Albanese, Palumbo, Cantoni, Nicolo, Manglante, 1992). Both smoking and betel nut chewing are risk factors for oral cancer. When the diets of betel nut chewers were supplemented with beta-carotene and vitamin A, the placebo group had triple the incidence of new lesions and nine times lower regression of existing lesions than the study group (Stich et al., 1988). Smokers supplemented with beta-carotene at the level of 30 mg/day for 6 months had 70% greater lesion remission than controls.

In humans, treatment of oral leukoplakia with 13-cis-retinoic acid led to a reversal of these precancerous lesions (Lippman, Benner, & Hong, 1993).

Vitamin C

Vitamin C prevents nitrosamines, which are carcinogens, from forming in the stomach. Vitamin C has also been shown to reduce some tumors in laboratory animals. Direct relationships between vitamin C and human cancers such as breast cancer have not been demonstrated, however, even when very large doses were employed (10-20 times the Recommended Dietary Allowance [RDA] of 45 mg), nor do large doses appear to be effective in decreasing precancerous colon polyps (Greenberg et al., 1994).

Vitamin E

Vitamin E is an important antioxidant and is a potential cancer-preventive compound, but is difficult to study because it is widespread and its content in foods varies widely. In epidemiological studies vitamin E has been associated with lower risk of several cancers. The results of controlled clinical trials of vitamin E have been conflicting, however (Rock, Jacob, & Bowen, 1996). Inadequate doses, confounding effects of other nutrients, and overpowering effects of carcinogens such as smoking have all been proposed as explanations for the conflicting results.

Selenium

Selenium is an essential trace element that functions as part of the peroxide -destroying enzyme glutathione peroxidase. It is also needed for optimal immune function. Because of its role in antioxidant processes, selenium deficiency may be associated with increased risk of cancer (Neve, 1991). In a 4-year study of over 1,000 women, however, those with the highest selenium intakes had no fewer cancers than those with the lowest intakes. Indeed, those who took selenium supplements had twice the risk of cancer of those who did not. Although these findings only represent correlations and not causal relationships, it seems wise to caution against megadoses of nutrients that may have toxic effects.

NUTRITION CONSEQUENCES OF CANCER AND ITS TREATMENT

Nutritional Consequences of Cancer

The leading cause of death in patients suffering from cancer is malnutrition (Feldman, 1988). This association was first noted in 1932, when autopsies of 500 patients with cancer showed that 22% had died from no other identifiable cause than malnutrition and cachexia, a state of general wasting. Cancer patients have the highest incidence of protein-calorie malnutrition of hospitalized patients, with overt malnutrition seen in about 40% of patients with advanced cancers (Smith, Dwyer, & Lafrancesca, 1990).

The incidence of malnutrition is related to the site of disease; upper gastrointestinal cancers are especially likely to cause malnutrition (Daly & Shinkwin, 1995). The obstructive, systemic, and psychological effects of the neoplasm itself and the side effects of treatment can cause changes in the desire and ability to eat and result in secondary malnutrition in patients whose progress is otherwise excellent. Changes in taste and smell often give rise to anorexia. The iatrogenic effects of cancer therapies often may undermine nutritional status (Williams & Meguid, 1989), and therefore nutrition surveillance and monitoring is especially critical in these patients.

Malnutrition undermines tumor response to treatment, increases the severity of toxicities, and increases the incidence of associated infection (Welch, 1981). Nutritional status also appears to influence prognosis. In one study, patients with a 20% preoperative weight loss from normal weight had a 30% mortality, whereas when weight loss was 50% or more, mortality approached 100% (Williams & Meguid, 1989). The problem with such observations is separating out cause and effect. Adequate nutrition may improve tolerance and response rate to radiation and chemotherapy, improve immune status, increase wound healing, reduce complications, for example, fistula formation and flap necrosis, and may potentially benefit cardiac and pulmonary status by improving the strength of respiratory muscles (Nayel, el-Ghoneimy, & el Haddad, 992; Williams & Meguid 1989).

Malnutrition also disrupts intestinal function and impairs food absorption (Feldman, 1988). Thus, a vicious cycle ensues; the disease causes tissue depletion, and decreased food intake and absorption further deplete nutrient stores. Metastatic cancer causes observable nutritional deterioration in patients, because the rapid uncontrolled growth of the neoplasm disrupts metabolism. This cancer cachexia syndrome is characterized by disturbances in protein, fat, carbohydrate, and mineral metabolism, early satiety, anorexia, anemia, weight loss, and wasting.

Nutritional Consequences of Cancer Treatment

Cancer treatment may consist of surgery, radiation, or a combination of therapies. Small tumors are often treated successfully by surgery or radiation alone. Advanced lesions usually require a combination of several approaches. Surgery, chemotherapy, and radiation may also be useful to relieve pain in patients with advanced cancers.

Present approaches to cancer treatment are designed to eliminate or palliate the disease. However, they often have side effects that can further contribute to malnutrition, undermine recovery, and diminish the quality of life (National Institutes of Health Consensus Development Panel, 1990). In addition, the physical disfigurement, speech problems, eating difficulties, and psychological and emotional problems associated with some cancers and their treatment can contribute to social withdrawal and to a decline in the ability or desire to eat (Holland, 1977; Schmale, 1979), thereby leading to additional declines in nutriture (Rosenthal et al., 1990).

SECONDARY PREVENTION: INITIAL SCREENING AND EDUCATION OF THE CANCER PATIENT

Diet is an adjunctive treatment that aids or assists other therapies to be more effective, but it is not curative in itself. Because diet therapy and nutrition support can help prevent secondary malnutrition and its sequelae, however, nutritional interventions should be initiated as early as possible (Smith et al., 1990).

The Process of Nutrition Care

Nutritive care of the cancer patient involves three phases: screening and assessment, development and implementation of a care plan, and monitoring and evaluation. These are summarized in Table 9.1. The care plan includes nutrition repletion (to improve diagnosed nutritional problems prior to treatment), anticipatory guidance (to help counteract expected side effects of treatment), and problem-oriented nutritional counseling during and after therapy (Dwyer, Golay, Malsch, & Palmer, 1986; Henshaw & Schloerb, 1983).

The goals of nutritional therapy for the cancer patient are:

- to prevent or reverse nutritional deficits,
- to support antineoplastic treatment,
- enhance treatment response rates and survival, and
- palliate symptoms and improve quality of life.

Table 9.1 The DETERMINE Checklist: Factors to Look for in Screening

Disease

Type and extent of lesions and ultimate prognosis are important. Side effects from surgical or radiation therapies that are nutritional implications also need to be looked for.

Eating poorly

Explore any difficulties in eating, including appetite. Cancer itself and the side effects of treatment can impact ability and desire to eat.

Tooth loss and mouth pain

This is especially relevant in head and neck cancers, but may also be a problem in other cancers.

Economic hardship

As many as 40% of older Americans have incomes of less than $6,000/year.
It is difficult to get a nutritious diet on less than $25-$30/week. It may be even more difficult if food choices are limited not only financially but also by food intolerances and anorexia.

Reduced social contact

Socialization benefits attitude and subsequent appetite. Social isolation increases the risk of poor diet and subsequent malnutrition.

Medications

Chemotherapy often causes nausea, vomiting, and other effects. Medications for symptom relief or disease control often have nutritional implications.

Involuntary weight loss

Initial low weight and precipitous involuntary weight loss are "red flags" that indicate major nutritional concerns. They must be avoided and addressed if optimal response to cancer and its treatment is to occur.

Needs assistance with self-care

If a patient is unable or unwilling to perform activities of daily living, this contributes to nutritional risk. This may be associated with depression or other emotional factors that inhibit eating.

Elderly over 80

Very old patients may have general frailty and compromised immunity. These conditions make good nutrition even more important, yet more difficult.

Nutrition Interventions Manual (1992).
Reprinted with permission by the Nutrition Screening Initiative, a project of the American Academy of Family Physicians, the American Dietetic Association and the National Council on the Aging, Inc., and funded in part by a grant from Ross Products Division, Abbott Laboratories.

The Nutrition Care Standards from the Joint Commission on Accreditation of Healthcare Organizations (JCAHO) outline the important considerations in nutrition management (*1995 Accreditation Manual for Hospitals*, 1995). They are as follows:

- plan care
- provide appropriate nutrition care including food and nutrition therapy and using all appropriate resources
- Integrate nutrition care with other aspects of patient care (this involves the physician, registered dietitian, nurse, pharmacist, and other professionals)

(Nutrition care includes screening, assessing, and reassessing needs; developing a plan for nutrition therapy; prescribing or ordering therapy; preparing and distributing or administering therapy; and monitoring the patient in relation to the nutritive-care process.)

An interdisciplinary team approach is essential to both the clinical assessment and management of cancer patients. The team should consist of members or consultants from medical and surgical oncology, radiation therapy, dentistry, nursing, nutrition and dietetics, social service, and possibly speech or occupational therapy, depending on the problems the patient experiences. The nutritive care of the cancer patient is not the sole responsibility of the nutritionist. Its planning must involve all members of the team who are in a position to ensure that appropriate nutritive care is provided.

Registered dietitians are available through the dietary departments in hospitals. Most hospitals, clinics, and health maintenance organization (HMOs) employ dietitians on a full- or part-time basis.

Nutrition counseling should be provided to cancer patients and their families prior to, during, and after therapy. Physicians, nurses, or other clinical personnel should be able to screen new patients for nutritional risk. Those judged at high risk should be referred for nutritive care so that problems can be rectified. Early intervention ensures that the patient is prepared for the treatment-induced changes that can further compromise nutritional status. Health care providers also can assure adequate follow-up nutritional care.

Anticipatory Guidance on Nutritional Quackery

Cancer patients are particularly vulnerable to nutrition quackery, questionable remedies, and "nontraditional" approaches to treatment, especially when traditional medical care is unable to cure the disease or relieve the symptoms. These questionable approaches may be costly and may detract from instead of enhancing quality of life and functional status (Cassileth et al., 1991; Montbriand, 1994; Zloznik, 1994). For cancers, such treatments include laetrile, immunoaugmentative therapy, chelation therapy, megavitamin therapy, and macrobiotic diets (Dwyer, 1986; Dwyer, Efstathion, Palmer, & Papas, 1991). Regulations governing the composition and sale of these products and food supplements over the counter are not as strictly enforced as those governing the sale and promotion of drugs. Some quite potent treatments are widely available. Anticipatory guidance alerts patients to the potential risks of such approaches and may lessen ill effects.

TERTIARY PREVENTION: PROBLEM-ORIENTED NUTRITIONAL COUNSELING AND SUPPORT

Today, nutritional approaches are available that can sometimes improve chances of survival, enable the implementation of aggressive therapy, reduce long-term medical costs, and improve quality of life. Nutritional support ranges from general counseling on food choices to aggressive implementation of state-of-the art approaches such as enteral hyperalimentation and total parenteral nutrition in selected cases.

Nutrition Monitoring, Surveillance, and Evaluation

Most cancers are chronic conditions. Because nutritional status changes over the course of time, continuous monitoring and surveillance are needed and dietary prescriptions must be altered as the situation changes.

PUBLIC HEALTH INITIATIVES FOR CANCER PREVENTION

Increasing evidence of relationships between nutrition and cancer has led to public health initiatives to reduce cancer risk by modifying eating patterns and other lifestyle factors. All such public health initiatives involve partnerships on a variety of levels.

For public health initiatives to be effective they must be carefully designed and have reasonable expectations, given the limitations of the research environment. Research designs that are the easiest to implement are those that improve knowledge (e.g., cancer/nutrition relationships). Changing group behavior (eating more fruits and vegetables) is a more complex goal. Intervention studies that aim to change health outcomes (such as those aimed at reduced cancer incidence) are the most difficult to accomplish of all.

Federal Initiatives

The Year 2000 goals for the nation (*Healthy People 2000*, 1991) was a step forward in American public health planning. They reflect consensus on specific risk-reduction goals for the nation, and on objectives and steps designed to achieve these goals. They are now being carried out in programs with local, state, and national health initiatives and are as follows:

- Reduce cigarette smoking to a prevalence of no more than 15% among people aged 20 and older.
- Reduce dietary fat intake to an average of 30% of calories or less and average saturated fat intake to less than 10% of calories among people aged 2 and older (1985 baseline levels were 36%).
- Increase complex carbohydrate and fiber-containing foods in the diets of adults to five or more daily servings for vegetables (including legumes) and fruits, and to six or more daily servings for grain products (1985–1986 baseline levels were 2.5 and 3.0, respectively).
- Increase to at least 69% the proportion of people of all ages who limit sun exposure, use sunscreens and protective clothing when exposed to sunlight, and avoid artificial sources of ultraviolet light.

At the federal level, the National Center for Health Statistics (part of the USDHHS's Centers for Disease Control) monitors the incidence and prevalence of cancers in the U.S. population. This agency collects and summarizes mortality and morbidity data.

The U.S. Public Health Service (USPHS) and the National Institutes of Health (NIH) both have a major commitment to health research. The National Cancer Institute of NIH has as its primary goal directing and overseeing initiatives that will prevent and reduce cancer in the U.S.

population. Research ranges from basic research on the molecular level to multisite intervention studies aimed at cancer prevention control, cancer etiology, and cancer treatment. The NCI funds both intramural and extramural research on cancer (Greenwald, 1993).

The National Health Interview Survey of 1987 contained a Cancer Control Supplement, funded by NCI, which queried the public on whether they had made dietary changes during the past 5 years for health reasons. More than 73% of respondents knew that diet and cancer were related, but 44% either did not believe that anything could be done to prevent it or did not know what to do to achieve preventive efforts. Income and education levels were the major determinants of knowledge, attitudes, and beliefs relevant to cancer prevention, indicating a need for cancer education and risk reduction at lower socioeconomic levels (Cotugna, Subar, Heimendinger, & Kahle, 1992).

The Women's Health Initiative is a multicenter clinical trial with three components: dietary modification, calcium/vitamin D supplementation, and hormone replacement therapy. The dietary modification arm is designed to determine whether low fat diets can reduce the risk of breast and colorectal cancer and heart disease in women. Other aims of the study focus on measures to reduce coronary artery disease, osteoporosis, and stroke (Cummings, 1993).

The National Polyp Prevention trial is designed to determine whether a diet high in fiber and low in fat can reduce the risk of intestinal polyp development in men.

The Five-A-Day Initiative provided grants to states for demonstration projects designed to increase fruit and vegetable consumption, with the hope that such diets may promote eating patterns that lower cancer risks (Clifford, & Kramer, 1993).

State and Local Initiatives

The state departments of public health monitor the incidence and prevalence of cancers in their states and provide direction for state-specific cancer prevention and intervention initiatives. These include developing state plans for cancer prevention and lobbying state legislatures to provide appropriate funding for cancer risk reduction and treatment programs. States are also the vehicles for allocating funds for specific national initiatives, such as the Five-A-Day Program, which is funded through the National Cancer Institute but provided and monitored through the states.

Voluntary Agencies

Voluntary agencies play an important role in promoting governmental initiatives, providing funding for smaller projects, and providing information and support. The American Cancer Society (ACS) was established in 1913 "to disseminate knowledge concerning the symptoms, treatment, and prevention of cancer, to investigate conditions under which cancer is found; and to compile statistics in regard thereto" (Cancer Facts and Figures—1996). Today, the ACS consists of a national society, 57 divisions, and over 3400 units. It is the largest private source of cancer research funds in the United States and is second only to the National Cancer Institute in total research funding. Public education programs focus on tobacco control, diet and cancer relationships, multiple risk reduction with programs such as "Changing the Course," school health education, and early detection.

ACS education directed at health professionals includes conferences and workshops, self-study materials, clinical awards, and educational materials, such as pamphlets and newsletters. Patient services include community programs such as transportation and home-care items, rehabilitation programs, such as the "Reach to Recovery" program for breast cancer patients, patient and family education programs, and group-support programs. The Society also has a strong public issues and governmental relations component that serves as an advocate for public policy initiatives relating to cancer. The American Institute for Cancer Research is a smaller voluntary organization that supports research projects and provides professional education and public organization.

Industry Alliances

Organizations such as state and local chapters of the American Dietetic Association or independent consultant agencies may develop alliances with industry to implement community initiatives. One common approach has been "point-of-purchase" supermarket-based intervention to encourage low-fat, high-fiber choices. In such an initiative, the "Eat for Health" program tested whether a supermarket-based program could change shoppers' knowledge, attitudes, and food-buying behavior to be consistent with nutrition and cancer-risk-reduction guidelines (Rodgers et al., 1994). Another effort used videotaped public service announcements in grocery stores to try to increase nutrition awareness and healthful dietary choices.

PLANNING NUTRITION POLICYMAKING FOR CANCER PREVENTION AND RISK REDUCTION

The planning process must be conducted in a deliberate and orderly fashion, taking into consideration those factors essential to successful program development and implementation. These principles, which are generic to all program development, will help guide the process of planning a cancer control program. The process is as follows (Herzog, 1989).

Problem Definition and Diagnosis

The first step in the planning process is to identify and diagnose the problem. Many programs are doomed to failure precisely because planners incorrectly diagnosed the problems and contributing factors for which they were planning solutions. Problem definition is the pattern of behavior that deviates from the implied standard. Problem diagnosis is the determination of the causal sequence leading to the problem defined. For example, in "Anystate, USA" the problem may be a lung cancer rate higher than in other states or higher than national guidelines say should exist. In order to plan an effective cancer-prevention program for such a state, the planners must first determine the extent of the discrepancy and analyze contributing factors.

Stakeholder Analysis

Stakeholders are people who have a vested interest in the issue and are essential to the process by their support or lack of it. As many types of stakeholders as possible should be involved in the process. This may include community activists, Department of Public Health administrators, health professionals in the community, parents, and so on. This step is essential because without it, planners can rely only on their own preconceived notions, which may be incorrect. It has been said that "people are always trying to help others solve problems that they don't think they have." For people whose support is essential, ways need to be found to help them become vested in the project. This can be done by appealing to their sense of values or by pointing out mandates from groups in authority. For example, groups of parents of cancer sufferers can be mobilized to make a direct appeal, or mandates for the development of state cancer control plans can be presented. For example, in "Anystate, USA," a series of background papers can be commissioned from outside professionals to document the role of nutrition in cancer development at the time the plan is to be presented to the legislature for approval.

Needs Assessment

Needs assessment involves data collection from a variety of sources in order to determine what the problems are, their prevalence and incidence, the contributing factors, the extent to which needs are being met, and potential barriers to improvement. Several data-collection methods should be employed, not just one. The needs assessment must be done by groups who are representative of all target constituents. Political pressures should not be allowed to determine need. Cancer data can be gathered from hospitals, clinics, private physicians, as well as from national sources, such as the Centers for Disease Control, USDHHS, and the American Cancer Society.

Setting Goals and Objectives

Setting goals and objectives helps in developing priorities. Goals are the end points to be attained. Objectives are the various steps achieved in the process of attaining the goals. In order to be effective, goals must be set high enough to require effort, but low enough to be attainable. It is important that the goals of the project be consistent with the mission of the greater organization, thus showing how the project can help in achieving the mission. For example, the mission of the Health Department of "Anystate" is to "ensure the general health of the state's people," the needs assessment can show the extent of the cancer problem, and the program goals should be targeted at preventing cancer. A sample goal might be: by the year 2000, the incidence of all cancers in "Anystate" will be reduced from 10% to 8%. Objectives must be designed with measurable outcomes. For example, every community health center will institute cancer screening routinely by 1997, or smoking-cessation programs will be implemented for all relevant groups to reduce the incidence of smoking from 30% of the population to no more than 10% by a certain target date.

Program Planning (Design)

Planning can go forward when a significant number of key people have reached consensus on values, recognized a discrepancy between what is and what should be, and agreed that the project is the right thing to do. From this point the design of the systems, structures, and procedures can go forward. Alternative approaches can be identified and analyzed. Cost/benefit analysis should be instituted to determine approaches to be used. For example, although a television nutrition and cancer educational campaign might seem desirable, a focused cable TV program targeted to a specific population (whose pre- and postviewing behaviors could be measured) might be more feasible and sound. It might be too costly to screen all people for cancers, but it may be feasible to screen those seen to be at particular risk for specific cancers.

Implementation

A well-designed plan does not necessarily ensure wide acceptance. Factors to consider in planning for program implementation include determining (Lewin, 1951):

- what organizational factors can influence the process and how to address them;
- which project characteristics are most likely to influence acceptance by stakeholders;
- what resources are available;
- what mix of strategies is most likely to succeed in promoting initial change and ultimate institutionalization of the effort (e.g., educating and informing, consulting, persuasion, power coercion);
- what forces , barriers, resistances or restraints can affect the process;
- what are the structural and systematic requirements for implementing the plan;
- what types of project management tools might be useful (e.g., flow charts, computer program management or spreadsheet programs).

Monitoring and Evaluation

Monitoring and evaluation are ongoing functions throughout the planning process. Evaluation, therefore, must be built into the system at the beginning. Continuous monitoring of progress allows for adjustment as needed and helps ensure successful outcomes. Evaluation methods should be keyed to objectives and may focus on structural aspects (e.g., improving staff qualifications), process aspects (improving systems of care), or outcomes (improved health status or audience knowledge or attitudes) (Donabedian, 1980).

Common failures of planning include:

- isolation from major organizational decisions;
- lack of management involvement;
- failure to manage agreement and disagreement;
- inadequate concern with implementation;
- inadequate attention to organizational complexity.

SUMMARY

Nutrition interventions can help prevent cancer, improve chances of survival, and improve quality of life. Today, nutritional approaches are available that can play a role in primary, secondary, and tertiary cancer prevention.

There has been modest improvement in the American diet in the past 20 years as regards decreasing fat and increasing the consumption of fruits and vegetables. Changes must be more rapid if Year 2000 goals are to be met, however. Better dietary surveillance is also essential to support the development and evaluation of more effective dietary interventions (Byers, 1993).

It behooves community members and health professionals at all levels to support public health initiatives for cancer prevention and to ensure that appropriate information and services are developed and made available to all citizens.

REFERENCES

Albanese, D., & Taylor, P. R. (1990). International differences in body height and weight and their relationship to cancer incidence. *Nutrition & Cancer, 14,* 69–77.

American Cancer Society Inc. (1996). *Cancer facts and figures.* Atlanta, GA: Author.

Bal, D. G., Nixon, D. W., Foerster, S. B., & Brownson, R. C. (1995). Cancer prevention. In G. Murphy, W. Lawrence, & R. J. Lenhard (Eds.), *American*

Cancer Society textbook of clinical oncology, (2nd ed., pp. 40–63). Atlanta, GA: American Cancer Society.

Bassett, M. R., & Dobie, R. A. (1983). Patterns of nutritional deficiency in head and neck cancer. *Otolaryngology Head and Neck Surgery, 91,* ll9–25.

Bendich, A. (1993). Clinical Importance of beta carotene. *Perspectives in Applied Nutrition, 1,* 14–22.

Block, G., Patterson, B., & Subar, A. (1992). Fruit, vegetables, and cancer prevention: A review of the epidemiological evidence. *Nutrition and Cancer, 18,* 1–29

Blumberg, J., & Block, G. (1994). The alpha-tocopherol, beta-carotene cancer prevention study in Finland. *Nutrition Reviews, 52*(7), 242–245.

Boffetta, P., Mashberg, A., Winkelmann, R., & Garfinkel, L. (1992). Carcinogenic effects of tobacco smoking and alcohol drinking on anatomic sites of the oral cavity and oropharynx. *International Journal of Cancer, 52,* 530–533.

Byers, T. (1993). Dietary trends in the United States: Relevance to cancer prevention. *Cancer, 72,* 1015–1018.

Byers, T., & Perry, G. (1992). Dietary carotenes, vitamin C and vitamin E as protective antioxidants in human cancers. *Annual Review of Nutrition, 12,* 139–159.

Cassileth, B. R., Lusk, E. J., Guerry, D., Blake, A. D., Walsh, W. P., Kascius, L., & Schultz, D. J. (1991). Survival and quality of life among patients receiving unproven as compared with conventional cancer therapy. *New England Journal of Medicine, 324*(17), 1180–1185.

Center for Disease Control. (1994, August). *Advanced data #254* (p. 8). National Center for Health Statistics, USDHHS. Washington, DC: U.S. Government Printing Office.

Clifford, C., & Kramer, B. (1993). Diet as risk and therapy for cancer. *Medical Clinics of North America, 77*(4), 725–744.

Cotugna, N., Subar, A. F., Heimendinger, J., & Kahle, L. (1992). Nutrition and cancer prevention knowledge, beliefs, attitudes, and practices: The l987 National Health Interview Survey. *Journal of the American Dietetic Association, 92*(8), 963–968.

Cummings, N. B. (1993). Women's health and nutrition research: US Governmental concerns. *Journal of the American College of Nutrition, 12*(4), 329–336.

Daly, J. M., & Shinkwin, M. (1995). Nutrition and the cancer patient. In G. P. Murphy, W. Lawrence, & R. E. Lenhard (Eds.), *American Cancer Society's textbook of clinical oncology* (pp. 580–597). Atlanta, GA: American Cancer Society.

Doll, R. (1994). The use of meta-analysis in epidemiology: Diet and cancers of the breast and colon. *Nutrition Reviews, 52*(7), 233–237.

Donabedian, A. (1980). *The definition of quality and its assessment.* Ann Arbor, MI: Health Administration Press.

Donaldson, S. S., & Lenon, R. A. (1979). Alterations of nutritional status: impact of chemotherapy and radiation therapy, *Cancer, 43,* 2036–2052.

Dwyer, J. T. (1986). Nutrition education of the cancer patient and family: Myths and realities. *Cancer, 58,* 1887–1896.

Dwyer, J. T. (1989). The spectrum of dietary and nutritional approaches to cancer. *Nutrition, 5*(3), 197–199.

Dwyer, J. T., Efstathion, A., Palmer, C. & Papas, A. (1991). Nutritional support in treatment of oral carcinomas. *Nutrition Reviews, 49*(11), 332–337.

Dwyer, J. T., Gallo, J. J., & Reichel, W. (1993). Assessing nutritional status in elderly patients [Review]. *American Family Physician, 47*(3), 613–620.

Dwyer, J. T., Golay, J., Malsch, K., & Palmer, C. (1986). Current management of feeding and ingestion problems in head and neck cancer patients. In *Rehabilitation and treatment of head and neck cancer* (pp. 101–118). U.S. Department of Health and Human Services, Public Health Service, National Institutes of Health, NIH Pub. No. 86-2762. Washington, DC: U.S. Government Printing Office.

Dwyer, J. T., & Roy, J. (1994). Diet therapy. In J. D. Wilson, E. Braunwald, K. J. Isselbacher, R. G. Petersdorf, J. B. Martin, A. Fauci, & R. K. Root, (Eds.) *Harrison's principles of internal medicine.* (13th ed., pp. 455–463). New York: McGraw Hill.

Feldman, E. B. (1988). *Essentials of clinical nutrition.* (pp. 538–544). Philadelphia: F. A. Davis Company.

Franceschi, S., Bidoli, E., La Vecchia, C., Talamini, R., D'Avanzo, B., & Negri, E. (1994). Tomatoes and risk of digestive-tract cancers. *International Journal of Cancer, 59*(2), 181–184.

Frentzel-Beyme, R., & Chang-Claude, J. (1994). Vegetarian diets and colon cancer: The German experience. *American Journal of Clinical Nutrition, 59*(5) (Suppl): 1143s–1152s.

Freudenheim, J., Marshall, J. E., Graham, S., Laughlin, R., Vena, J. E., Muti, P., Swenson, M. A., & Nemoto, T. (1994). Exposure to breastmilk in infancy and the risk of breast cancer. *Epidemiology, 5*(3), 324–331.

Gaby, S. K., Bendich, A. Singh, V. N. & Machlin, L. J. *Vitamin intake and health: A scientific review* (pp. 29–57). New York: Marcel Dekker.

Gaby, S. K., & Singh, V. N. (1991). Beta carotene. In S. K. Gaby, A. Bendich, V. N. Singh, & L. S. Machlin (Eds.), *Vitamin intake and health: A scientific review* (pp. 29–57). New York: Marcel Dekker.

Ganz, P. A., & Schag, A. C. (1993). Nutrition and breast cancer. *Oncology, 7*(12), 71–75; 78–80.

Garewal, H. S., (1992). Potential role of beta carotene and antioxidant vitamins in the prevention of oral cancer. *Annals of the New York Academy of Science, 669,* 261–267.

Gaziano, J. M., Manson, J., Buring, J. E., & Hennekens, C. H. (1992). Dietary antioxidants and cardiovascular disease. *Annals of the New York Academy of Science, 669,* 249–259.

Ghadirian, P., Ekoe, J. M., & Thouez, J. P. (1992). Food habits and esophageal cancer: An overview. *Cancer Detection and Prevention, 16*(3), 163–168.

Goldin, B. R., Woods, M. N., Spiegelman, D. L., Longcope, C., Morrill-LaBrode, A., Dwyer, J. T., Gualtieri, L. J., Hertzmark, E., & Gorbach, S. L. (1994). The effect of dietary fat and fiber on serum estrogen concentrations in pre-menopausal women under controlled dietary conditions. *Cancer 74*(3), 1125–1131.

Goodwin, W. J., & Torres, J. (1984). The value of the prognostic nutritional index in the management of patients with advanced carcinoma of the head and neck. *Head and Neck, 6,* 932–937.

Greenberg, E. R., Baron, J. A., Tosteson, T. D., Freeman, D. H., Beck, G. J., Bond, J. H., Colacchio, T. A., Coller, J. A., Frankl, H. D., & Haile, R. W. (1994). A clinical trial of antioxidant vitamins to prevent colorectal adenoma. *New England Journal of Medicine, 331,* 141–147.

Greenberg, E. R., Baron, J. A., Stukel, T. A., Stevens, M. M., Mandel, J. S., Spencer, S. K., Elias, P. M., Lowe, N., Nierenberg, D. W., & Bayrd, G. (1990). A clinical trial of beta carotene to prevent basal cell and squamous cell cancers of the skin. *New England Journal of Medicine, 323,* 789–795.

Greenwald, P. (1993). NCI cancer prevention and control research. *Preventive Medicine, 22,* 642–660.

Hankin, J. H. (1993). Role of nutrition in women's health: Diet and breast cancer. *Journal of the American Dietetic Association, 93*(9), 994–999.

Healthy People 2000. (1991). National Health Promotion and Disease Prevention Objectives, U.S. Department of Health and Human Services, Public Health Service DHHS Publ.# (PHS) 91-50212.

Helzlsouer, K., Block, G., Blumberg, J., Diplock, A., Levine, M., Marnett, L., Schulplein, R., Spence, J., & Simic, M. (1994). Summary of the round table discussion on strategies for cancer prevention: diet, food, additives, supplements , and drugs. *Cancer Research, 54,* (Suppl). 2044s–2051s.

Henderson, J. C. (1995). Breast cancer. In G. W. Murphy, W. Lawrence, R. Lenhardt, (Eds.). (pp.198–219). *American Cancer Society textbook of clinical oncology* (2nd ed.), Atlanta GA: American Cancer Society.

Henderson, J. C. (1995). Paradigmatic shifts in the management of breast cancer [editorial; comment]. *New England Journal of Medicine, 332*(14), 951–952.

Henshaw, E., & Schloerb, P. (1983). Nutrition and the cancer patient, In P. Rubin, (Ed.), *Clinical oncology: A multidisciplinary approach*, (6th ed.). New York: American Cancer Society.

Herzog, W. T. (1989). Action planning for health organizations. In workshop proceedings: *Empowering nutritionists for leadership in public health*. Meeting held at the University of North Carolina, Chapel Hill, NC, June 4–7.

Hooley, R., Levine, H., Flores, T. C., Wheeler, T., & Steiger, E. (1983). Predicting head and neck complications using nutritional assessment: The prognostic nutritional index. *Archives of Otolaryngology, 109,* 83–85.

Holland, J. C. B. (1977). Anorexia and cancer: Psychological aspects. *Cancer, 27,* 363–367.

Hong, W. K., Endicott, J., Itri, L. M., et al. (1986). 13-cis-retinoic acid in the treatment of oral leukoplakia. *New England Journal of Medicine, 315*(24), 1501–1505.

Howard, L., Heaphey, L. L., & Timchalk, J. (1986). A review of the current nutritional status of home parenteral and enteral nutrition from the provider and consumer perspective. *J P E N, 10,* 416.

Hwang, H., Dwyer, J. T., & Russell, R. M. (1994). Diet, helicobacter pylori infection, food preservation and gastric cancer risk: Are there new roles for preventative factors. *Nutrition Reviews, 52,* 75–83.

Kaugars, G. E., Brandt, R. B., Carcaise-Edinboro, P., Strauss, R., & Kilpatrick, J. (1990). Beta carotene supplementation in the treatment of oral lesions (Abstr). *Oral Surgery, Oral Medicine, Oral Pathology, 70,* 607–608.

Kodama, M., Kodama, T., Miura, S., & Yoshida, M. (1991). Nutrition and breast cancer risk in Japan. *Anticancer Research, 11*(2), 745–754.

Koren, M. J. (1986). Home care-who cares? *New England Journal of Medicine, 314,* 917.

Lawton, M. P., & Brody, E. M. (1969). Assessment of older people: Self-maintaining and instrumental activities of daily living. *Gerontologist, 9*(3), 179–186.

Lee, H. P. (1993). Diet and cancer: A short review. *Annals of the Academy of Medicine, 22*(3), 355–59.

Lewin, K. (1951). *Field theory in social sciences.* New York: Harper and Row.

Lippman, S. M., Benner, S. E., & Hong, W. K. Retinoids in chemoprevention of head and neck carcinogenesis. *Preventive Medicine, 22*(5), 693–700.

Maki, P. A., & Newberne, P. M. (1992). Dietary lipids and immune function. *Journal of Nutrition, 122* (3 Suppl.), 610–614.

Meister, K. (1994). Antioxidants: What the conflicting reports mean. *Priorities, 6*(3), 7–11.

Mills, P. K., Beeson, W. L., Phillips, R. L., & Fraser, G. E. Cancer incidence among California Seventh-Day Adventists, 1976–1982. *American Journal of Clinical Nutrition, 59*(5 Suppl), 1136S–1142S.

Mobarhan, S., & Trumbore, L. S. (1991). Enteral tube feeding: A clinical perspective on recent advances. *Nutrition Reviews, 49,* 129–140.

Montbriand, M. (1994). An overview of alternative therapies chosen by patients with cancer. *Oncology Nursing Forum, 21,* 1547–1554.

Muller, J M,, Dienst, C., Brenner, U., & Pichlmaier, H. (1992). Pre-operative parenteral feeding in patients with gastrointestinal carcinoma. *Lancet 1*(8263), 68–71.

National Institutes of Health Consensus Development Panel. (1990). Consensus statement: Oral complications of cancer therapies. *NCI Monograph #9,* pp. 3–8.

Nayel, H., el-Ghoneimy, E., & el Haddad, S. (1992). Impact of nutritional supplementation on treatment delay and morbidity in patients with head and neck tumors treated with irradiation. *Nutrition, 8*(1), 13–18.

Neve, J. (1991). Physiological and nutritional importance of selenium. *Experientia, 47*(2), 187–93.

1995 Accreditation Manual for Hospitals. (1995). Oakbrook Terrace, IL: Joint Commission on the Accreditation of Hospitals Publications.

Nutrition Screening Manual for Professionals Caring for Older Americans: Nutrition Screening Initiative. (1992). Executive summary. Nutrition Screening Initiative. 2626 Pensylvania Ave. NW. Suite 301. Washington, DC 20037.

Palmer, C. (1984). The team approach to the care of the patient with head and neck cancer. *American Journal of Intravenous Therapy and Clinical Nutrition, 1*, 12–18.

Risch, H. A., Jain, M., Marrett, L. D., & Howe, G. R. (1994). Dietary fat intake and risk of epithelial ovarian cancer. *Journal of National Cancer Institute, 86*(18), 1409–1415.

Rock, C. L., Jacobs, R. A., & Bowen, P. E. (1996). Update on the bioligical characteristics of the antioxidont micronutrients: Vitamin C, vitamin E, and the caroternoids. *Journal of the American Dietetric Association, 96*, 693–702.

Rodgers, A. B., Kessler, L. G., Portnoy, B., Potosky, A. 1., Patterson, B., Thompson, F. E., Krebs-Smith, S. M., Breen, N., & Mathews, O. (1994). "Eat for Health" a supermarket intervention for nutrition and cancer risk reduction. *American Journal of Public Health, 84*(1), 72–76.

Rosenthal, P., Griffin, T., Dow, K., Lingos, T., Macewicz, R., & O'Connor, L. (1990). Complications of cancer and cancer treatment. In *Cancer manual.* (8th ed., pp. 420–449). Boston: American Cancer Society.

Schapira, D. V. (1992). Nutrition and cancer prevention. *Primary Care; Clinics in Office Practice, 19*(3), 481–491.

Schmale, A. H. (1979). Psychological aspects of anorexia. *Cancer, 43*, 2087–2092.

Smith, T. J., Dwyer, J. T., & Lafrancesca, J. P. (1990). Nutrition and the cancer patient. In *Cancer manual*, (8th ed., pp. 485–497). Boston: American Cancer Society.

Steele, G. (1995). Colorectal cancer. In G. W. Murphy, W. Lawrence, R. Leuhart, (Eds.). *American Cancer Society textbook of annual ocology,* (2nd ed., pp. 236–250). Atlanta: American Cancer Society.

Stich, H. F., Rosin, M. P., Hornby, A. P., Mathew, B., & Sankaranarayanan, R. (1988). Remission of oral leukoplakias and micronuclei in tobacco/betel chewers treated with beta carotene and with beta carotene plus vitamin A. *International Journal of Cancer, 42*, 195–199.

Taylor, P. R., Li, B., Dawsey, S. M., Li, J. Y., Yang, C. S., Guo, W., & Blot, W. J. (1994). Prevention of esophageal cancer: The nutrition intervention trials in Linxian China. Linxian Nutrition Intervention Trials Study Group. *Cancer Research, 54*(7 Suppl.), 2029s–2031s.

Toma, S., Benso, S., Albanese, E., Palumbo, R., Canton, E., Nicolo, G., & Mangionle, P. (1992). Treatment of oral leukoplakia with beta carotene. *Oncology, 49,* 77–81.

Tominaga, S., & Kato, I. (1992). Diet, nutrition, and cancer in Japan. *Nutrition and Health, 8*(2-3), 125–132.

U.S. Department of Health and Human Services, Food and Drug Administration. (1989). Food labeling: Advance notice of proposed regulations. *Federal Register, 54,* 32610–32615.

Welch, D. (1981). Nutritional consequences of carcinogenesis and radiation therapy. *Journal of the American Dietetic Association, 78,* 467–471.

Weisburger, J. H., & Williams, G. M. (1995). Causes of cancer. In G. Murphy, W. Lawrence, & R. W. Leihend (Eds.), *American Cancer Society textbook of clinical oncology* (2nd ed., pp. 10–39). Atlanta: American Cancer Society.

Weisburger, J. H., & Wynder, E. L., (1991). Dietary fat intake and cancer. *Hematology-Oncology Clinics of NA, 5*(1), 7–23.

Willett, W. C., Stampfer, M. J., Colditz, G. A., Rosner, B. A., Hennekens, C. H., & Speizer, F. E. (1987). Relation of meat, fat, and their fiber intake to the risk of colon cancer in a prospective study among women. *New England Journal of Medicine, 323,* 1664.

Williams, E. F., & Meguid, M. M. (1989). Nutritional concepts and considerations in head and neck surgery. *Head and Neck Surgery, 11,* 393–399.

Wilson, P. R., Herman, J., & Chubon, S. J. (1991). Eating strategies used by persons with head and neck cancer during and after radiotherapy. *Cancer Nursing, 14,* 2, 98–104.

Winn, D. M. (1995). Diet and nutrition in the etiology of oral cancer. *American Journal of Clinical Nutrition, 61*(2), 437s–445s.

Ziegler, R. G., Subar, A. F., Craft, E. N., Ursin, G., et al. (1992). Does beta-carotene explain why reduced cancer risk is associated with vegetable and fruit intake? *Cancer Research, 52*(7 Suppl), 2060s–2066s.

Zloznik, A. J. (1994). Unproven (unorthodox) cancer treatments. *Cancer Practice, 2*(1), 19–24.

CHAPTER 10

Osteoporosis

Felix Bronner

O steoporosis, also termed osteopenia, may be defined as a condition of the skeleton characterized by diminished bone mass per unit volume. Characteristically, it affects women beginning in the decade after menopause, therefore it is often termed postmenopausal osteoporosis. It also affects men, however, though later in life, typically beginning in their eighth decade. Persons afflicted with this condition are subject to vertebral compression, leading to back pain, shortened stature, and spinal buckling, that is, the well-known "widow's hump." As long bones thin, they are subject to readier fracture, so that falls or other incidents can lead to major invalidism that would not have been incurred at a younger age. Hip fractures in women in their seventies are common and often force major changes in living arrangements, from independence to unhappy dependence. It is thus clear that as the proportion in the population of people beyond their sixth decade increases, osteoporosis and its sequelae become a major public health concern.

Bone mass increases from birth to approximately the end of the third decade in both women and men. Thereafter, it decreases quite gradually to the age of 50. In women, as they undergo menopause, there is a marked and rapid drop in bone mass over the decade that follows. That drop severely affects trabecular bone, which constitutes about 20% of all bone, whereas the decrease in cortical bone is much more gradual. Trabecular bone, also known as cancellous bone, is formed largely in the metaphyses of long bones, whereas cortical bone forms the outer wall of all bones and is largely responsible for the supportive and protective function of the skeleton. Cancellous bone contains the bone marrow, responds to structural stress, and carries out the homeostatic functions of the skeleton, as contributing to the maintenance of the very stable plasma calcium level (Bronner, 1995). For details of bone structure and function, see Jee (1991).

In both men and women, the drop in bone mass parallels the drop in gonadal hormones, gradual in men, abrupt in women at the menopause, becoming comparably gradual in women in their seventh decade (Bronner, 1994). It is now generally accepted that gonadal hormones, probably together with cytokines and other local factors released by bone and precursor cells in response to stimulation by or interaction with gonadal hormones, play a major regulatory role in bone metabolism (Bronner, 1994). Thus the age-dependent drop in gonadal hormones is primarily responsible for the age-dependent diminution in bone mass. Moreover, the rate of bone mass diminution, when expressed as a function of the bone mass, is constant. In other words, the larger the bone mass in the fifth decade of life, the longer it will take before the bone mass decreases to the point where it fractures readily. This means that a menopausal woman with a small bone mass would likely be subject to debilitating fractures at a younger age than a menopausal woman with a large bone mass.

Skeletal size and mass are genetically programmed. To attain the programmed size and mass, it is necessary to have available the raw materials that make up the skeleton, calcium and phosphorus in particular. It is therefore obvious that attaining the programmed skeletal size and mass in the first two decades of life will assure that the risk of osteoporosis and fracture has been delayed as long as is naturally possible. Further delay will require restoring gonadal hormone levels to where they were before the abrupt fall in women undergoing the menopause or in men before their fourth decade. Alternative therapeutic approaches involve slowing bone resorption rates (Osteoporosis, 1984) or stimulating bone formation rates. In this connection, it must be remembered that after the fourth decade, both formation and resorption rates decrease, but that without therapeutic intervention, bone formation decreases faster than resorption (Bronner & Stein, 1995). When resorption exceeds formation, there is net loss of bone mass, the situation that characterizes most individuals past 50 years of age. This loss may be small, but over the years can amount to a third of the total bone mass.

It is generally thought that there is linkage between bone formation and resorption, but the mechanism of linkage is not known. Attempts to influence either bone formation or resorption singly entail the risk of ultimately altering also the opposite process. Current therapeutic interventions have involved three approaches (Bronner, 1994; Osteoporosis, 1984) (1) gonadal hormone replacement; (2) inhibition of bone resorption by means of fluoride, biphosphonate or calcitonin treatment; and (3) calcium and vitamin D supplementation.

Hormone treatment and calcium supplementation are frequently combined and should be if the patient's habitual calcium intake is significantly below that of the Recommended Daily Allowance (RDA). Vitamin D supplementation alone has not proved effective (Bronner, 1995), but may be of help with calcium supplementation, particularly in the elderly whose vitamin D intake or exposure to sunlight is inadequate. Calcium supplementation alone or with vitamin D has not been shown to be efficacious in postmenopausal women if the latter do not also receive hormone replacement (Bronner, 1994; Bronner & Stein, 1995). Calcium supplementation in the elderly (>70 years) of both sexes seems beneficial, as it may slow cortical bone loss (Bronner & Stein, 1995).

Although calcium and vitamin D intake can be increased by individual decision, other therapeutic interventions require medical supervision and prescription. The nutritional component of skeletal health relates primarily to adequate calcium intake throughout life and it is toward that aim that nutritional policy must be directed. In the United States, easily two-thirds of calcium intake is from dairy products (Bronner, 1995). The current availability of milk and milk products that are low in fat makes it possible for individuals who do not suffer from lactose deficiency to consume 1g of calcium per day without increasing fat intake, inasmuch as 1L of skim milk provides 1.2 g of elemental calcium. Lactose-treated milks are now commercially available.

Because osteoporosis is so widespread and because appropriate nutritional practice can help in achieving a skeleton of optimum size and mass, nutrition officers in public health settings need to develop educational programs directed at good bone health. Such programs should include pamphlets for general distribution; contact with journalists to help spread information on bone health via television, radio, and print media; occasional symposia or update meetings directed at and addressed by appropriate health professionals; in-service programs for hospital dietitians and dietary personnel in schools and in facilities for the elderly. Emphasis should be placed on the importance of adequate calcium intake throughout life and on the importance of appropriate medical intervention at menopause. Intervention in men will undoubtedly become an option in the next several years. National Institute of Health (NIH) statements on osteoporosis and calcium intake can serve as authoritative references (Optimal Calcium Intake, 1994; Osteoporosis, 1984).

To what extent nutrition policy should also contemplate specific interventions so as to make calcium-containing foods more available or to encourage calcium supplementation of existing foods is as yet controversial. Grocery stores and supermarkets can be encouraged to stock dairy foods at reasonable prices that are acceptable to lactase-deficient individuals. Food processors can include additional calcium in processed foods at minimal added cost. Breakfast cereals in particular often already contain added calcium. Calcium can also be readily added to bread flour and baked goods.

The message of appropriate calcium intake needs to be spread to the population as a whole, but has particular relevance for girls just before and after the menarche, periods when the calcium deposition rate is particularly high (Abrams, Schanler, Yergey, Vieira, & Bronner, 1994). Moreover, the calcium intake of U.S. women tends to be below the Recommended Daily Allowance (Bronner, 1994). For this reason, women and their daughters should constitute the major targets of the educational efforts of nutrition officers.

A number of environmental factors modulate the risk of osteoporosis. *Exercise* that strengthens muscles has a beneficial effect on bone strength. Contrariwise, when, as in space flight, the body is subjected to hypogravity, bone mass is diminished. Excessive exercise, however, as encountered in some female runners, leads to amennorhea and subsequent bone thinning.

Smoking, *alcohol* consumption, and *coffee* drinking have been identified as risk factors for good bone health (Bronner & Stein, 1995). The extent and manner in which these activities contribute to the risk of osteoporosis is as yet unsettled, however.

REFERENCES

Abrams, S. A., Schanler, R. J. Yergey, A. L. Vieira, N. E. & Bronner, F. (1994) Compartmental analysis of calcium metabolism in very-low-birth-weight infants. *Pediatric Research, 36,* 424–428.

Bronner, F. (1994). Calcium and Osteoporosis. *American Journal of Clinical Nutrition, 60,* 831–836.

Bronner, F. (1995). Function of calcium in the mammalian organism. In G. Berthon, (Ed.), *Handbook on metal-ligand interactions in biological fluids* (Vol. 1, pp. 161–185). New York: Marcel Dekker.

Bronner, F., & Stein, W. D. (1995). Calcium nutrition and osteoporosis. In F. Bronner (Ed.), *Nutrition and health—Topics and controversies* (pp.113–136). Boca Raton: CRC Press.

Jee, W. S. S. (1991). Introduction to skeletal function: Structural and metabolic aspects. F. Bronner & R. F. Worrell, (Eds.), *A basic science primer in orthopaedics* (pp. 3–34). Baltimore: Williams & Wilkins.

Optimal Calcium Intake. (1994). *National Institutes of Health Consensus Development Conference Statement, 12,* 1–3.

Osteoporosis. (1984). *National Institutes of Health Consensus Development Conference Statement, 5,*(3), 1–6.

CHAPTER 11

Dental Caries Prevention

Martin S. Giniger

T his chapter provides a comprehensive review of the benefits and risks of dental caries prevention through the public health policy of community water fluoridation. Fluoridation has long been recognized as one of the most reliable, cost-effective public health policy interventions instituted in this century. Yet despite the ensuing marked reduction in caries that has resulted from this initiative, antifluoridation activity is still widespread in the United States (Mandel, 1985; Public Health Service, 1991).

Prevention is generally considered to be preferable to treatment for almost any disease. Preventive medicine and dentistry not only save considerable time and suffering, but also reduce the expense associated with treatment of a more advanced disease process. Dental caries are, simply put, the most persistent and widespread chronic disease affecting children in the United States and the world. Although 90% of the U.S. population suffers from its effects, only 50% of these people seek out dental care in a given year. In addition, the effects of dental caries go beyond the oral cavity. Cavities can progress from a minute incipient area of enamel decalcification to large areas of decay that can then spread infection to associated areas of the head and neck. In fact, if left untreated in a susceptible host, dental caries will lead to general systemic infection and even death. More commonly, dental caries can also adversely affect eating and speech patterns, nutritional adequacy, and facial appearance with associated loss of self-esteem.

If the above medical concerns are considered together with the fact that Americans are now spending more than $20 billion annually on dental services, it is little wonder that local and state governments have campaigned so actively for communal water fluoridation. This nutrition policy remains the safest, most cost-efficient, most effective public health measure available to prevent and control disease (Easley, 1985).

In the past 50 years, thousands of reports have been published that prove that community fluoridation is safe, has a high benefit-to-cost ratio, and can effectively prevent or minimize disease. Nevertheless, antifluoridation activity is on the rise and one of the United States' most successful community-based nutrition policies is under attack. This chapter therefore attempts to define the benefits, risks, and consequences of fluoridation, as well as to provide historical and scientific perspective to the claims that have been made on both sides of the issue. The gains made over the last 5 decades are threatened if fluoride use is curtailed because of the lack of knowledge, apathy, or inadequate involvement of nutrition and public health officers to educate and set the public record straight (Mandel, 1985; Public Health Service, 1991).

DEFINITION OF "FLUORIDATION"

Fluoridation is the deliberate upward adjustment of the natural trace element, fluoride, in public water supplies for the purpose of promoting the public's health through the prevention of tooth decay. Fluoride is present in small, but widely varying amounts in all soils, water supplies, plants, and animals. Thus it can be considered to be a normal constituent of all diets. The fluoride ion itself comes from the element fluorine; fluorine is the 13th most abundant element in the earth's crust. Fluorine is never found in its free state, however, but only in combination with other elements as a "fluoride" compound (Largent, 1987; Safe Drinking Water Committee, 1977). In fact, the need for fluoride as a trace nutrient is set out in the Recommended Dietary Allowances (RDA) (National Research Council, 1980).

The highest concentrations of fluoride in the human body are found in bones and teeth. All public water supplies in this country contain a least a small amount of natural fluoride. For the purpose of preventing dental caries, the optimal concentration in public water supplies has been found

Table 11.1 Recommended Optimal Drinking Water Fluoride
Concentrations According to Climate

Annual Average Maximum daily air TEMP (°F)	Recommended fluoride concentration (PPM)
40.0–53.7	1.2
53.8–58.3	1.1
58.4–63.8	1.0
63.9–70.6	0.9
70.7–79.2	0.8
79.3–90.5	0.7

Source: Centers for Disease Control, 1991.

to be between 0.7 to 1.2 parts per million, or 0.7 to 1.2 milligrams per liter (Table 11.1; Centers for Disease Control, 1986, 1991).

HISTORY OF DENTAL CARIES PREVENTION

Fluoride was first added to this country's public drinking water in the 1940s to prevent tooth decay (Public Health Service, 1991). At the beginning of the twentieth century a young dentist named Frederick S. McKay had moved from the East Coast to Colorado Springs, Colorado and had noticed that many of his new patients' teeth exhibited a condition he called "Colorado Brown Stain." The people in the community had been unaware that anything was wrong because so many were affected. Because this condition was not described in the scientific literature, Dr. McKay set out to investigate the phenomenon and found that dental fluorosis (i.e., "brown stain" or "mottled enamel") was prevalent throughout the surrounding El Paso County (Murray & Rugg-Gunn, 1982a).

In the late 1920s, Dr. McKay made another major discovery. The mottled teeth he had been observing over the preceding decade were essentially free of dental decay. In 1931, with the advent of a new scientific technique called spectrographic analysis, Dr. McKay and an Alcoa Company chemist, Dr. H. V. Churchill, identified fluoride as the element in the Colorado Springs drinking water that caused the brown stain and also inhibited dental caries (Murray & Rugg-Gunn, 1982a).

In the 1930s Dr. H. Trendley Dean, of the United States Public Health

Service, and Dr. McKay collaborated to determine if fluoride could be added to the drinking water to prevent cavities. Their studies established a community fluorosis index but were incomplete and were interrupted by World War II. In 1945 and 1947 four classic studies were begun that proved the benefits of adding fluoride to the drinking water of several communities. Fluoridation began in January 1945 in Grand Rapids, Michigan; in May 1945, in Newburgh, New York; in June 1945 in Brantford, Ontario; and in February 1947 in Evanston, Illinois. Together these studies firmly established fluoridation as a practical and effective public health measure that would prevent dental caries (Murray & Rugg-Gunn, 1982a).

Today more than 10,000 U.S. communities and numerous foreign countries use adjusted and naturally fluoridated water (Centers for Disease Control and Prevention, 1991). Over the past 50 years, continuous studies have been conducted on fluorides and fluoridation. Since 1970 alone there have been hundreds of studies on fluoride. Clearly therefore the safety and effectiveness of water fluoridation have been extensively researched and documented over the past several decades. Several thousand references on the biological effects of fluoride on bones and teeth now exist. To date, no harmful effects have been found at the concentrations recommended for dental health. Studies have repeatedly shown that drinking fluoridated water from birth, in the range of 0.7–1.2 parts per million (ppm) of fluoride, can reduce the incidence of tooth decay by as much as 65% (Council on Community Health, 1989).

STATUS OF COMMUNITY WATER FLUORIDATION

Throughout the world, over 320 million people receive the benefits of water fluoridation as a way to prevent dental caries. In the United States, there are approximately 144 million persons served by water supplies whose fluoride content has been adjusted to the recommended optimum levels, or whose natural fluoride content is dentally significant (0.7 ppm or greater). Among our 50 largest cities, 42 now have fluoridated water. Internationally, fluoridation is practiced in over 30 countries, with extensive fluoridation in Asia, Australia, North and South America, and New Zealand. Many European countries, which do not currently fluoridate their water supplies, provide "alternative fluoride programs," such as fluoride supplement tablets and fluoridated table salt.

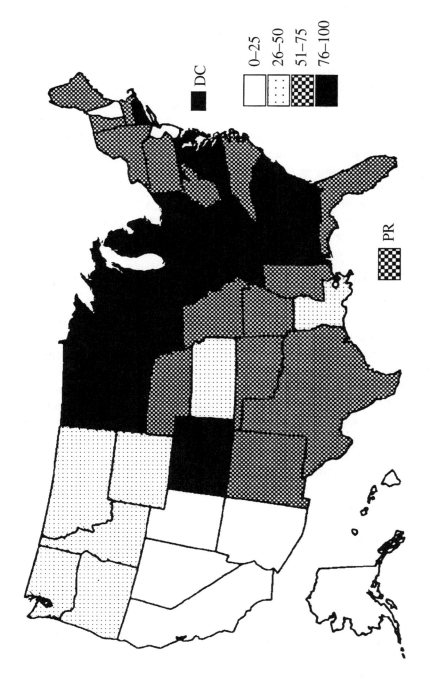

DC ■

☐ 0–25

▦ 26–50 (dotted)

▩ 51–75 (checkered)

■ 76–100

PR ▩

Figure 11.1 Percentage of U.S. population who receive fluoridated drinking water according to 1989 fluoridated Census (Centers for Disease Control, 1991).

Only 55.8% of the United States' population receive fluoridated water. There is a large disparity in the proportion of the population served by fluoridated water in different regions of the country, however (Hinman, 1995).

In virtually all states east of the Rocky Mountains more than half the population receives optimally fluoridated water, with more than 90% in the Great Lakes States (Figure 11.1). By contrast, only 45% of the population of the northwestern states and 18% of the southwestern states are currently served by fluoridated water systems. The state of California ranks 48th in the nation in terms of the percentage of the population receiving fluoride benefits, with only 15.7% of the state's population on-line with fluoridated public water supplies. In fact, California has 60% of the 150 largest nonfluoridated cities in the United States (Hinman, 1995).

HOW FLUORIDE PREVENTS DENTAL CARIES

There are three basic compounds commonly used for fluoridating drinking-water supplies in the United States: sodium fluoride, sodium silicofluoride, and hydrofluosilicic acid (Centers for Disease Control and Prevention, 1986, 1991). All of them must meet the American Water Works Association's standards for use in water fluoridation (Centers for Disease Control and Prevention, 1986). Like numerous other compounds, all three have a number of industrial uses. It should be noted, however, that the U.S. Environmental Protection Agency no longer lists sodium fluoride as a registered rodenticide (Environmental Protection Agency, 1986).

When water containing fluoride is ingested, about 20% is retained by the saliva in the mouth and exerts a topical effect on the teeth. About 80% of the fluoride is absorbed in the gastrointestinal tract. Plasma levels of fluoride peak in about 30 minutes. The major organ involved with the removal of fluoride from the body is the kidney. Within 24 hours, 50% of the absorbed fluoride is excreted in the urine, 10% is excreted in the feces, and 40% gets deposited in the skeletal system (Whitford & Pashley, 1984; Whittford, Pashley, & Stringer, 1976).

The bones, teeth, and other parts of the skeleton tend to attract and retain fluoride, whereas the soft tissues do not. Incorporation of fluorides is most rapid during a child's first 12 years of life. Erupted teeth differ from other parts of the skeleton in that there is not much remodelling due to a lack of cellular activity. Therefore, it is important that children drink optimally fluoridated water during the development of their teeth, starting at birth, so that the unerupted teeth can incorporate as much fluoride as possible (Whitford, Pashley, & Reynolds, 1979).

Only soluble and inorganic fluorides (e.g., CaF_2) can be incorporated into tooth structure. Organic fluorides are not used by the body (Guy, 1979). The mechanism for the incorporation of the fluoride ion into teeth and bones is not fully understood. The fluoride ion is known to replace the hydroxyl ion (OH-) in the crystal lattice of enamel (hydroxyapatite), this, in turn, results in stronger teeth that are comprised of fluoroapatite.

Recent literature indicates that the mechanisms by which fluoride provides caries resistance can be grouped into five categories: (1) increased enamel resistance to acid attack through formation of fluoroapatite; (2) increased rate of mineralization immediately following eruption; (3) increased remineralization of early lesions; (4) interference with bacterial metabolism to produce acid; and (5) changes in the bacterial composition of plaque. Furthermore it is customary to classify the mechanisms as resulting from fluoride–tooth interaction that is either topical or systemic. Systemic processes are those in which fluoride is ingested and the unerupted teeth are the targets of the fluoride activity. Topical fluoride action can only occur on erupted teeth. Optimally fluoridated water provides both a topical and systemic effect. Fluoridated water provides topical contact to erupted teeth as it passes through the oral cavity. After the water is absorbed by the gastrointestinal tract, the fluoride is circulated and deposited systemically in developing, unerupted teeth (Melberg & Ripa, 1983; Murray & Rugg-Gunn, 1982b; Newbrun, 1989b).

Decades ago, when community water fluoridation first began, most scientists believed that the anticavity activity of fluoride was primarily the result of the incorporation of fluoride into the apatite crystals of developing enamel. This increased the stability of the tooth enamel by reducing the solubility of the apatite structure when under acid attack. Since then, however, it has been learned that the correlation between enamel fluoride concentration and caries experience is not very consistent. It is now believed that the observed reduction of dental decay is due to *both* preeruptive (systemic) and posteruptive (topical) influences (Beltran & Burt, 1988; Ripa, 1993). These may be summarized as follows:

1. Incipient enamel lesions are barely affected by water fluoridation. The progression of these lesions into clinical cavities that need to be filled is slowed by the topical effect of 1.0 ppm fluoride contact, however.

2. For adolescents exposed to 1.0 ppm fluoride in their drinking water for their entire lives, the reduction in dental caries was 50% due to the topical effect and 50% due to the systemic effect.

3. The best protection against cavities is achieved if exposure to community water fluoridation starts at birth. However, 85% of maximal protection can be achieved if exposure begins between ages 3 and 4.

4. Prevention of cavities between teeth and on smooth tooth surfaces is due to both a systemic and topical mechanism of action. The preeruptive effect accounts for 25% to 50%. Alternatively, caries protection in the pits and fissures of teeth accounts for nearly two thirds of the cavity protection due to the systemic effect of drinking an optimally fluoridated water supply (Groeneveld, Van Eyck, & Backer-Dirks, 1990; Ripa, 1993).

REVIEW OF FLUORIDATION IN DENTAL CARIES PREVENTION

The inverse relationship between increasing fluoride concentrations of the drinking water and decreasing incidence of dental caries continues to be as true today as 50 years ago (Ripa, 1993). Since the Grand Rapids experiment, there have been dozens of comprehensive reviews that have summarized the results of community water fluoridation studies over the past half century (Ripa, 1993). The reports of the first fluoridation studies conducted in the United States, Canada, the United Kingdom, and New Zealand between 1945 and 1965 were reviewed by McClure (1970). In the second edition of *Fluorides in Caries Prevention*, published in 1982, Murray and Rugg-Gunn reviewed the literature through 1980 and summarized the results of 95 fluoridation studies conducted in 20 countries (Murray & Rugg-Gunn, 1982a). Most recently, Newbrun, participating in a University of Michigan Workshop on the cost-effectiveness of caries prevention in public health, reviewed the results of water-fluoridation studies published between 1979 and 1988 (Newbrun, 1989a; Ripa, 1993). Sufficient clinical evidence now exists to conclude that there are decided benefits to all teeth from water fluoridation.

Although children are often thought of as being the primary beneficiaries of communal water fluoridation, adults also reap benefit. Often in studies of adults, the comparison is between those living in fluoride-deficient or optimally fluoridated communities and those adults living in cities where the drinking water fluoride content is higher than 1.2 ppm. More adult studies are needed in which the conventional comparison is made between residents of optimally fluoridated communities and adults living in areas that are fluoride deficient (Ripa, 1993). The existing evidence clearly shows reductions in dental caries in the adult population, however.

In the few "traditional" studies that have been published in the United States and Canada (Burt, Eklund, & Loesce, 1986; Newbrun, 1989a; Ripa, 1993), an effect has been shown on both coronal and root surface cavities. The coronal and root surface caries prevalence rates of adults living in cities with higher fluoride concentration in the drinking water have consistently shown to have fewer cavities than adults living in communities with lower levels of fluoride in the drinking water. In a recent study (Grembowski, Fiset, & Spadafora, 1992) of 600 adults ranging in age from 20 to 34 years, investigators have found that the cavity incidence was reduced by about 25% in people who lived in cities with water that had optimal fluoride levels.

COST ASPECTS OF COMMUNITY WATER FLUORIDATION

The cost of adding fluoride to the water supply is usually expressed as the annual cost per capita of the total population being served. The costs include: (1) amortization of initial capital expenditures, (2) the annual cost of supplies, and (3) the annual operating costs for maintenance, rent, and salaries. The annual cost of community water fluoridation will vary according to a plant's capacity, type of equipment and fluoride compound used, the number of injection points and the natural concentration of fluoride in the water. A universal economic tenet is that cost usually varies inversely with the size of the population being served (Ripa, 1993).

In the late 1970s, Newbrun (1978) estimated that the approximate annual cost of water fluoridation was 20¢ per capita in the United States. He also estimated that after 12 years of water fluoridation, a typical community would recognize an average annual savings of $10.00 in dental treatment expenditure per capita. Therefore he concluded that the approximate cost–benefit ratio for water fluoridation would be 1:50. In 1988 a Michigan Workshop on Community Water Fluoridation (Burt, 1989) concluded that the average annual cost of fluoridation was between $0.12 to

$0.21 in cities with populations greater than 200,000; between $0.18 and $0.75 in cities and towns with populations ranging between 10,000–200,000; and cost would range between $0.60 and $5.41 in small towns and villages with populations of less than 10,000. The reason for the large cost variability in small towns results from their sensitivity to changes in the variables that comprise the analysis.

In a recent review that compared eight published reports that measured the cost of fluoridation with its benefits, the overall cost–benefit ratio varied from 1:2.5 to 1:11.5. In their cost-effectiveness analysis, White, Antczak-Boukom, and Weinstein (1989) looked at studies published between 1973 and 1987, used "caries prevention" as the measure of effectiveness and concluded that cost effectiveness of community water fluoridation is influenced by at least three variables: (1) the baseline caries rate and disease pattern fluctuation over time; (2) the mobility of the population in the community; and (3) the number of people at risk for caries. Of these, the most important variable is the baseline caries rate and disease pattern fluctuation over time, a factor that was not well examined in many of the earlier studies. Although the cost–benefit ratio calculated by White and colleagues (1989) was considerably less than Newbrun's and that of many others, water fluoridation was nevertheless found to be one of the most cost–effective preventive dental programs and the most cost–effective preventive nutrition program in health care (Ripa, 1993).

SAFETY

In reference to the claim that fluoride causes cancer, independent studies conducted in the United States by the National Cancer Institute, the National Heart, Lung, and Blood Institute, and the Centers for Disease Control found no relationship between fluoridation and cancer mortality. Since 1977, at least 17 reports have refuted claims that there is any association between the fluoridation of community water supplies and cancer (Council on Community Health, 1989; National Cancer Institute, 1975).

The most recent analysis of the effects of fluoride in animals and humans was released in February 1991 by the U.S. Public Health Services (Public Health Service, 1991). This report reviewed virtually all studies on the effects of fluoride in animals and humans and concluded that "if fluoride presents any risks to the public at the levels to which the vast majority of us are exposed, those risks are so small that they have been impossible to detect in the epidemiological studies to date. In contrast, the benefits are great and easy to detect." The report also failed to find any data establishing an association between fluoride and cancer in humans.

With respect to recent studies published regarding the relationship between fluoride and bone health, there is no evidence that drinking optimally fluoridated (0.7–1.2 ppm) water has any adverse effect on bone. Current research indicates that osteoporosis is found less frequently where the drinking water contains naturally high (approximately 4.0–8.0 ppm) concentrations of fluoride. The data from this research are not conclusive and further research is planned. Individuals who currently live in communities with optimally fluoridated water have no need for concern, however, and may even reap some beneficial effect (Bernstein, Sadowsky, Hegsted, Guri, & Stare, 1966; Council on Community Health, 1989; Leone, 1955).

The claim that fluoride inhibits or impairs the activity of enzymes, has no relevance to fluoridated water. The World Health Organization Report, "Fluorides and Human Health" states that there is no evidence that has ever been provided to suggest that fluoride ingested at 1 ppm in the drinking water affects intermediary metabolism of food, vitamin utilization, or either hormonal or enzymatic activity (Health, 1989; Jenkins, Venkateswarla, & Zipkin, 1970).

Fluoridation should not be considered a form of medication because it cannot treat or cure tooth decay. The National Research Council has recognized fluoride as an essential dietary ingredient for the growth and development of teeth and bones (National Research Council, 1980). The 1988 Surgeon General's Report on Nutrition and Health recommends that water systems contain fluoride at optimum levels for the prevention of tooth decay. Fluoride adjustment in a public water supply is undertaken to provide the necessary amount of this essential nutrient to help the body resist disease (Public Health Service, 1988).

Fluorosis, a developmental disorder of the enamel, occurs only if high levels of fluoride are ingested while the teeth are developing. Optimum levels of fluoride in the range of 0.7–1.2 parts per million of fluoride will not cause unsightly staining of the teeth in the vast majority of individuals. At the concentration recommended for protection against dental decay, mild degrees of dental fluorosis may occur in 10%–15% of children who consume fluoridated water from birth. This degree of fluorosis does not cause dark staining or impair appearance. Therefore there is no need to modify the recommended optimum fluoride concentration of drinking water (Council on Community Health, 1989; Driscoll, 1986).

Although enamel fluorosis does not directly affect oral health or esthetics except in its severest forms, a 1991 United States Public Health Service Review of Fluoride Benefits and Risks concluded that an increase in the prevalence of enamel fluorosis indicates that "total" fluoride exposure may be more than is necessary to prevent tooth decay (Public Health Service, 1991). Continued research is, therefore, needed to monitor the prevalence and severity of enamel fluorosis in both fluoridated and nonfluoridated populations so that regimens of fluoride administration can be tailored to reduce the prevalence and severity of decay to a maximum while minimizing the risk of dental fluorosis.

EPIDEMIOLOGY OF DENTAL CARIES PREVENTION

Epidemiological evidence of studies through the 1980s has indicated that dental caries are declining throughout the United States. Figure 11.2 demonstrates that, on average, nearly 36% more children were caries free in 1987 as compared to 7 years earlier. This is a major change that can be attributed in large part to increased availability of community water fluoridation (Figure 11.3). From 1971 through 1987, three national surveys of U.S. children demonstrated a continued decrease in cavity prevalence (Morbidity and Mortality Weekly Report, 1992; National Center for Health Statistics, 1979; National Institute of Dental Research, 1981, 1989). In the national survey conducted from 1986–1987, it was concluded that prevalence of caries among children with a history of lifelong exposure to optimally fluoridated water decreased 18% when compared to the prevalence among children with no exposure to optimally fluoridated water (Table 11.2; Figure 11.4; National Institute of Dental Research, 1989). In fact, dental-caries prevalence declined to 25% when the analysis factored out children with history of fluoride therapy (e.g., dietary supplements or professionally applied topical gels) (Newbrun, 1989a).

Recent epidemiological studies have also found a consistently lower incidence of dental caries, both on coronal and root surfaces, among adults who live in cities with optimal or greater fluoride content when compared to adults who live in communities with lower concentrations of fluoride in the water supply (Newbrun, 1989a). Epidemiological studies of dental caries prevalence in U.S. citizens aged 60 or older show that there is evidence of 17% to 35% less coronal and root surface dental caries in those

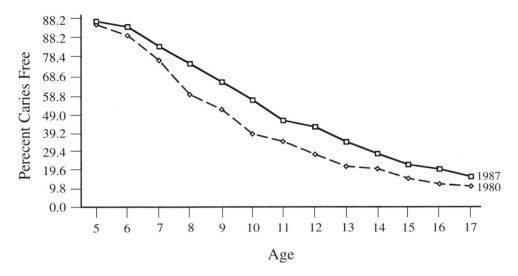

Figure 11.2 Percentage of U.S. children completely free of dental caries.

Sources: N.I.D.R., 1981, 1989.

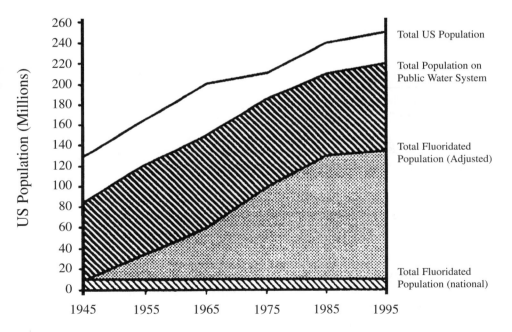

Figure 11.3 U.S. population receiving water fluoridation.

Source: Centers for Disease Control, 1991.

Table 11.2 Mean DMFS of U.S. Children with Permanent Teeth by Age and Water Fluoridation Exposure

Age	Life-long water fluoridation exposure mean DMFS	No water fluoridation exposure mean DMFS	Percentage difference (%)
5	0.03	0.10	70
6	0.14	0.14	0
7	0.36	0.53	32
8	0.64	0.79	19
9	1.05	1.33	21
10	1.64	1.85	11
11	2.12	2.63	19
12	2.46	2.97	17
13	3.43	4.41	22
14	4.05	5.18	22
15	5.53	6.03	8
16	6.02	7.41	19
17	7.01	8.59	18
All ages	**2.79**	**3.39**	**18**

Source: National Institute of Dental Research, 1989.
DMFS = Decayed missing filled surfaces.

seniors with a history of continuous, long-term residence in optimally fluoridated communities (Brustman, 1986; Hunt, Eldredge, & Beck, 1989).

ALTERNATIVE METHODS OF CARIES PREVENTION WITH FLUORIDE

In general there are five alternatives to community water fluoridation: (1) dietary supplementation, (2) fluoride dentifrices (toothpaste and mouthwash), (3) professionally applied topical fluoride, (4) self-applied topical fluoride, and (5) school water fluoridation. Table 11.3 demonstrates the effectiveness of these various methods of fluoride administration determined

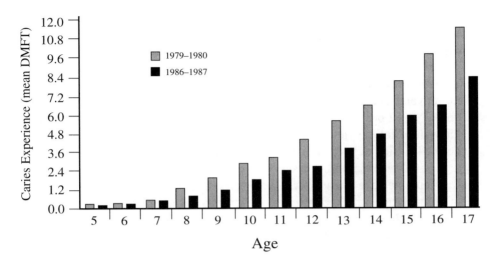

Figure 11.4 Mean number of dental caries in U.S. children.

Based on two national surveys.

DMFT=Decayed missing filled teeth.

Table 11.3 The Effectiveness of Various Methods of Fluoride
Administration in Reducing Dental Caries

Method of fluoride administration	Mean percentage of reduction of dental caries
Public water supply	Up to 65% reported
School water program	Up to 40% reported
Dietary supplements	Up to 65% reported
In-office fluoride	Up to 40% reported
Home brush-on gel	Up to 50% reported

from studies from 1950 to 1980. Those data show that community water fluoridation is as effective as dietary supplements and more effective than the other three alternative methods of fluoride administration in the reduction of dental caries (Miller & Truhe, 1995).

Fluoridation of municipal water supplies is by far the most cost-effective and practical means for reducing the incidence of dental caries in the population, costing on the average about $0.50 to $0.60 per person annually.

It has been calculated that the average overall cost of fluoridation to an individual over a 75-year life span amounts to the equivalent cost of a single surface dental restoration.

For purposes of cost comparison, the mean annual cost of school-based topical fluoridation is $2.53 per child per year (Garcia, 1989), a procedure moreover that excludes adults. Fluoride toothpastes and mouthrinses cost about $2.00 per tube or bottle, but even a conservative estimate of 100 tubes in a lifetime yields a very expensive alternative. Other possible methods of fluoride delivery are even more costly.

Compliance is another issue. Although Table 11.3 shows that fluoride supplements have been shown to achieve effectiveness comparable to that of fluoridation under controlled conditions, usage of tablets and drops yields much lower percentages. Even in a study that used highly motivated and educated groups of parents (physicians and dentists), only half continued to give their children supplements for the necessary number of years (Newbrun, 1980). Therefore, there are three barriers to considering fluoride supplements as an equivalent alternative to community water fluoridation: (1) poor compliance on a daily basis in children from birth until age 12; (2) the overall annual cost of supplements per child is much greater; and (3) the poorest children in our society have the least access, although they may be the most needy.

In countries other than the United States there are two additional alternatives to community water fluoridation: fluoridated salt and fluoridated milk. Fluoridated salt has been sold in Switzerland since 1955 and recently has been introduced in other countries, for example, France and Mexico. This method is believed to be as effective as community water fluoridation and fluoridated salt is useful in countries where a lack of a centralized water supply makes fluoridation of water difficult and expensive. However the addition of fluoride to salt is not indicated in the United States because of its well-developed network of municipal water systems. Other obstacles would be the propriety of promoting salt ingestion with its known link to hypertension (Ripa, 1993; World Health Organization, 1986b).

Milk has also been used as a vehicle for fluoride. It has been proposed for use by children in areas where the water supply is fluoride deficient (Murray & Rugg-Gunn, 1982c; Ripa, 1993; World Health Organization, 1986c). Studies of this particular method are limited, however, and it certainly would not be as cost-effective as communal water fluoridation. Another problem is that milk consumption typically decreases with age. Finally, regulation would be difficult, because fluoridated milk would have to be kept out of communities that already have naturally or adjusted optimal levels of fluoride in the water supply, so as to avoid the risk of dental fluorosis.

THE ANTIFLUORIDE MOVEMENT

Opposition to community water fluoridation as a nutrition-based, public health policy goes back 50 years or more. Since Grand Rapids, Michigan became the first to adjust the fluoride content of its water supply, individuals and groups have opposed water fluoridation for a variety of reasons. Many early opponents of fluoridation were associated with the health-food industry and made claims that fluoride would "poison the food and water supply." Chiropractors have traditionally opposed fluoridation as an infringement on personal freedom, as a dictate from organized medicine, and as incompatible with chiropractic nutritional policy. Individual Christian scientists have often challenged the measure as forced mass medication and the John Birch Society has linked water fluoridation to Communism (Barrett, 1980b; Bernhardt & Sprague, 1980; Easley, 1985).

Eventually the above-mentioned groups began exchanging ideas and experiences and formed local groups for the purpose of fighting fluoridation. The early local organizations usually lacked funding and experience to have an impact beyond the communities where they were based. However within a few years, well-funded national multi-issue organizations began to include in their goals the elimination of the use of community water fluoridation. Through exploitation of our society's current concerns about health and disease, these national groups have become increasingly successful in negatively influencing the public about the effectiveness, safety, and economy of community water fluoridation. Their tactics have ranged from community actions aimed at local governmental agencies, to organized referenda, to litigation in the federal courts, and lobbying directed at state legislators and the U.S. Congress (Easley, 1985).

Although the traditional emphasis of antifluoridation groups has been on litigation, there has been a recent shift in emphasis to grass-roots political campaigns. Therefore individuals involved in health and nutrition policy issues on a regular basis, whether employed in the public sector, academic centers, insurance companies or hospitals, must be made aware of the activities of these groups in order to be in a position to continue promoting scientifically based dental disease prevention through community water fluoridation.

There exists a small cadre of professional propagandists who serve as the driving force behind many local and state-level lawsuits and referenda. These professional propagandists act as legal strategists for local attorneys representing the antifluoride movement, serve as "expert witnesses" during litigation or legislative hearings, and often initiate fund-raising activities to support local legal or legislative activities. Three major groups currently involved in the antifluoridation movement largely control the flow of information and propaganda to individuals on a local basis (Easley, 1985):

1. National Health Federation (Monrovia, California). This organization was one of the first antifluoridation groups to have promoted the mistaken notion that fluoride in the community water supply causes cancer. More recently this group has placed less emphasis on the antifluoride movement and has shifted its interest to the promotion of laetrile and other questionable nutritional practices (Barrett, 1980a; Easley, 1985; Herbert, 1982; Herbert & Barrett, 1982).

2. Center for Health Action (Springfield, Massachusetts). Headquartered in a private home, the Center for Health Action was formed through a merger of two Ohio antifluoride groups. This group claims it is interested in the broad "health food movement," although its primary activity appears to be fighting established community water fluoridation programs. More recently the group opposed the use of fluoride in all forms, whether fluoride toothpastes, fluoride supplements obtained on proscription, or topical fluoride preparations used in dental offices (Barrett, 1980a; Easley, 1985; Yiamouyiannis, 1984).

3. National Fluoridation News (Gravette, Arkansas). Publishes and distributes a quarterly, the *National Fluoridation News,* which contains antifluoridation articles, promotes other antifluoride publications, contains antifluoride cartoons, and markets home water-distilling equipment (Easley, 1985).

These activities and the existence of these organizations clearly indicate that fluoridation is no longer just a scientific or legal issue, but has also become a volatile political issue. Although the U.S. judicial system has continued to support the concept of fluoridation as safe, effective, economical and legal, most efforts to bring community water fluoridation to the people via referenda have failed (Easley, 1985).

Moreover, there has been increasing political pressure on local and state governments to prevent implementation or stop existing fluoridation programs. Reason and moderation seem to have been pushed aside as even voluntary uses of fluorides are no longer considered acceptable alternatives by the antifluoride groups (Easley, 1985).

POLITICAL ISSUES

It would be ideal if health issues were decided by health experts; however, for water fluoridation this is rarely the case, as this issue has found its way into the political arena (Horowitz, 1990; Ripa, 1993). Authorization to fluoridate a public water supply can be made by an administrative decision, by voter initiative, or by legislative action. Eight states, plus the District of Columbia and Puerto Rico, have mandatory laws requiring the fluoridation of public water supplies. Unsuccessful attempts have been made over the last several years by Pennsylvania and Hawaii (Easley, 1990). In addition there are three states (Massachusetts, Alaska and Nevada) that have "enabling" fluoridation legislation that empowers local authorities to institute fluoridation under certain circumstances (e.g., by administrative decision or local referendum) (World Health Organization, 1986a).

Referenda have been the nemesis of fluoridation. Between 1980 and 1989, 63% of community fluoridation referenda failed to pass. Where fluoridation was considered by legislative initiative only, however, 78% of bills were passed (Easley, 1990; Ripa, 1993). The reasons for the public's rejection of a proven health benefit have proven a quandary for public health officials. To explain this phenomenon, a World Health Organization publication lists three factors (Ripa, 1993; World Health Organization, 1986a):

1. Ignorance and confusion about the dental health benefits of fluoridation. Voters are confused by exposure to conflicting arguments.
2. Ambivalence of the public toward science with greater reservations about scientific findings that concern the human body.
3. Misrepresentation of the scientific and technical information involved, allowing the opposition to distort the issues and frighten the public.

A fourth factor not listed by the WHO, but that may be of great importance in the United States, is the issue of controlling one's destiny. This sentiment is echoed in the statement of the leader of a successful 1983 campaign to defluoridate Levittown, NY, who explained that "We are skeptical of government—we want control over what our children consume" (McNeil, 1985).

INFRINGEMENT OF INDIVIDUAL RIGHTS

A frequent objection to community water fluoridation is that it infringes on individual rights and freedom of choice. The United States court system, however, has ruled consistently in favor of fluoridation, ruling that fluoride is a nutrient, not a medication, that it is naturally present in the environment and essential for overall health. Moreover, no one is actually forced to drink fluoridated water, as fluoride-free sources are available (Council on Community Health, 1989; Roemer, 1965; Strong, 1968).

In cases where a person feels that fluoridation interferes with religious beliefs, the United States' highest courts believe that there is a difference between "freedom to believe," which is absolute, and the freedom to practice these beliefs, which in some cases may have to be restricted to protect the public's interest. Furthermore, in this regard, the courts often cite that no objections have been raised regarding the addition of other substances to the drinking water, such as copper sulfate, chlorine, and other antibacterial agents. Therefore ruling against, and singling out, fluoride would be hypocritical (Council on Community Health, 1989; Roemer, 1965; Strong, 1968).

Suits against fluoridation have also been brought on the basis of the right of parents to decide what is beneficial for their children. Decisions ensuring the health of minors are often determined and supervised by society, however.

During the past 40 years the legality of community water fluoridation in the United States has been thoroughly tested in the court system and no court of last resort has rendered an opinion against fluoridation. In fact, the Supreme Court has denied reviews of fluoridation cases at least twelve times, citing that no constitutional questions were involved (Block, 1986; Council on Community Health, 1989; Sfikas, 1983).

CONCLUSIONS

Beginning with Leonard A. Scheele in 1951, every Surgeon General has strongly endorsed water fluoridation as a preventive, nutrition-based public health policy. In 1983, then-Surgeon General Dr. C. Everett Koop stated that this preventive measure is the single most important commitment that a community can make to the oral health of its citizens and future generations. He urged all health officials and concerned citizens to join him in supporting this commitment.

Community water fluoridation is unquestionably effective in preventing dental caries at minimal cost although there is a risk of very mild fluorosis under certain circumstances. A careful and objective analysis of all available evidence indicates, however, that the benefits of fluoridation far outweigh the risks.

Unfortunately, the controversy over fluoride hazards will continue because it has become a political issue, more than a scientific or legal issue. Also risk evaluation is always a matter of personal interpretation. The data clearly indicate that fluoride, at the dosages found in drinking water, is not carcinogenic.

Although increasing numbers of Americans are exposed to fluoridated municipal water supplies, there is still much work to be done. The first and most immediate challenge is the expansion of the role of the health professional in the political arena promoting community water fluoridation as essential public health policy. The goal set by the United States Public Health Service *Healthy People 2000* is that 75% of the population will be served by fluoridated water supplies by the year 2000 (Public Health Service, 1990). Considering that the current percentage is only 62%, there is a long way to go.

A second challenge must be the continued commitment to improve community water fluoridation methods through the replacement of aging fluoridation equipment. And it is also necessary to reassess the 50-year old national policies on optimal levels of fluoride in the drinking water.

The most important challenge is the continued education of the public regarding the overall societal benefits of fluoridation. Public health and nutrition specialists, as well as dentists and physicians, must continue to retell the story that community water fluoridation is the most reliable, cost-effective, safe measure to prevent dental disease. The lifetime cost of water fluoridation is less than the cost of a single dental restoration and the health and economic benefits of water fluoridation accrue to individuals of all ages and socioeconomic groups. Water fluoridation is a shining example of success of nutrition public health policy, but one that must be safeguarded by continued research and activism.

REFERENCES

Barrett, S. (1980a). *The health robbers.* Philadelphia: G. F. Stickley.

Barrett, S. (1980b). The unhealthy alliance. In S. Barrett & S. Rovin (Eds.), *The tooth robbers* (pp. 9–16). Philadelphia: G. F. Stickley.

Beltran, E., & Burt, B. (1988). The pre- and posteruptive effects of fluoride in the caries decline. *Journal of Public Health Dentistry, 48,* 233–240.

Bernhardt, M., & Sprague, B. (1980). The poisonmongers. In S. Barrett & S. Rovin (Eds.), *The tooth robbers* (pp. 1–8). Philadelphia: G. F. Stickley.

Bernstein, D. S., Sadowsky, N., Hegsted, D. M., Guri, C. B., & Stare, F. J. (1966). Prevalence of osteoporosis in high and low fluoride areas in North Dakota. *Journal of the American Medical Association, 198,* 499–504.

Block, L. (1986). Antifluoridationists persist: The constitutional basis for fluoidation. *Journal of Public Health Dentistry, 46*(4), 188–98.

Brustman, B. (1986). Impact of exposure to fluoride-adequate water on root surface caries in elderly. *Gerodontics, 2,* 203–207.

Burt, B. (1989). Results of the workshop. *Journal of Public Health Dentistry, 49*(Special Issue), 331–337.

Burt, B., Eklund, S., & Loesce, W. (1986). Dental benefits of limited exposure to fluoridated water in childhood. *Journal of Dental Research, 61,* 1322–1325.

Centers for Disease Control and Prevention. (1986, September). *Water fluoridation: A manual for engineers and technicians.* United States Department of Health and Human Services. Washington, DC: U.S. Government Printing Office.

Centers for Disease Control and Prevention. (1991, July). *Fluoridation census 1989.* United States Department of Health and Human Services.

Council on Community Health. (1989). *Fluoridation facts.* American Dental Association pub. no. W120. Chicago, IL: American Dental Association Press.

Driscoll, W. (1986). Prevalence of dental caries and dental fluorosis in areas with negligible, optimal and above-optimal fluoride. *Journal of the American Dental Association, 113,* 29–33.

Dunning, J. (1986). *Principles of dental public health (4th ed).* Cambridge, MA: Harvard University Press.

Easley, M. (1985). The new antifluoridationists: Who they are and how they operate. *Journal of Public Health Dentistry, 45,* 133–141.

Easley, M. (1990). The status of community water fluoridation in the United States. *Public Health Report, 105,* 348–353.

Environmental Protection Agency. (1986, June). *EPA statement on fluoridation in public water supplies to prevent tooth decay.* Washington, DC: United States Environmental Protection Agency.

Garcia, A. (1989). Caries incidence and costs of preventive programs. *Journal of Public Health Dentistry, 49*(Special Issue), 259–271.

Grembowski, D., Fiset, L., & Spadafora, A. (1992). How fluoridation affects dental caries. *Journal of the American Dental Association, 123,* 49–54.

Groeneveld, A., Van Eck, A., & Backer-Dirks, O. (1990). Fluoride in caries prevention: Is the effect pre- or posteruptive. *Journal of Dental Research, 69*(Special Issue), 751–755.

Guy, W. (1979). Inorganic and organic fluoride in human blood. In E. Johansen & T. Olsen (Eds.), *Continuing evaluation of the use of fluorides* (pp. 125–147). Boulder, CO: Westview Press.

Hardwick, J., Teasdale, J., & Bloodworth, G. (1982). Caries increments over 4 years in children age 12 at the start of water fluoridation. *British Dental Journal, 153,* 217–222.

Herbert, V. (1982). *Nutrition cultism: Facts and fictions.* Philadelphia: G. F. Stickley.

Herbert, V., & Barrett, S. (1982). *Vitamins and health foods: The great American hustle.* Philadelphia: G. F. Stickley.

Hinman, A. (1995, April 18). *A public health view of community water fluoridation.* California General Assembly. Atlanta, GA: Centers for Disease Control.

Horowitz, H. (1990). The future of water fluoridation and other systemic fluorides. *Journal of Dental Research, 69*(Special Issue), 760–764.

Hunt, R., Eldredge, J., & Beck, J. (1989) Effect of residence in a fluoridated community on the incidence of coronal and root caries in an older population. *Journal of Public Health Dentistry, 49,* 138–141.

Jenkins, G., Venkateswarla, P., & Zipkin, I. (1970). Physiological effects of small doses of fluoride. In *Fluorides and human health* (monograph no. 59, pp. 163–224). Geneva: World Health Organization.

Largent, E. (1987). The supply of fluoride to man. In *Fluorides and human health* (monograph no. 59, pp. 17–18). Geneva: World Health Organization.

Leone, N. (1955). Roentgenologic study of a human population exposed to high fluoride domestic water. A 10 Year Study. *American Journal of Roentgenology, 74,* 874–875.

Leske, G. (1983). Water Fluoridation. In J. Melberg & L. Ripa (Eds.), *Fluoride in preventive dentistry. Theory and clinical application* (pp. 103–123). Chicago: Quintescence.

Mandel, I. (1985). A symposium on the new fight for fluorides. *Journal of Public Health Dentistry, 45*(3), 133.

McClure, F. (1970). *Water fluoridation. The search and the victory.* Washington, DC: U.S. Government Printing Office.

McNeil, D. (1985). America's longest war: The fight over fluoridation. *Wilson Quarterly, 9,* 140.

Melberg, J., & Ripa, L. (1983). Anticaries mechanisms of fluoride. In J. Melberg & L. Ripa (Eds.), *Fluoride in preventive dentistry. Theory and clinical applications* (pp. 41–80). Chicago: Quintescence.

Miller, M., & Truhe, T. (1995). *Fluoride: An update for the year 2000.* Princeton, NJ: Center for Dental Information.

Morbidity and Mortality Weekly Report (1992, May 29). Public health focus: Fluoridation of community water supplies. pp. 372–381.

Murray, J., & Rugg-Gunn, A. (1982a). A history of water fluoridation. In *Fluorides in cavity prevention. Dental practitioners handbook no. 20* (pp. 1–30). Boston, MA: Wright PSG.

Murray, J., & Rugg-Gunn, A. (1982b). Modes of action of fluoride in reducing caries. In *Fluoride in caries prevention. Dental practitioner handbook no. 20* (pp. 222–232). Boston, MA: Wright PSG.

Murray, J., & Rugg-Gunn, A. (1982c). Other methods of systemic administration of fluoride. In *Fluorides and caries prevention. Dental practitioners handbook no. 20* (pp. 74–84). Boston, MA: Wright PSG.

National Cancer Institute. (1975). *Statement on fluoride studies by National Health Federation.* United States Department of Health, Education, and Welfare, pub. no. FL-76. Washington, DC: U.S. Government Printing Office.

National Center for Health Statistics. (1979). *Basic data on dental examination findings of persons 1–74 years: United States 1971–1974* United States Department of Health, Education and Welfare pub no. (PHS) 79–1662.

National Institute for Dental Research. (1981). *The prevalence of dental caries in United States children. 1979–1980: National caries prevalence study.* United States Department of Health and Human Services. NIH pub no. 82–2245. Washington, DC: U.S. Government Printing Office.

National Institute for Dental Research. (1989). *Oral health of United States children: The national survey of dental caries: 1986–1987: National and Regional Findings.* United States Department of Health and Human Services, NIH pub no. 89–2247. Washington, DC: U.S. Government Printing Office.

National Research Council, Food and Nutrition Board (1980). *Recommended daily allowances.* Washington, DC: National Academy of Science.

Newbrun, E. (1978). Cost effectiveness and practicality features in the systemic use of fluorides. In B. Burt (Ed.), *The relative efficiency of methods of caries prevention in dental public health* (pp. 27–48). Ann Arbor, MI: University of Michigan.

Newbrun, E. (1980). Systemic fluoride: An overview. *Journal of the Canadian Dental Association, 1980,* 31–37.

Newbrun, E. (1989a). Effectiveness of water fluoridation. *Journal of Public Health Dentistry, 49,* 279–289.

Newbrun, E. (1989b). The use of fluorides in preventive dentistry. In *Cariology* (pp. 331–355). Chicago: Quintescence.

Public Health Service. (1988). *The Surgeon General's report on nutrition and health.* United States Department of Health and Human Services. Washington, DC: U.S. Government Printing Office.

Public Health Service. (1990). *Healthy People 2000: National health promotion and disease prevention objectives.* United States Department of Health and Human Services, pub. no. PHS 91–50212.

Public Health Service. (1991). *Executive summary: Review of fluoride benefits and risks* (p. 1). United States Department of Health and Human Services, pub. no. PHS 91–3520. Washington, DC: U.S. Government Printing Office.

Ripa, L. (1993). A half century of community water fluoridation in the United States: Review and commentary. *Journal of Public Health Dentistry, 53,* 17–44.

Roemer, R. (1965). Water fluoridation: Public health policy and the democratic process. *American Journal of Public Health, 55*(9), 1337–1348.

Safe Drinking Water Committee, National Research Council. (1977). *Drinking water and health* (pp. 369–400). Washington, DC: National Academy of Sciences.

Sfikas, P. (1983). The litigation battle: Past and present. In *Fluoridation Litigation and Changing Public Policy: Proceedings of a Workshop at the University of Michigan* (pp. 3–16). Ann Arbor: MJ Argus.

Strong, G. (1968). Liberty, religion and fluoridation. *Journal of the American Dental Association, 76,* 1398–1409.

White, B., Antczak-Boukom, A., & Weinstein, M. (1989). Issues with the economic evaluation of community water fluoridation. *Journal of Dental Education, 53,* 646–657.

Whitford, G., & Pashley, D. (1984). Fluoride absorption. The influence of gastric acidity. *Calcified Tissue International, 36,* 303–307.

Whitford, G., Pashley, D., & Reynolds, K. (1979). Fluoride tissue distribution: Short term kinetics. *American Journal of Physiology, 236,* F141–F148.

Whitford, G., Pashley, D., & Stringer, G. (1976). Fluoride renal clearance: A pH dependent event. *American Journal of Physiology, 230,* 527–532.

World Health Organization. (1986a). Community water fluoridation. In J. Murray (Ed.), *Appropriate use of fluoride in human health* (pp. 38–37). Geneva: World Health Organization.

World Health Organization. (1986b). Salt fluoridation. In J. Murray (Ed.), *Appropriate use of fluoride in human health* (pp. 74–83). Geneva: World Health Organization.

World Health Organization. (1986c). School water and milk fluoridation. In J. Murray (Ed.), *Appropriate use of fluoride in human health* (pp. 84–99). Geneva: World Health Organization.

Yiamouyiannis, J. (1984). Prospectus and update fluoridation reports (pp. 1–8). Delaware, OH: Center For Health Action.

CHAPTER *12*

Selected Disease Entities: AIDS, Alcoholism, Diabetes Mellitus, Lead and Lead Poisoning, Neural Tube Defects, Nutritional Anemias

Felix Bronner

T his chapter discusses several nutrition-related conditions and illnesses with public health significance. Although no one of these may constitute a major component of the tasks of a nutrition officer and although some may be dealt with in separate programs, their relative importance and relationship to nutrition justify inclusion.

AIDS

The acquired immunodeficiency syndrome (AIDS), caused by the human immunodeficiency viruses, HIV-1 and HIV-2, by the end of 1994 had caused disease in some 500,000 people in North America, with a cumulative death rate for about two-thirds of this number. Moreover, the number of people who may be infected with HIV has been estimated as 1 million.

The challenge that this disease and its sequelae present is virtually unmatched in modern times and represents a severe test for all parts of the health care system. Prevention of the disease and "prevention and prompt treatment of opportunistic infections are the first line of defense against rapid weight loss and lean body mass loss seen with HIV and AIDS" (Anonymous, 1994, p.1042).

Nutritional problems have been part of the clinical aspects of AIDS from the beginning (Keusch & Thea, 1993). Chronic weight loss and diarrhea have now become part of the case description of AIDS and will occur in essentially all patients. Indeed when lean body mass has dropped to 55% of what is normal for the age and weight of a patient, death is imminent (Keusch & Thea, 1993), regardless of the cause of wasting. As yet, it is unclear whether wasting in AIDS patients is merely that of individuals who become malnourished or whether immunosuppression increases specific wasting. Patients with AIDS develop sores in their mouth, muscular weakness that makes swallowing difficult, general loss of appetite, so that their wasting can be attributed to both starvation—that is, inadequate food intake—and cachexia, that is, generalized disease leading to malnutrition.

Patients with AIDS often appear to have protein-energy malnutrition and may have micronutrient deficiencies, particularly of thiamin, vitamin A, and vitamin B_{12}, though the specifics are in dispute. Clearly, nutritional deficiencies or abnormalities that affect patients with AIDS are multifactorial, including reduced and altered food intake, intestinal malabsorption, increased catabolism and nutrient redistribution (Keusch & Thea, 1993). For this reason, nutritional support must include high-energy and high-protein foods, frequent small meals rather than fewer large meals, vitamin and perhaps also mineral supplements, and scrupulous attention to good sanitation practices in the preparation and serving of foods, as AIDS patients are particularly susceptible to opportunistic infections. In the later stages, moreover, such opportunistic infections characterize the disease and may be the cause of death. In the late stages of the disease, when it becomes difficult for patients to take food by mouth, enteral or parenteral nutrition may become a necessity. Throughout the period of illness, as patients with AIDS are being treated, often with a variety of drugs, attention must be paid to possible drug–nutrient interactions and, in consultation with the treating physician, the avoidance of undesirable interactions must be weighed against the benefit thought to be derived from the drug.

Because treatment of AIDS has not been curative, patients, out of desperation, have opted for so-called alternative treatments, including diet fads. Health professionals must understand the drive that leads afflicted individuals to these steps, but at the same must be prepared to discuss and discourage irrational and potentially harmful treatments and food practices.

Nutrition officers in public health agencies and public health officials with nutrition responsibilities need to be aware of the profound role that nutrition support can play in slowing the course of the disease or buffering the severity of the illness. They therefore should develop education programs directed at health professionals and also at the public at large. Such programs should use specialists in AIDS and deal with all aspects of food preparation and nutrition. Special programs may be usefully addressed to nutritionists in both the public and private sectors, particularly in food processing. There is undoubtedly a need for highly digestible, energy-rich, protein-rich and vitamin-enriched foods that can readily be swallowed and that are attractive in appearance. Obviously such foods can also find use in other wasting conditions. Recently it has been proposed that supplementation with antioxidants, for example, beta-carotene, selenium, or vitamin E, may extend the period between HIV infection and the appearance of the clinical signs and symptoms of AIDS. As yet, no results are available from large-scale clinical trials to substantiate these effects, suggested on the basis of limited in vitro and in vivo studies (Vitamin E Research Summary, 1995).

Antianorexia drugs are now being developed or tested (Keusch & Thea, 1993) and may find a place in the nutritional management of the AIDS patient. Nutrition officers in public health agencies must learn to keep up with newly developing information in this explosive field. Contact with specialists in the AIDS field and in-service seminars are obvious methods used to keep abreast of the field and to be able to share new and relevant information with other nutritionists or the public.

ALCOHOLISM

Alcohol consumption is extremely widespread in the population, with perhaps no more than 10% of the total population practicing complete abstinence (Scheckit, 1994). Alcohol-induced problems are encountered in nearly half of the population's men at one time or another, with alcohol addiction afflicting between 5%–10% of the people.

Ethanol, the chemical responsible for most effects of drinking wine, beer, and spirits, is a central nervous system depressant, although at low concentrations it may act as a stimulant.

One drink can provide close to 100 kcal and substantial consumption, for example, three to four bottles of beer while watching television during an evening, can provide some 600 kcal or one-fourth of a typical daily energy requirement. Thus, abundant alcohol consumption can lead to obesity.

Many chronic alcoholics, on the other hand, tend to consume less than needed in terms of other foods, that is, proteins, fats, minerals and vitamins. For this reason, they may in fact be malnourished, particularly if they are poor and/or homeless. Three disease conditions with a specific nutritional basis that are associated with high alcohol consumption are Wernicke's syndrome—essentially a deficiency of thiamin (vitamin B_1), the encephalopathy of alcoholics who have a niacin deficiency, and peripheral neuropathy in which supplemental multivitamins are effective. Indeed, polyvitamin, polyprotein, and carbohydrate supplements are medically indicated to help overcome the nutritional depletion of the chronic alcoholic and can be life saving.

Alcohol education programs or public health campaigns to combat alcoholism will usually place only a limited emphasis on nutrition and nutrition aspects. Nutrition officers of public health departments or administrators responsible for nutrition programs should be informed about the existence of such programs and be prepared to contribute to them. The most common misunderstanding to combat is that alcohol does not contribute calories. As pointed out above, a heavy drinker may derive a substantial fraction of caloric intake from alcohol, but these are "empty" calories, that is, they do not contribute essential nutrients. A drinking binge may contribute significantly to caloric intake, so that frequent consumption of significant quantities of alcoholic beverages may contribute to overweight and its attendant problems.

Moderate consumption of alcohol, the equivalent of one drink per day, may in fact be beneficial in terms of minimizing the likelihood of cardiovascular disease. Alcohol consumed in the company of others contributes to sociability, so that alcohol consumption in moderation may deserve encouragement in settings like old age homes or residencies, provided the individual is not on medically prescribed drugs with counterindication to alcohol consumption. Moderate alcohol intake often also acts as an appetite stimulant and may therefore be beneficial in institutional settings of the elderly. For these reasons, the nutrition officer, when dealing with dietitians and nutrition personnel in institutions for the elderly, should inquire about the availability and policy regarding alcohol consumption.

Alcohol consumption is not a value-neutral subject. Many individuals and groups oppose alcohol consumption on moral and/or religious grounds. Therefore, public advocacy of even moderate alcohol consumption is likely to encounter vociferous opposition, may provoke political fights and polarization and may consequently compromise other nutrition programs that are more nearly value neutral. In discussing alcohol consumption in the field, the nutrition officer should therefore deal with the nutritional and public health concerns, but should refrain from taking on an advocacy role. This differs from other nutrition concerns, for example, multivitamin supplementation, which, even when not indicated, is rarely harmful and even more rarely is perceived as such.

DIABETES MELLITUS

Primary diabetes mellitus is a disease characterized by relative or absolute insulin deficiency, relative or absolute glucagon excess, and the metabolic consequences thereof (Foster, 1989). Two types of diabetes mellitus are distinguished—the insulin-dependent type, with susceptibility genetically determined and incidence usually triggered by an environmental cause, initiating an autoimmune response—and the noninsulin-dependent type. In the noninsulin dependent type, it is insulin release by the beta cells of the pancreas that is interfered with, leading to a defect in glucose production by the liver and in glucose disposal by muscle and fat tissue. Obesity is the most common cause of the noninsulin-dependent type.

Diabetes is fairly prevalent in the general population, probably affecting between 1% and 2% of the population (Foster, 1994), with the insulin-dependent type affecting perhaps one-fourth of diabetics: this type is more prevalent in the young. Noninsulin-dependent diabetes usually begins in middle life or later and, if weight reduction can be achieved, can be treated by diet alone, whereas insulin is needed by the insulin-dependent diabetic. Because many patients with noninsulin-dependent diabetes do not respond sufficiently to diet therapy, they also are treated with insulin.

Devising an appropriate diet for patients with diabetes has been an ongoing occupation of health professionals concerned with diabetes and diabetics and has been dealt with in detail in the relevant literature (American Diabetes Association, 1994; Foster, 1994; Franz et al., 1994). In general, some caloric restriction is recommended, with 10%–20% of the energy intake derived from protein, with less than 10% of calories from saturated fat, up to 10% from polyunsaturated fats, with the remainder, 60%–70% of total energy intake, to be derived from monounsaturated fats and carbohydrates. It has generally been thought that diabetics should avoid or minimize the ingestion of simple sugars, to be replaced by complex carbohydrates, but there is little evidence to support this and the general recommendations now tend to deal with total carbohydrate intake rather than particular constituents. The emphasis today in diet treatment of diabetes is individualized nutrition therapy, based on treatment goals, and desired outcome, as evaluated by available tests, body weight, and quality of life. Inasmuch as diet therapy of diabetes may last many years, even a lifetime, treatment must enable the patient to sustain the diet with a minimum of stress. Quick diet therapy is not feasible. At the same time, approaches tend to vary. For example, diets high in monounsaturated fat and low in carbohydrate have been reported (Sheard, 1995) to produce more desirable plasma glucose, lipid, and insulin profiles in noninsulin-dependent diabetes than the older diet regimes.

In light of the above, the public health nutritionist and nutrition officer need to develop mechanisms for keeping up to date on developing information on diabetes and its treatment. This can be done via the literature and networking with health care personnel involved in diabetes therapy. In turn, this information needs to be shared with the public and other nutrition-oriented health professionals. By helping to spread information, the nutrition officer can contribute to disease control. This can be done by specific education, by pamphlets, seminars and the judicious use of the media.

Inasmuch as noninsulin-dependent diabetes is so frequently an outcome of obesity, it is important to emphasize the relationship between obesity and diabetes in all campaigns directed to combat overweight and obesity. Nutrition policy that emphasizes moderation in total caloric intake, reduction of calories derived from fat to 30%, and emphasis on fruit and vegetables will, as overweight is reduced, also reduce the incidence of noninsulin diabetes. Nutrition policy of this type can therefore play a significant role in disease prevention.

LEAD POISONING

Lead toxicity is ancient (Wedeen, 1992). Roman water pipes and drinking vessels contained lead and symptoms afflicting Romans have since been diagnosed as caused by lead poisoning. Exposure to lead dust in lead mines and of workers in lead smelters has been a major cause of occupational lead poisoning. Two other important sources of lead toxicity in the 20th century are lead-containing gasolines and lead-containing paint. Incomplete combustion of lead-containing gasoline, in wide use in the decades between 1920 and 1980, caused lead to become deposited along roadways and ultimately to enter acquifers. Consequently, persons who lived in city sections where automobile traffic was heavy were exposed to lead dust in the air and, in suburban or rural areas, to lead contamination of drinking water. This exposure has been of particular concern in the case of children who have a high rate of bone growth compared to that of adults, who have a mature skeleton, inasmuch as lead follows the path of calcium in the body (Bronner, 1992). This reasoning also applies to lead paint, which becomes a source of lead when ingested. Ingestion of paint is possible when paint is peeling, often true of substandard housing inhabited by the poor, or if baby furniture has been painted with lead-containing paint. In the case of peeling paint, ingestion tends to be casual and occasional by small children; lead pica is quite rare. Baby furniture, especially guard rails of cribs, are often chewed by babies or small children, either because they are teething or out of boredom or hunger. Again, these are conditions more frequently encountered among the poor. The general use of lead-containing gasoline or paint is now prohibited and these are no longer acute sources. Lead that has entered the environment still constitutes a danger, however, particularly in areas of dense automobile traffic.

Lead enters the body either via the intestine or the lungs. Lead absorption is likely to parallel calcium absorption (Fullmer, 1992), competing with calcium for binding to calbindin D_{9k}, the molecule that assures transcellular calcium absorption. In addition, lead, like calcium, moves down its chemical concentration gradient and enters the body fluids via the intercellular spaces (tight junction) between intestinal cells. Once inside the body fluids, it has a 45% chance of being excreted in the urine and a 55% chance of becoming deposited in bone (Jones, Bockman, & Bronner, 1992). Its overall return back into the blood from bone is much slower, with only a 9% chance to be released from bone. With time, most of the lead in bone will be in segments of bone with the slowest turnover. The true health hazard stems from lead that enters and accumulates in soft tissue, as in the brain where, in sufficient but poorly known amounts, it can cause mentation defects (Wedeen, 1992).

The public health concerns that stem from lead are often handled by special staff in state or municipal health departments, with separate support from the U.S. government. Nutrition officers need to know who their colleagues are who deal with these problems, so that they can refer concerns and complaints to the appropriate individuals. At the same time, they need to be aware of the principal sources of lead in the food chain and in the environment. Above all, dietitians and those working in food processing and distribution need to be made aware of the need to avoid lead contamination. Nutrition officers working with women and children should be particularly alert to the need to avoid lead contamination. At the same time, it is important to be aware that the principal danger from lead ingestion is due to chronic rather than acute exposure. Lead intake in adults from the diet has been estimated as 0.2–0.4 mg per day (Underwood, 1973), an amount that is not considered harmful even over a person's lifetime. Thus, public health concern should be directed to sources of lead contamination.

NEURAL TUBE DEFECTS

The formation of the neural tube occurs during gatrulation, that is, the period in embryonic development when the ectoderm, an epithelial sheet on the outside of the embryo, is induced to form the neural plate (Papalopalu & Kintner, 1994). Three general types of neural tube defects are encountered (Lemire, 1986). The first type occurs in the early stages of the human embryo, when the neural plate forms, folds, and initially fuses into a neural tube. The second type, "anencephaly," occurs when the embryo is slightly older (23–76 days gestational age). The third type, "meningomyelocele," arises when the gestational age of the embryo is 26–30 days. Neurulation defects do not occur after this stage.

Neural tube defects have multiple etiologies, are multifactorial in origin, with both genetic and environmental factors playing a role (Seller, 1994). Manipulation of the diet of the mother has been shown both in animal models and in human studies to affect the environmental factor, thereby reducing the likelihood that an embryo would be pushed beyond the threshold and develop the malformation (Seller, 1994).

It is now known that neural tube defects arise when there is a defect in the metabolic pathway of folic acid (Papalopulu & Kintner, 1994), but the exact mechanism is not known. What is known is that folic acid supplementation prevents three out of four neural tube defects in humans (Seller,

1994). Although the mechanism is not yet known, the introduction of preventive measures, of supplementing the diets of pregnant mothers with 0.4 to 0.8 mg folic acid per day, has been shown to exert a substantial protective effect (Wald, 1994). This is particularly important because nearly all infants with neural tube defects are born to mothers who have not previously had an affected pregnancy (Wald, 1994). Prevention of neural tube defect is thus a prime example of the important public health effect proper nutrition can have.

Possible Hazards of Folic Acid Supplementation

At one time, pernicious anemia was treated with high doses of folic acid (Wald, 1994). This resolved the megaloblastic anemia, but tended to mask or even precipitate the neurological signs of pernicious anemia. Current treatment of pernicious anemia is with vitamin B_{12} and folic acid. With supplementation of 0.4 to 0.8 mg folic acid, there seems to be no danger of exacerbating undetected pernicious anemia in pregnant mothers.

Another potential complication of folic acid supplementation arises in women who have epilepsy and are being treated with anticonvulsants. Folic aid may counteract the anticonvulsant therapy. It has been suggested that pregnant women who have epilepsy be advised to take folic acid but be warned that their epilepsy may be less well controlled (Wald, 1994).

A major difficulty of a supplementation program is that neural tube defects arise, as indicated above, in the first month of pregnancy, that is, at a time when most women are unlikely to know whether they are pregnant. Thus it is desirable that all women who can have children ingest a folic acid supplement to guard against a neural tube defect in their future children. Suppplements of 0.4 to 0.8 mg have been shown to have no undesirable side effects (Wald, 1994).

Including folic acid in multivitamin tablets is technically simple. Neural tube defects are more common among the socioeconomically disadvantaged sectors of society, however, precisely because individuals in those sectors are least likely to take multivitamin supplements on a regular basis. For this reason, enrichment of ordinary foods with folic acid seems the most logical step. Currently, many breakfast cereals are fortified with folic acid, but the range of fortified foods needs to be extended.

Nutrition officers working in public helath agencies need to make the public and other health professionals aware of the need to supplement with folic acid. Campaigns to that end need to concentrate in particular on health programs directed to women of child-bearing age and also to women's groups in general, for example, League of Women Voters, women's social and church organizations, and so on. Although it is desirable to emphasize the need for folic acid supplementation to women who plan to become pregnant and therefore to direct special campaigns also to obstetricians, gynecologists, nurse midwives, and others involved with women of reproductive age, the greatest effect in reducing the incidence of neural tube defect is by fortification of common foods (cereals, bread, flour, etc.). Current evidence suggests that fortification should provide 0.6 mg of folic acid per day per individual. Wald (1994) has calculated that if bread were fortified with 0.3 mg of folic acid per 100 g, the median additional folic acid intake per individual (over the current population mean) would be 0.2 mg/day; even individuals consuming eight slices of bread per day would be at no risk.

The effectiveness of a supplementation policy can be evaluated by analyzing serum levels of folic acid. Thus, if the median folic acid serum concentration were to rise significantly from 5 mg/ml (Wald, 1994), the policy can be considered successful. Such analyses would also permit modifying the policy to increase or decrease folic acid supplementation or to verify whether a given public health strategy was working.

NUTRITIONAL ANEMIAS

Anemia may be defined as a state in which red blood cell values are less than normal (Moore, 1963). Iron deficiency is the most common cause of anemia, but vitamin B_{12}, folic acid, and protein deficiencies are other causes of anemias, as are lead poisoning, radiation, or toxins such as benzol. In addition, anemias occur in a variety of diseases, such as leukemia, Hodgkins disease, certain splenic disorders, and so on. From the point of view of nutrition policy, the principal focus is on iron-deficiency anemias.

In the United States, iron deficiency can be encountered during four periods of life (Recommended Dietary Allowances, 1989): (1) in the infant between 0.5 and 4 years of age, because milk is a poor source of iron and the iron reserves accumulated during the first 6 months of life are insufficient to meet the needs associated with rapid growth; (2) during early adolescence, when rapid growth and the need for iron for both muscle and blood may exceed intake; (3) in women during their reproductive period, that is, between menarche and menopause, when they lose red blood cells at the menstrual period; and (4) during pregnancy, because of the demands of the fetus and the loss of blood during childbirth.

The incidence of iron deficiency according to U.S. surveys (Recommended Dietary Allowances, 1987) is fairly wide, affecting perhaps 5% of the total population and involving easily twice as great a percentage of groups 1, 2, and 3, above. For this reason, nutritional anemia is a clear concern of the public health community and needs to be part of the program of the nutrition officer. Moreover, there is no special professional group that deals with anemia. To be sure, pediatricians, gynecologists, and obstetricians are likely to be concerned with the hemoglobin status of their patients, but the latter constitute only a portion of the population at risk.

It is essential, therefore, that appropriate public health campaigns be organized to make both the public and health professionals aware of the risk of iron deficiency and how to overcome it. Literature directed at professionals and separate literature for the public at risk needs to be available and distributed periodically. Potential iron deficiency as a topic needs to be included in various education campaigns that are undertaken in the community or region. At the same time, support needs to be extended to programs that include concern with anemia, as in the Women, Infants, and Children (WIC) program (see Chapter 13) and in school nutrition programs.

Whether or not dietary sources are sufficient to provide the needed iron intake is not clear. In a survey (cited in Recommended Dietary Allowances, 1989), it was found that about one-fourth of dietary iron was derived from cereals fortified with iron. Heme iron, as found in animal tissues, is an excellent source of dietary iron, fruits and vegetables are also good sources. Mothers should be encouraged to increase their consumption of good sources of iron and that of their young and adolescent children. Physicians need to be alerted to the need for increased iron intake, but must know that dietary iron deficiency is only one cause of anemia.

Excessive iron intake is unlikely to lead to toxicity in adults, but can do so in young children. Hence the need to minimize the likelihood that young children have access to iron-containing medication intended for adults. Nutrition policy with respect to iron needs also to take into account the incidence of hemochromatosis, due either to iron overload as in thalassemia major, or as an idiopathic hemochromatosis, which results from an inborn error of metabolism. Although the true incidence of this genetic disease has not yet been established, homozygotes may constitue 4% of the population. Thus iron fortification may also constitute a risk for some people. This is turn illustrates the complexity of aiming at a nutrition policy that benefits many, but poses some risk for a minority of the population.

REFERENCES

American Diabetes Association. (1994). National recommendations and principles for people with diabetes mellitus. *Diabetes Care, 17,* 519–522.

Anonymous. (1994). Position of the American Dietetic Association and the Canadian Dietetic Association: Nutrition intervention in the case of persons with human immunodeficiency virus infection. *Journal of the American Dietetics Association, 94,* 1042–1045

Bronner, F. (1992). Bone and calcium homeostasis. *Neurotoxicology, 13,* 775–782.

Foster, D. (1989). Diabetes mellitus. In C. R. Scriver, A. L. Beaudet, W. S. Sly & D. Valle (Eds.), *The metabolic basis of inherited disease* (Vol., 1, pp.375–397). New York: McGraw-Hill.

Foster, D. (1994). Diabetes mellitus. In K. J. Isselbacher, E. Braunwald, J. O. Wilson, J. B. Martin, A. S. Fauci, & D. L. Kasper (Eds.), *Harrison's principles of internal medicine*, (13th ed., pp. 1979–2000). New York: McGraw Hill.

Franz, M. J., Horton, E. S., Bantle, J. P., Beebe, C. A., Brunzell, J. D., Coneston, A. M., Henry, R. R., Hoogwerf, B. J., & Stacpoole, P. W. (1994). Nutrition principles for the management of diabetes and related complication. *Diabetes Care, 17,* 490–518.

Fullmer, C. S. (1992). Intestinal interactions of lead and calcium. *Neurotoxicology, 13,* 799–808.

Jones, K.W., Bockman, R. S., & Bronner, F. (1992). Microdistribution of lead in bone: a new approach. *Neurotoxicology, 13,* 835–842.

Keusch, G. T., & Theam, D. M. (1993). Malnutrition in AIDS. *Medical Clinics of North America, 77*(4), 795–814.

Lemire, R. J. (1986). Causes of neural tube defects. In R. L. McLaurin, S. Oppenheimer, L. Dias, & W. E. Kaplan (Eds.), *Spina bifida. A multidisciplinary approach* (pp. 2–7). New York: Praeger.

Moore, C. V. (1963). The anemias. In P. B. Beeson & W. McDermott (Eds.), *Cecil–Loeb textbook of medicine* (llth ed., pp. 1071–1186). Philadelphia: Saunders.

Papalopulu, N., & Kintner, C. R. (1994). Molecular genetics of neurulation. In G. Bock & J. Marsh (Eds.), *Neural tube defects* (pp. 90–98). Ciba Foundation Symposium 181. New York: Wiley.

Recommended Dietary Allowances. (1989). *Recommended dietary allowances* (10th ed., p. 284). Washington, DC: National Academy Press.

Scheckit, M. A. (1994). Alcohol and alcoholism. In K. J. Isselbacher, E. Braunwald, J. O. Wilson, J. B. Martin, A. S. Fauci, & D. L. Kasper (Eds.), *Harrison's principles of internal medicine*, (13th ed., pp. 2420–2425). New York: McGraw-Hill.

Seller, M. J. (1994). Vitamins, folic acid and the cause and prevention of neural tube defects. In G. Bock & J. Marsh (Eds.). *Neural tube defects* (pp. 161–172).

Ciba Foundation Symposium 181. New York: Wiley.

Sheard, N. (1995) The diabetic diet: Evidence for a new approach. *Nutrition Reviews, 53,* 16–18.

Underwood, E. J. (1973). Trace elements. In *Toxicants occurring naturally in foods* (2nd ed., pp. 61–64). Committee on Food Protection. Food and Nutrition Board. National Research Council. Washington, DC: National Academy of Sciences.

Vitamin E Research Summary. (1995). LaGrange, IL: VERIS, Vitamin E Research and Information Service.

Wald, N. J. (1994). Folic acid and neural tube defects: The current evidence and implications for prevention. In G. Bock & J. Marsh (Eds.) *Neural tube defects* (pp. 192–207). Ciba Foundation Symposium 181. New York: Wiley.

Wedeen, R. P. (1992). Removing lead from bone: Clinical implications of bone lead stores. *Neurotoxicology, 13,* 843–852.

PART 3

Nutrition Policies and Approaches Targeted at Populations at Risk

CHAPTER 13

Pregnant Mothers and Their Young Children—The WIC Program

Alma W. Cain

A growing number of mothers and their children are at risk for malnutrition or undernutrition. This group is culturally diverse including many Blacks, Hispanics and Asians who live in urban areas. Moreover, undernutrition and much malnutrition is particularly prevalent among the poor who tend to be concentrated in inner cities. Indeed, in the United States, one in five children lives in poverty.

It is appropriate to consider the nutrition of pregnant and lactating women along with that of their children. Egan (1991), in a historical perspective of the maternal and child health programs, has shown that nutrition services have developed in parallel with general health care programs. For example, in the early 1900s, when the American Child Health Association and the Commonwealth Fund developed child health demonstration projects, nutrition clinics were established at the same time. This close association continues today, primarily because in our society, the mother's traditional role is that of nurturing her young child and taking care of the responsibilities associated with those functions.

There exists adequate evidence that well nourished mothers produce healthier children. Appropriate weight gain during pregnancy leads to improved infant birth weights and reduced infant mortality and morbidity (Surgeon General's Report, 1988).

Factors that place women at nutritional risk include: adolescence, short interconceptional period, poor reproductive performance, economic deprivation, food faddism, substance abuse, chronic systemic disease, and inadequate or excessive prepregnant weight (below 85% or above 120% of standard weight for height).

Focusing on child nutrition as a public health issue commands attention. As early as 1897, the Henry Street Visiting Nurse Association of New York City included milk stations in its program for those in need (Egan, 1994). Later, when the U.S. Office of Education was established, it was given responsibilities for nutrition in public schools. Under the Social Security Act of 1935, the federal Food Distribution Program authorized grants to states for nutrition services to mothers and children. In the 1960s and 1970s, child nutrition was to receive even more public attention.

The 1969 White House Conference on Food, Nutrition and Health followed the Child Nutrition Act that was passed in 1966. In their Report to the President (1970) delegates of the conference called for expansion of existing food programs and for providing quality nutrition education to all school children. Subsequently, the U.S. Department of Agriculture established the Food and Nutrition Service to administer federal food-assistance programs.

This same period was characterized by a great deal of turmoil. The war in Southeast Asia; civil rights unrest; poverty and hunger; access to health care; increasing environmental pollution; a rising prevalence of behavior-related problems, such as substance abuse, adolescent pregnancy, and sexually transmitted disease captured the attention of the general public and those responsible for health and safety. At the same time, many cities experienced an increase in infant mortality; this was particularly true for African Americans.

These events led President Johnson to declare a "War on Poverty." With the enactment of enormous amounts of social legislation, several new health programs targeted to low-income, high-risk populations were established (Table 13.1).

The late 1980s and 1990s saw worsening economic conditions for the poor. As a result, the number of homeless people, particularly in the major cities, began to increase. Among the homeless were families, mothers, and children. Wiecha and Palombo (1991) have described the nutrition and health services requirements of the homeless. Common in this population is hunger, lack of food, inadequate diets, poor nutritional status, and nutrition-related health problems, such as stunted growth, failure to thrive, low-birth-weight, infant mortality, anemia, and compromised immune systems.

Table 13.1 Special Projects—War on Poverty

Project	Year initiated
Maternity and Infant Care (M & I)	1963
The Comprehensive Health Projects for Children and Youth (C & Y)	1965
Community health centers	1965
Migrant health programs	1965
Family planning program	1969
Head Start program	1965
Medicare and Medicaid	1965
University-affiliated centers program	1963

Adapted from Egan, M. C., (1994), Public health nutrition: A historical perspective. *Journal of the American Dietetic Association, 94,* 298-304.

THE SPECIAL SUPPLEMENTAL NUTRITION PROGRAM FOR WOMEN, INFANTS, AND CHILDREN

In 1972 Congress enacted legislation establishing the Special Supplemental Food Program for Women, Infants, and Children (WIC). The WIC program is administered by state health departments. Using federal regulations as a guide, state agencies retain substantial flexibility in program operations, including setting specific eligibility requirements, allowable foods, and the delivery of those foods. WIC services are provided at approximately 9,000 clinic sites by over 1,800 local agencies around the country. Most of these are state or local agency public health clinics. WIC services are also provided to migrant and community health centers, community action agencies, and nonprofit organizations. At the federal level, WIC is overseen by the Food and Consumer Service of the Department of Agriculture.

WIC is primarily federally funded, but some states allocate additional funds for program operations. Unlike the Food Stamp Program, WIC is not an entitlement program, but a discretionary program. It is funded through annual Congressional appropriations. These have increased significantly, rising from $736 million in 1980 to nearly $3.21 billion in 1994, when some 9.5 million persons were eligible for the program. Only about 65% of eligible women, infants and children in the U.S. are actually served by the WIC program, however.

The Special Supplemental Food Program for Women, Infants, and Children provides food and nutrition screening and education for at-risk, low-income pregnant women, postpartum and breastfeeding women, infants and children under 5 years of age. Eligibility is determined by income and nutritional and medical risk. Each state has its own definition of risk, with risk assessment made by a health professional. Families become eligible if their gross income equals or is below 185% of the federal poverty guidelines (Table 13.2).

Designed to be an adjunct to good health, WIC participation is closely linked with routine pediatric and obstetric care. States are required by federal regulations (Federal Register, 1994) to have health referral mechanisms in place for both social services and health care services, if these are not provided by the agencies themselves. In addition referrals can include drug abuse and smoking cessation for women, and immunization assurances for children.

The program provides supplemental foods to women who are pregnant, postpartum through 6 months, and those who breastfeed their infants, with the maximum supplementation period of 1 year. Infants and children are served up to 5 years of age. Foods provided include cereals fortified with iron, fruit juice high in vitamin C, eggs, infant formula, dried peas or beans, and peanut butter. For women who breastfeed, canned tuna fish and carrots are available. These foods have been selected because of their nutrient content, as they are good sources of protein, of vitamins such as A and C, and of the minerals calcium and iron, as well as other nutrients that may be lacking in the diets of this low-income group.

States differ in how they administer their programs, but all are subject to the same federal regulations. Eligibility determination is one such element. Eligibility assessment begins with income screening and an evaluation of household income of those individuals living as a family or as one economic unit. Income standards may vary from state to state. The maximum permissible family income is 185% of the federal poverty income guidelines. Documentation such as pay stubs, public-assistance cards, or income tax statements may be required as proof of income.

A health assessment to determine nutritional risk or nutritionally related medical conditions is made by a health professional. At a minimum, height, weight, and a hemoglobin or hematocrit analysis are required. Using nutritional risk criteria established by the state WIC agency and other health-assessment data, a dietitian, nutritionist, physician, nurse, or other medically trained professional ascertains the priority placement of

Table 13.2 Annual Poverty Guidelines, 1996*

Household size	Poverty Guideline (100% poverty)
1	$7,740
2	10,360
3	12,980
4	15,600
5	18,220
6	20,840
7	23,460
8	26,080
For each additional family member add	2,620

* This table shows income levels equal to the poverty line (100% of the poverty line). Programs sometimes set program income eligibility at some point above the poverty line. For example, if a program sets income eligibility at 185% of the poverty line, then the cutoff for a family of two living in the 48 contiguous states is $10,360 x 185% = $19,166.

Adapted from Department of Agriculture Food and Nutrition Service. *Federal Register*, March 1996.

the person, and certifies or authorizes the enrollment (Table 13.3). When a person has been certified as eligible, the WIC nutritionist prescribes a combination of allowable supplemental foods tailored to meet the person's specific nutritional needs.

Nutrition education is a key component of any food assistance program. The United States Department of Agriculture programs aim to produce nutritionally literate consumers who can make informed decisions when selecting, handling, and consuming foods in ways that improve their nutritional health and well-being.

WIC program regulations have undergone a number of amendments since the program began. In April of 1995 (Department of Agriculture Food and Consumer Service, 1995), the WIC Program's nutritional risk priority system was amended allowing categorical and income-eligible homeless or migrant individuals to receive WIC Program assistance solely due to homelessness of migrancy.

In the same legislation, the name of the program was changed from the Special Supplemental Food Program for Women, Infants, and Children to the Special Supplemental *Nutrition* Program for Women, Infants, and Children.

Table 13.3 The WIC Priority System

Priority I	Pregnant and breastfeeding women
	Based on nutritionally related medical conditions
	Infants
	Based on nutritionally related medical conditions
Priority II	Infants to 6 months of age
	Whose mother participated in WIC during pregnancy
	Whose mothers would have been eligible due to medical conditions
Priority III	Children up to age 5
	Based on nutritionally related medical conditions
Priority IV	Pregnant women, breastfeeding women, and infants
	Inadequate dietary pattern
Priority V	Children up to age 5
	Inadequate dietary pattern
Priority VI	Postpartum women
	At nutritional risk
Priority VII	Previously certified participants who might regress in nutritional status without continued provision of supplemental foods

Adapted from Department of Agriculture, Food and Nutrition Service. *Federal Register*, 1990.

A food-delivery system is the end point in the WIC process. The WIC state agency uses a variety of methods in supplying foods to participants. Supplemental foods may be purchased by participants with a WIC voucher, a coupon, or a WIC check. Foods may be delivered to the individual's home as in Vermont. In Chicago, WIC foods are "bought" with WIC vouchers in a WIC supermarket that sells WIC foods exclusively. In most states, however, supplemental foods are purchased by the client in retail food markets.

In recent years, the nutrition-counseling requirements of the program have been expanded to include counseling such as substance abuse, smoking, and alcohol prevention. Because WIC reaches a large population at heightened risk, the need to assess the immunization status of children and to refer them if needed has broadened the program's focus, accelerated coordination with other health services, and strengthened referral mechanisms. In one study in Massachusetts in an urban setting (Sargent, Attar-Abate, Meyers, Moore, Kocher-Ahern, 1992) researchers found that approximately 61% of the referrals made by the WIC nutritionists to other services were for supplemental foods, 20.5% were for non-nutrition related medical and dental services, whereas developmental and educational services accounted for 12.5%, and social services 5.4%. For women, the non-nutrition related referrals included referrals for family planning, substance abuse, job training, parenting for teenagers, and education programs. For infants and children, referrals were mainly for dental care, growth failure, to the Head Start Program, kindergarten enrollment, early intervention, and protective services.

BREASTFEEDING

Meeting the basic nutritional needs of the infant is a key element of the supplemental nutrition program. Human milk can provide most of the nutritional needs of the infant for the first 6 months of life. When WIC infants are breastfed the diet of the breastfeeding mother is supplemented; alternatively, the infant receives infant formula. It is also possible for the mother to receive some quantity of infant formula while breastfeeding, to be used during her absence or in emergency situations.

In their 1993 survey, Ross Laboratories (1993a) looked at breastfeeding trends from the 1970s to 1993 and found that breastfeeding has risen steadily from 1991–1993. In the general population of mothers surveyed, 55.9% reported breastfeeding their newborns in the hospital, with 19 percent reporting that they were still breastfeeding 6 months after birth.

The desire to increase breastfeeding in the United States to ensure the health and well-being of infants is well recognized. The Department of Health and Human Services (Healthy People, 1990) established the year 2000 as a national objective to increase the percentage of women who breastfeed their infants to at least 75% at hospital discharge, and a minimum of 50% at 5 to 6 months postpartum.

A smaller fraction of low-income women breastfeed than women in the population as a whole. The 1989 data (Ross, 1993b) show that 35% of WIC participants breastfed when discharged from the hospital and 9% were breastfed 6 months later. This compares with 52% of all women when discharged from the hospital and 18% 6 months later.

Since its inception, controversy has surrounded the effect the WIC program has had on infant-feeding practices. Schwartz, Popkin, Tognetti, and Zohoori (1995) report that providing breastfeeding advice to pregnant women in the WIC program may significantly improve initiation of breastfeeding, but was found to have had no effect on breastfeeding duration.

REBATING

Since its beginning, the number of people likely to need the program has exceeded the funding available. In an effort to serve more clients, states began in the early 1980's to look for ways to reduce food costs. Because infant formula prices had risen substantially, infant-formula expenditures became the main focus of cost-reduction efforts. Thus began a trend that USDA later termed cost containment.

In 1990 WIC regulations were amended, mandating that states seek food cost-reduction measures. Infant formula rebating by major manufacturers, and on a more limited basis, cereal rebating by cereal manufacturers soon became standard practice in all states. These procedures have significantly contributed to the expansion of the program nationwide. In 1993, rebate dollars amounted to approximately $1.1 billion, resulting in an additional 2.1 million people receiving benefits.

WIC Farmer's Market Nutrition Program

The WIC Farmer's Market Nutrition Program (FMNP) was created in 1992 to allow WIC program participants to purchase fresh fruits and vegetables at authorized farmers' markets. With coupons of $10 to $20, the program is designed to increase fresh fruit and vegetable consumption among the population (Catalog, 1993).

The National Association of Farmers' Market Nutrition Programs has reported (National Association, 1996) that 71% of participants surveyed stated they ate more fresh fruit and vegetables as a result of the FMNP. In addition, 40% reported having bought fruits or vegetables they had never tried before, and another 77% said they plan to eat more fresh fruits and vegetables all year round.

The farmers' market program is an example of the dynamic nature of the WIC program. It continues to change in response to identified needs of its high-risk clients, particularly needs of a health or nutrition nature.

WIC EVALUATIONS

The WIC program has grown tremendously since its inception in the mid-1970s and a number of studies have been conducted to look at its effectiveness. From 1970 until about 1987, WIC funding and participation in the program steadily increased. The large increases were primarily due to the annual increases in WIC appropriations and to the infusion of infant formula rebate dollars. According to a USDA study (WIC Dynamics, 1995, p. I-2), which looked at WIC operations between 1988 and 1993, "WIC evolved from being an adjunct to maternal and child health services to becoming the gateway program through which many low-income households enter the public health system."

A series of medical evaluations has shown that WIC improves the health of participating women, infants, and children. Rush (1986) has reported that WIC contributed to a reduction of 20%–33.33% in the late fetal death rate; increased head size of infants; that women had longer pregnancies leading to fewer premature births, and participation appeared to lead to better cognitive performance. Improvements in dietary intake among women were seen in more consumption of key nutrients such as iron, protein, calcium, and vitamin C. The average intake of iron and vitamin C among infants was increased and the frequency of low consumption of iron and vitamins A and C diminished. The diets of older preschool children improved as well. In this group, the average consumption of iron, vitamin C, thiamine, and niacin increased and the frequency of low intakes of vitamins A and B and riboflavin were decreased.

In a study released by the United States General Accounting Office (GAO, 1992), it was found that providing WIC benefits and services to low-income pregnant women had a marked impact, reducing the number of infants born with low birthweights by 25% and very low birthweight births by 44%.

Based on 105,000 medical records of mothers and babies in five states, the Devaney, Bilheimer, and Shore study (1991) found that WIC decreased the risk of low birthweight by increasing weights of infants covered by Medicaid by 51 to 117 grams. Preterm infants experienced even greater weight improvements. For every dollar invested in WIC for pregnant women, GAO estimates $1.92 to $4.21 in Medicaid savings were achieved for newborns and their mothers in the first 60 days after birth. And, for every pregnant woman who receives WIC benefits some time during her pregnancy, Medicaid costs were reduced between $376 to $753.31.

In a study conducted over a 10-year period by the Centers for Disease Control, it was found that a two-thirds reduction in childhood anemia occurred among children enrolled in the Pediatric Nutrition Surveillance System (Leads from the MMWWR, 1986). Additionally, the study found that those children not enrolled in WIC had significantly higher prevalence of anemia than those who are enrolled.

OTHER NUTRITION PROGRAMS

A number of other nutrition programs are available in the U.S. to mothers and their young children. Some are designed to increase food-purchasing power, whereas others have broader goals of education, health prevention, and skill development directed toward self sufficiency.

The Food Stamp Program

The Food Stamp Program dates back to the Great Depression, when thousands of people stood on bread lines and farmers experienced a surplus of crops they could not sell to the consuming public (Food & Nutrition, 1992). The purpose of the program is to improve the diets of low-income households by increasing their food-purchasing power. Coupons are issued directly to families for the specific purpose of buying food. House-hold eligibility and allotments are based on household size, income, assets, housing costs, work requirements, and other factors (Catalog, 1993).

Child and Adult Care Food Program

Federal funds and USDA-donated foods are provided to nonresidential child care and adult day-care facilities and to family day-care homes for children. These are aimed at improving the nutrient quality of meals and snacks served in public or private nonprofit child-care centers, Head Start centers, neighborhood centers, some for-profit child-care centers, and licensed or approved day-care centers for small groups of children (Catalog, 1993).

Commodity Supplemental Food Program

The Commodity Supplemental Food Program, administered by the U.S. Department of Agriculture, donates supplemental foods for distribution to low-income pregnant, postpartum, and breastfeeding women, infants, children up to 6 years of age, and elderly people who have been determined to be at nutritional risk by a health professional. The program has both age and income requirements (Catalog, 1993).

The Expanded Food and Nutrition Education Program

The Expanded Food and Nutrition Education Program is designed to improve the nutritional status of low-income families with children under the age of 18. Through education, EFNEP offers knowledge and skills development that assists families in understanding the relationship of food and nutrition to health and fitness, to get the most value for their food dollars and to select and prepare nutritious foods (Catalog, 1993).

Head Start

The Head Start Program was initiated by the Office of Economic opportunity in 1965. Head Start provides 3- to 5-year-old children from low-income families with comprehensive education, health, and nutrition services.

In 1981 The Select Panel for the Promotion of Child Health reported that children participating in Head Start have a lower incidence of anemia, are better immunized, and have better nutrition and improved overall health than children who do not participate (Select Panel, 1981).

National School Lunch and Breakfast Programs

The National School Lunch Program and the School Breakfast Program (Catalog,1993) provide financial assistance to schools so that students receive a nutritious lunch and breakfast. Those schools participating in the program receive both food commodities and cash payments from the federal government. Payments are based on the number and proportion of meals served either free, at a reduced price, or at full price, with low-income children eligible for free and reduced-price meals.

Special Milk Program

The Special Milk Program sponsored by the United States Department of Agriculture provides for a cash reimbursement for each half-pint of milk served to children in schools that are not participating in the National School Lunch Program.

Summer Food Service Program for Children

The Summer Food Service Program funds meals and snacks during school vacation for eligible children. Operating in low-income areas, more than half of the children are from households with incomes at or below 185% of the poverty level. Local schools as well as government units, such as park and recreation departments, community action agencies, and non-profit organizations act as sponsors of the programs.

Emergency Food Assistance Program

Begun as the Temporary Emergency Food Assistance Program (TEFAP), The Emergency Food Assistance Program has been operating since 1982. Originally, the program was designed to reduce the level of government-held surplus commodities by distributing them to low-income households as a supplement to their purchased foods. Subsequently in 1988 with the enactment of the Hunger Prevention Act, the federal government was authorized to purchase commodity foods, expanding both the quantity and variety of foods made available to these families (Levedahl & Matsumoto 1990).

Food-assistance programs make a significant contribution to the nutritional well-being of low-income mothers, young children, and their families by providing the necessary dollars to increase their food-purchasing power, by distributing foods to them or by providing meals or snacks. Participation in federally funded food-assistance programs is not necessarily mutually exclusive. For example, a family can be enrolled in the Food Stamp Program while the pregnant mother and her infant receive WIC and the school-age children in the family receive free or reduced-price lunches. In a community where the Commodity Supplemental Food Program and WIC are both available to the pregnant woman and small children, however, no family member can be enrolled in both programs simultaneously.

Table 13.4 Federally Funded Nutrition Assistance Programs, 1994

Program	Participation	Funding
Food Stamp Program[a]	27,465,654	24,490,517,704
Avg. benefit/person ($)	69.02	
National School Lunch Program	25,280,251	4,954,561,769
School Breakfast[b]	5,835,911	958,987,351
Special Milk Program	601,689	17,793,530
Summer Food Serv Program[c]	2,187,200	225,126,514
Child/Adult Care Food[d]	2,187,663	1,355,137,618
Comm.Supplemental Food Program[e]	363,059	107,362,091
Special Supplemental Food Program for Women, Infants and Children[e]	6,477,189	3,164,717,562
Avg. Food Cost/Person ($)	29.91	
The Emergency Food Assistance Program	2,287,645	200,657,001

a. Includes benefits costs and the federal share of state administrative expenses.
b. Includes all cash-reimbursement costs.
c. Includes all cash reimbursements, food costs, and administrative costs.
d. Includes all cash reimbursements (meal earnings), food costs (value of entitlement and bonus commodities), SF-269 cash-in-lieu of commodities, and SF-269 administrative costs.
e. Includes all food costs and administrative costs. WIC total also includes Program Studies (U.S. level only) and WIC FMNP costs.

Source: National Data Bank. Data Base Monitoring Branch, Program Information Division, Food and Consumer Service, USDA. July 1995.

In federal fiscal year 1994, funding of the Food Stamp Program was in excess of $24 billion dollars with approximately 27 million people participating. The average monthly benefit per person was $69.02. During the same period, the WIC Programs' supplemental food cost averaged $29.91 (Table 13.4). The combined food cost in 1994 for a low income pregnant woman enrolled in both the Food Stamp and WIC programs would have been $98.93 each month.

SUMMARY

The health officer is challenged at several levels. Beginning with the immediate community, an assessment of health and nutritional status of the most vulnerable population is essential in determining the nutritional programming required. Data exist at the state and federal levels that give information on the extent of poverty and that provide criteria that aid in determining the at-risk population in the community.

The availability of state and federal funds to alleviate conditions of hunger, malnutrition, and food insecurity must then be determined and sought out. Funding for food-assistance programs is always limited and falls short of need. Programs such as the Food Stamp Program are entitlement programs. The dollars spent on this type of program are based on the number of individuals who apply, how many of these meet the program's eligibility criteria, and the benefits to which they may be entitled. Nutrition and health officers should encourage the maximum number of families to apply. An investment in outreach efforts can produce returns when more individuals apply for the program, are enrolled, and receive benefits.

Discretionary or nonentitlement program funding is controlled by the United States congress through its annual appropriations process. Both these funding mechanisms impose limits. By identifying needs and by means of advocacy at all levels, it is possible to exert a positive influence on the appropriation of public funds directed to nutrition programming.

An understanding of the internal as well as the external factors that affect the lives of a disadvantaged group can be the basis for establishing efficient and effective food-assistance and nutrition programs. This requires both planning, collaboration, and coordination at various levels of government, including those agencies responsible for the social services and the health care systems as well.

REFERENCES

Catalog of Federal Domestic Assistance and Food Assistance Programs. (1993). *Food program facts 1993.* Washington, DC: U.S. General Services Administration.
Department of Agriculture, Food and Nutrition Service. (1990). Consolidation of WIC regulations, *Federal Register,* September, 261–449/20879. Washington, DC: U.S. Government Printing Office.

Department of Agriculture, Food and Nutrition Service. (1994). Special supplemental food program for women, infants, and children (WIC). Coordination rule: Mandates of child nutrition and WIC reauthorization act of 1989. *Federal Register,* Vol. 59, # 48 March. Washington, DC: U.S. Government Printing Office.

Department of Agriculture, Food and Consumer Service. (1995). Special supplemental food program for women, infants, and children (WIC): Homelessnesss/ Migrancy as Nutritional risk conditions. *Federal Register,* Vol. 60, # 75 April. Washington, DC: U.S. Government Printing Office.

Department of Agriculture, Food and Consumer Service (1996). Special supplemental food program for women, infants, and children (WIC): Poverty income guidelines. *Federal Register,* Vol. 61, # 53 March. Washington, DC: U.S. Government Printing Office.

Devaney, B., Bilheimer, L., & Schore, J. (1991). *The savings in Medicaid cost for newborns and their mothers resulting from prenatal participation in the WIC program. Addendum.* Princeton, NJ: Mathematica Policy Research.

Egan, M. C. (1991). *Nutrition services in the Maternal and Child Health program: A historical perspective. Call to action: Better nutrition for mothers, children, and families.* Washington, DC: National Center For Education in Maternal & Child Health.

Egan, M. C. (1994). Public health nutrition: A historical perspective. *Journal of the American Dietetic Association, 94,* 298–304.

Healthy people 2000: National health promotion and disease prevention objectives (1990). U.S. Department of Health and Human Services, Public Health Service. Washington, DC: U.S. Government Printing Office.

Leads from the MMWR. (1986). Declining anemia prevalence among children enrolled in public nutrition and health program selected states, 1975–1985. *Journal of the American Medical Association, 256,* 2165.

Levedahl, J., & Matsumoto, M. (1990). *U.S. domestic food assistance programs: Lessons from the past.* U.S. Department of Agriculture, Economic Research Service, Agriculture Information Bulletin no. 570. Washington, DC: U.S. Government Printing Office.

National Association of Farmers' Market Nutrition Programs. (1996). *Program impact report for the 1995 WIC farmers' market nutrition program.* Washington, DC.

National Data Bank. (1995). *Data Base Monitoring Branch, Program Information Division.* Food and Consumer Service, U.S. Department of Agriculture. Washington, DC: U.S. Government Printing Office.

Ross Laboratories. (1994). *The Ross mothers survey.* Ross Products Division of Abbott Laboratories. Columbus, OH.

Rush, D. (1986). *The national WIC evaluation: An evaluation of the special supplemental food program for women, infants and children.* US Department of

Agriculture, Food, and Nutrition Service. Washington, DC: U.S. Government Printing Office.

Sargent, J., Attar-Abate, L., Meyers, A., Moore, L., & Kocher-Ahern, E. (1992). Referrals of participants in an urban WIC program to health and welfare services. *Public Health Reports, 107,* 173–178.

Select Panel for the Promotion of Child Health. (1981). *Better health for our children: A national strategy.* U.S. Department of Health and Human Services, DHHS Pub. No. 79-55071. Washington, DC: U.S. Government Printing Office.

Schwartz, B., Popkin, B., Tognetti, J., & Zohoori, N. (1995). Does WIC participation improve breastfeeding practices? *American Journal of Public Health, 85,* 729–731.

The Surgeons Generals' Report on Nutrition and Health. (1988). *U.S. Department of Health and Human Services.* Washington, DC: U.S. Government Printing Office.

U.S. Department of Agriculture, Food and Consumer Service, (1995). *The WIC dynamics study, volume I final report,* Washington, DC: U.S. Government Printing Office.

White House Conference on Food, Nutrition and Health. (1970). *Final report.* Washington, DC: U.S. Government Printing Office.

Wiecha, J. L., & Palombo, R. (1989). Multiple program participation comparison of nutrition and food assistance program benefits with food costs in Boston, Massachusetts. *American Journal of Public Health, 79,* 591–594.

CHAPTER 14

Issues in Development of a Nutrition Policy for Preschool and School-Aged Children

Aryeh D. Stein

C hildhood is a time of physical and educational development. Habits, attitudes toward preventive lifestyles, and risk factors for future health and disease are being developed; once established, these may persist for decades. Although adequate supplies of nourishing food are a basic right of childhood, children have limited autonomy in their ability to select their own foods, though this increases with age. Restrictions on food selection are imposed by geography and climate; by economic, social, or cultural constraints; and by choices imposed by parents and other providers. As infants, children are either breast- or formula-fed, then weaned onto those solid foods chosen by caregivers. Toddlers and school-age children are better able to articulate their desires and obtain food independently of parental supervision; nevertheless, providers set bounds on choice by limiting the selection of foods found in the house or selected while eating elsewhere, and by establishing family norms. Public health nutrition aims to influence these choices through a combination of public education and government regulation.

Food and nutrition policy as it relates to children is guided by both short- and long-term objectives. In the short term, nutrition policy focuses on the need to ensure that the child is healthy. Acute, clinical undernutrition in early childhood is common in populations subject to periodic food shortages. Common syndromes include protein-energy malnutrition, hypovitaminosis A, and iron-deficiency anemia: these may result in growth retardation, increased frequency and severity of infection, and reduced educational attainment. These syndromes are characterized by a relatively short latent period. Therefore, a clear relationship between food intake and clinical manifestation is often readily discernible. Moreover, these conditions are often amenable to short-term therapeutic interventions. Screening and programs to provide appropriate foods to high-risk populations are key in reducing the prevalence of these conditions.

Nutrition policy is also driven by long-term objectives, to ensure that the child grows into a healthy adult. This chapter examines the rationale and implications of a policy to encourage healthy eating by children, focusing on issues of increased importance in affluent societies where overall food availability is not a primary constraint. These societies are characterized by extremely high child survival and good measures of health status in young adulthood, coupled with a high incidence of cardiovascular disease, cancer, diabetes, and other conditions in later adult life. The focus is on precursors of adult disease, particularly atherosclerosis and hypertension, conditions for which a dietary etiology has been established.

The evidence relating childhood nutrition to adult disease is weaker than the evidence relating acute undernutrition to disease in childhood. This is inherent in the nature of the adult diseases, which are characterized by multiple causes, long latent periods and clinical onset in late middle age. Studies of childhood precursors of adult disease are inherently difficult, as they require a longitudinal approach. One or more cohorts of children need to be enrolled and their diet assessed periodically. For a more powerful study design, children would be randomly assigned to one of several nutritional regimens to be maintained for life. The children would then be monitored for the onset of disease. Unfortunately, such studies are not practical, as the target diseases are exceedingly rare in early life and the study would have to be continued for 60 or 70 years. For this reason, most research into diet in childhood and chronic disease risk has focused on the effect of nutrients or dietary patterns on precursor states.

RECOMMENDED DIETARY PATTERNS FOR CHILDREN

The ninth revision of the U.S. Recommended Daily Allowances (RDA) for children and youth still reflected the long-standing philosophy of deficiency prevention (Food and Nutrition Board, 1980). In other words, the recommended intakes represented minimum levels designed to ensure that intakes meet physiological needs for the vast majority of the population. This policy is appropriate for nutrients, including most micronutrients, the deficiency of which would result in disease, but overabundance of which is unlikely to lead to deleterious effects. Recommendations in the tenth revision are designed to balance the need for sufficiency without encouraging excess nutrient consumption associated with future disease (Food and Nutrition Board, 1989). The primary recommendation, that children eat a diverse diet, remains a key component of these new guidelines.

Energy

Energy is required for basic metabolism, activity, and (among children) growth, and is provided by the oxidation of proteins, fats, carbohydrates, and alcohol. Energy requirements vary widely in individuals of the same body size and activity levels, so that it has generally not been possible to develop a single benchmark to assess adequacy, without anthropometric assessment. Insufficient energy intake is characterized by growth failure, with chronic marginal deficiency resulting in stunting and acute deficiency resulting in wasting. Conversely, excess energy intake results in excess weight gain, manifested by increases in body fat and obesity. Energy balance is maintained by altering total caloric intake and physical activity. Adequacy of energy intake is best assessed through sequential growth monitoring, which should focus on steady increases in height, but ensure that weight gain is not excessive. Reference growth standards can be found in any textbook of nutritional assessment (e.g., Gibson, 1990).

Fat

In adults, variation in fat intake is strongly implicated as causing differences in the risk for atherosclerotic disease, with saturated fat appearing to be the primary agent (e.g., Keys, 1980). Of the three principal macronutrients, protein, carbohydrate and fat, it is fat that is the most energy-dense, providing 9 kcal/g. Differences in fat intake are also major determinants of variation in total energy intake. Therefore, a reduction in saturated and total fat intake in childhood would benefit adult health in two ways, by reducing atherosclerosis and by preventing obesity. Most expert commissions have adopted the view that diets of adults should contain less than 30% of energy from fat, and less than 10% of energy from saturated fat (National Research Council, 1989). These recommended intake levels have also been adopted for children past their second birthday (American Academy of Pediatrics, 1986). Before age 2, overall fat restriction to below 30% may not provide enough calories to promote optimal growth.

Saturated fats in the diet are obtained primarily from meat and dairy sources. Several groups of researchers have tried to identify key foods that could form the focus of campaigns to reduce fat intake in children. Characteristics of these foods would be that they are widely consumed, but that the additional nutrients provided by the food could be adequately obtained by other foods. One such food appears to be whole liquid milk. Although it is a source of many nutrients, including calcium, phosphorus, protein, and vitamins, all these are also provided in identical concentrations by skim and low-fat milk (Table 14.1). The need for substitution, rather than elimination, of whole milk, is illustrated in two reports. Shea, Stein, Basch, and Zybert (1992), studying Hispanic children in New York City, found that diets lower in fat also tended to be lower in calcium and phosphorus. Basch, Shea, and Zybert (1992) reported that the major source of variation in fat intakes in this same study population was the extent to which the children drank whole milk (none of the children consumed skim or low-fat milk). They concluded that one simple substitution, that of low-fat (0.5–1%) or skim milk for whole milk, would result in the attainment of the recommended goal of no more than 30% of calories from fat by almost all children in their study. In a computer simulation based on diets of a nationally representative sample of children aged 6 months to 5 years, Sigman-Grant, Zimmerman, and Kris-Etherton (1993) reached the same conclusion for 4–5-year-old children, but felt that it would be difficult to meet all the recommendations for 2–3-year-olds by substituting low-fat or skim milk for whole milk, as diets with low-fat milks tended to be deficient in energy and other nutrients. Different populations differ in the sources of fat in the diet, with implications for the potential benefits and risks of dietary modification. Nicklas, Koschak, Webber, and Berenson (1992), in their analysis of diets of Black and white children in Bogalusa, Louisiana, found that the major source of variation in fat intake was caused by differences in meat consumption and that children with lower fat intake were also more likely to have diets low in the B vitamins and in iron. The differences between the findings of Basch et al. (1992) and Nicklas et al. (1992) point to the importance of identifying key sources of fat in the target population before an intervention is initiated.

Table 14.1 Composition of whole, 2%, 1%, and Skim Milk, per 1-Cup Serving.

Nutrient	Unit	Whole milk [a]	2% milk [a]	1% Milk [a]	Skim milk [a]
Calories	kcal	150	120	100	85
Protein	g	8	8	8	8
	% USRDA [b]	20	20	20	20
Carbohydrate	g	11	12	12	12
Fat	g	8	5	3	0
Sodium	mg	120	122	123	126
Potassium	mg	370	377	381	406
Vitamin A	% USRDA	4	10	10	10
Vitamin C	% USRDA	4	4	4	4
Vitamin D	% USRDA	25	25	25	25
Vitamin B_4	% USRDA	0	0	0	4
Vitamin B_6	% USRDA	4	4	4	0
Vitamin B_{12}	% USRDA	15	15	15	15
Calcium	% USRDA	30	30	30	30
Thiamin	% USRDA	6	6	6	6
Riboflavin	% USRDA	25	25	25	25
Phosphorus	% USRDA	20	20	20	20
Magnesium	% USRDA	8	8	8	8
Zinc	% USRDA	4	4	4	4
Pantothenic acid	% USRDA	6	6	6	6

a. Vitamin D added to all forms of milk. Vitamin A added to 2%, 1%, and skim milks.
b. Percentage of US recommended daily allowance. All forms of milk provide less than 2% of the USRDA per serving of iron and niacin.

Adapted from Gebhardt, S. E., & Matthews, R. H. *Nutritive value of foods.* Washington, DC: U.S. Government Printing Office, 1986. US Department of Agriculture, *Home and Garden Bulletin,* 72.

Micronutrients

Except for sodium, implicated in the etiology of hypertension, the RDA guidelines do not specify maximum recommended intakes of micronutrients (minerals and vitamins). Within the range of normal human diets, it is unlikely that toxic levels of these nutrients will be ingested. Some studies in adults have suggested that very high intakes of the fat-soluble antioxidant vitamins alpha-tocopherol and beta-carotene may reduce the risk for cardiovascular disease. Beneficial effects have been observed primarily among adults taking supplemental vitamins; this suggests that minor modifications in food intake alone are unlikely to alter the disease risk substantially. These antioxidants are thought to prevent the accumulation of oxidized low-density lipoprotein (LDL) cholesterol, a compound that appears to be particularly atherogenic. If these effects are substantiated, antioxidant supplementation in children may be indicated. Supplementation studies have not been conducted in children, and it is not known whether rare side effects occur in long-term supplementation.

DIETARY PATTERNS OF THE PRESCHOOL AND SCHOOL-AGED POPULATION OF THE U.S.

The dietary habits of the U.S. population are monitored periodically through the Health and Nutrition Examination Surveys (HANES). HANES is a large, extensive, nationally representative survey, conducted approximately every 10 years. As part of the examination, 24-hour dietary recalls are obtained from all survey respondents (by proxy for respondents below age 11).

The most recent HANES (HANES III) was conducted between 1988 and 1994. Results from the first phase, conducted between 1988 and 1991, have become available. Among children, total fat intakes varied from 32.9% of calories (at 3–5 years) to 34.5% of calories (16–19 years), whereas saturated fat intakes ranged from 12.2% of calories (at age 12–15 years) to 13.9% of calories (at age 1-2 years). Distribution of total and saturated fat intakes by age, gender, and ethnic origin is presented in Table 14.2. Further details are provided by McDowell et al. (1994). These intake levels suggest a modest decline in fat intakes over the past decade, although mean intakes of all population subgroups still exceed the dietary objectives. It appears that some progress is being made in the general population toward a lower fat diet, but it must be remembered that all dietary intake data are self-reported (or, in the case of young children, proxy reporting by parents and other caregivers), so there is always the

Table 14.2 Total and Saturated Fat Intakes (Percentage of Calories) Among Children 2 Months–19 Years, United States, 1988–1991, by Age, Sex, and Race

	Total fat (percent of calories)						Saturated fat (percent of calories)					
	White		Black		Hispanic		White		Black		Hispanic	
	Boys	Girls	Boys	Girls	Boys	Girls	Boys	Girls	Boys	Girls	Boys	Girls
2–11 months	35.8	37.1	39.8	38.2	38.0	39.8	15.6	15.9	15.9	15.8	16.6	16.4
1–2 years	33.1	33.8	35.2	36.0	35.3	34.2	13.7	13.9	13.6	13.9	14.4	14.0
3–5 years	32.7	32.7	35.2	35.2	32.2	34.3	12.7	12.4	13.0	12.7	12.2	13.1
6–11 years	33.8	34.2	35.6	35.5	34.1	34.7	12.9	12.8	12.8	12.5	12.8	13.0
12–15 years	32.7	32.5	34.9	37.9	35.2	34.8	12.4	11.6	12.2	13.3	13.2	13.1
16–19 years	34.4	34.1	36.8	36.2	34.8	35.0	12.8	12.2	12.8	12.7	12.3	12.5

Adapted from McDowell, M. A., Briefel, R. R., Alaimo, K., et al., Energy and macronutrient intakes of persons aged 2 months and over in the United States: Third National Health and Nutrition Examination Survey, Phase 1, 1988–91. Advance data from Vital and Health Statistics; No 255. Hyattsville, MD: National Center for Health Statistics, 1994.

possibility that survey respondents are being less than totally candid about their dietary habits.

DEVELOPMENT OF A PRUDENT LIFESTYLE

Tracking of Diet Over Time

The preceding discussion has described the dietary habits of groups of children of different ages, each measured on a single occasion. One important question is whether, in fact, an individual child's dietary pattern is consistent over time. If there is no consistency, then one would not try to effect a change from an existing pattern, as it would tend to change by itself regardless of educational interventions. On the other hand, if stable dietary habits do develop in childhood, and if these can be modified, then there may be scope for intervention. Thus there may be an educational role for encouraging prudent diets in childhood, if it can be shown that children exposed to these diets maintain prudent diets later in life. To study the persistence of dietary habits, researchers normally use a tracking index, such as the correlation coefficient, which measures the extent to which a group of people, monitored over time, maintain the relative distribution of the parameter of interest. It is a common observation that children who are heavy for their age at one point in time are likely to continue to be heavy for their age in later years as well. Similarly, children with elevated blood pressure are more likely to have elevated blood pressure as adults than are children with lower blood pressure levels (Levine et al., 1979; Nishio et al., 1989; Palti, Gofin, Adler, Grafstein & Belmaker, 1988; Shear, Burke, Freedman, & Berenson, 1986).

Studies of Tracking of Diets in Childhood

Young children are often described as being both picky eaters, that is, as always eating only a few foods, and at the same time as binge eaters, whose tastes and desires shift dramatically from one week to the next. As most children grow normally, however, these changes in dietary habits must, in the long run, balance each other out. Variability in intakes can occur over several time frames. When diets are carefully assessed over a period of several days, a negative correlation between intake at one meal and intake at a subsequent meal appears; this indicates that children self-regulate their intake, even though mean caloric intake at any one meal (breakfast, for example) can vary widely from one day to the next (Birch, Johnson, Andresen, Peters, & Schulte, 1991; Shea et al., 1992).

There is also variability in daily intakes from one day to another. One indicator of this short-term variability is the number of days of measurement required to estimate mean intake with a desired degree of precision. Miller, Kimes, Hui, Andon, and Johnston (1991) obtained multiple 24-hour recalls over 2 years from 70 children aged 5–14 years. These authors concluded that seven dietary recalls would be required to estimate energy intake with reasonable precision, that over 20 dietary recalls would be required to estimate vitamin intakes; and that other nutrients would require an intermediate number of recalls. Nelson et al. (1989) analyzed 7-day dietary records obtained in several settings in England. For the toddlers (ages 1–5 years), 7 days were required to estimate energy intake with an attenuation of 10%, whereas most nutrients could be estimated to this degree of accuracy using 12 or less dietary records. Differences in the stability of dietary patterns between the English toddlers and the American children and methodological differences between the two studies may have contributed to these divergent results. Treiber et al. (1990), in a study of preschool children in Georgia, found low to moderate correlation between two administrations of the 24-hour recall to the child's parent, spaced one week apart. These results highlight the large short-term variability in dietary patterns. In turn, this short-term variability is an unavoidable source of error when one tries to relate dietary intake at two points in time, or tries to relate dietary intake with clinical outcomes.

In considering the effect of habitual diet over the life span, these short-term fluctuations are only of moderate interest, however. Several studies of the stability of dietary habits over childhood, involving repeated assessment of the same children as they grow older, have been conducted. Most have been concerned with intakes of nutrients, rather than with specific foods.

The Bogalusa Heart Study, perhaps the most important study of the early etiology of cardiovascular disease, is a long-term study in a biracial community in Louisiana. Since the early 1970s, children have undergone regular physical examinations and they and their parents have completed questionnaires concerning lifestyle, diet, and other factors. One component of the study is the repeated examination of all children born over a 12-month period. In this birth cohort little correlation was observed between intakes of protein, carbohydrate, fat, and cholesterol, measured with the aid of single 24-hour dietary recalls at 6 months and 4 years of age. Correlation was found between intakes at 3 and 4 years of age, however; this suggests that intake levels may start to stabilize by age 3 years (Nicklas et al., 1987).

Our own data indicate that despite considerable day-to-day variability of dietary intakes, there is substantial tracking of underlying diets among Hispanic preschool children followed over a 19-month period (Stein, Shea, Basch, Contento, & Zybert, 1991). From 1986 to 1989 24-hour dietary recalls were administered on seven occasions (four times in year 1 and three times in year 3) to the children's mothers. Correlations between mean energy and unadjusted nutrient intakes at year 1 and year 3 ranged from 0.27 to 0.45. Correlations were attenuated when intakes were adjusted for energy intake; this suggests that overall energy intake is a consistent source of variation between children. In other words, and as many parents will recognize, some children consistently eat more than others overall, and hence also consume more of specific nutrients.

WHY BE CONCERNED ABOUT INTAKES OF CHILDREN?

In the United States (and in other industrialized societies), one goal of nutrition policy for children is to encourage dietary habits that might prevent or retard the development of the common diseases of adulthood (cardiovascular disease, cancer, diabetes, and others), while permitting the child to grow and achieve his or her full potential (National Research Council, 1989). With respect to the prevention of adult-onset chronic diseases, which are characterized by a long latent period in which subclinical precursor conditions develop and increase in severity, the underlying model governing the formulation of such a policy can be understood in terms of a clinical threshold of disease (see Figure 14.1). One might consider the gradual buildup of atherosclerotic plaque as an example. Fatty streaks have been observed in the arteries of children and young adults who died of other causes and were autopsied (Enos, Holmes, & Beyer, 1953; Holman, McGill, Strong, & Geer, 1958; McNamara, Molot, Stremple, & Cutting, 1971; Strong & McGill, 1962). These streaks increase in density with age, gradually covering greater and greater portions of the arterial wall. Eventually these fatty deposits calcify, resulting in atherosclerotic plaque. This plaque contributes to narrowing of the arterial lumen and

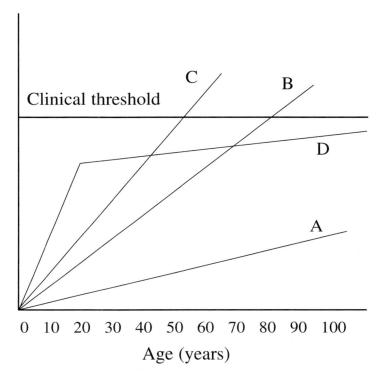

A: Consistent, low-risk throughout life—no symptomatic disease by age 100

B: Consistent, moderate-risk throughout life—symptomatic disease experienced late in life

C: High risk: symptomatic disease experienced in middle adulthood

D: Altered risk: Individual is at high risk initially, but modified risk successfully such that symptomatic disease is not experienced by age 100

Figure 14.1 The Clinical Threshold model of chronic disease risk.

restriction of blood flow, and rupture of the plaque may result in thrombosis and acute myocardial infarction. The clinical-threshold model suggests that this progression occurs over time, at a rate influenced by genetic and environmental factors, with clinical disease (experienced as angina pectoris, peripheral vascular disease, acute myocardial infarction) occurring once the atherosclerotic buildup reaches a critical level or threshold.

In some people, the threshold will be reached earlier in life, whereas for others the threshold will never be crossed; the latter will not experience clinical disease.

The important question is whether diet has an impact on this progression. In other words, can an individual reduce the slope of the progression line to a point at which clinical disease does not appear until very late in life? And if the slope can be modified, does the age at which intervention commences play an important role? In adults, there is consistent, strong evidence that dietary fat and cholesterol intakes have an impact on the process of atherosclerotic progression to clinical disease, and that risk-factor modification reduces disease risk (National Research Council, 1989). These findings have led to strong recommendations to reduce fat and cholesterol intakes.

From the perspective of formulation of nutrition policy for children, the main question is whether these same recommendations should cover childhood, or whether it is enough to encourage adults to consume a heart-healthy diet. There is no reason to assume that the underlying biological process of atherosclerosis is age-dependent. This assumption needs to be tested, however. Children, moreover, lack full autonomy. Widespread dietary change for children should not be prescribed until it is clear that the recommendations are safe and efficacious. This means that the resulting diet should be safe for children, and there should be a benefit to adult health over and above that due to diet modifications that occur in adulthood. With respect to precursors of cardiovascular disease, many studies have examined the relations between dietary fats and serum cholesterol, between dietary minerals and blood pressure levels, and in at least one study, the relation between dietary fat and atherosclerosis. Some of these studies are reviewed in the next section.

Dietary Fat and Serum Cholesterol

The relationship between dietary fat and serum cholesterol in adults has been demonstrated conclusively, and is reviewed elsewhere (National Research Council, 1989). In children, several studies have examined this question.

Observational Studies

Several investigators have used data from the Bogalusa study. Infants fed cow's milk (which is high in fat) had higher serum total cholesterol (TC) than infants fed lower fat formula (Farris, Frank, Webber, Srinivasan, & Berenson, 1982). By the age of 1, correlations were observed between total fat, animal fat, and dietary cholesterol and serum TC level (Berenson et al., 1979). At age 4, dietary cholesterol was associated with TC and low-density lipoprotein cholesterol (LDL-C). At age 7, dietary cholesterol was associated with LDL-C (Nicklas et al., 1988), and at age 10, those in the highest third of serum TC had higher intakes of total fat, animal fat, and saturated fat, but lower intakes of unsaturated fat (Berenson et al., 1989).

Shea et al. (1991) studied a group of 108 5-year-old Hispanic children in New York City. They found that LDL-cholesterol was highest among the children in the upper tertile of fat intake (expressed as nutrient density). Taken together, these studies show a consistent relationship between diet and serum cholesterol levels, in concordance with the association previously demonstrated among adults. The effects may be more marked at the extremes of dietary intake.

Experimental Studies

The Dietary Intervention Study in Children (DISC) is a randomized trial of family-based nutrition education (DISC Collaborative Research Group, 1995). Children 8-10 years of age with moderately elevated serum cholesterol were identified through mass screening, and were entered into a dietary intervention study. At baseline, these children were consuming typical U.S. diets, with 33.4% of energy coming from total fat and 12.6% of energy from saturated fat. Half of the children were encouraged to reduce total and saturated fat intake to 28% and 8% of total calories, respectively. By the end of the third year, mean total fat intake was 28.6% of energy, and mean saturated fat intake was 10.2% of energy in the intervention group, whereas the control group reported no change in mean intakes. At baseline, LDL-cholesterol levels were 130 mg/dl in both groups. In the intervention group, this declined to 115 mg/dl, whereas the control group experienced a slightly smaller decline, to 119 mg/dl. The overall difference, while small, was statistically significant ($p=0.02$).

Dietary Intakes and Blood Pressure

In adults, strong evidence associates blood pressure levels positively with sodium intake, and negatively with potassium and calcium intakes (National Research Council, 1989). The evidence associating blood pressure levels with intakes of other nutrients is less consistent.

In children, association between mineral intakes, as estimated by electrolyte excretion, and blood pressure was either weak or absent in studies conducted in Missisippi (Watson et al., 1980), China (Zhu, He, Pan, Zheng, & Gu, 1987), or Holland (Geleijnse, Drobbee, & Hofman, 1990).

In what is probably the best-designed study using a food-frequency questionnaire, 89 white, middle-class children 3–6 years of age living in Framingham, MA, were found to exhibit a statistically significant effect of calcium (0.19 mmHg reduction per mmol per 1000 kcal) for systolic, but not for diastolic blood pressure; a 6 mmHg difference in systolic blood pressure was observed between the children in the highest and lowest quartiles of calcium intake (Gillman, Oliviera, Moore, & Ellison, 1992).

We have examined associations between intakes of energy, sodium, potassium, calcium, magnesium, and fiber, and blood pressure level and trend in our study of 188 preschool children (48% male, aged 45–61 months at baseline, 91% Hispanic) in New York City (Stein, Shea, Basch, & Zybert, 1995). Increased potassium intake (estimated by dietary recall but not food frequency) was associated with increased systolic (difference between tertiles of energy-adjusted intake 3.8 mmHg) and diastolic (difference between tertiles 1.4 mmHg) blood pressure; this association disappeared after adjusting for other predictors of blood pressure. Energy-adjusted intakes of potassium, magnesium, and calcium were all associated ($p \leq 0.05$) with decreased slope of blood pressure change; again, these associations disappeared after covariate adjustment. We have previously shown that level and trend of stature, obesity, and fitness (all indirectly related to diet through energy adequacy and physical activity) are all determinants of blood pressure level and trend, respectively, in this cohort of preschool children (Gutin et al., 1989; Shea et al., 1994).

Dietary Fat and Atherosclerosis

Until recently it was not possible to obtain measures of atherosclerotic development without autopsy. Recent imaging techniques, such as quantitative coronary arteriography used by Gould et al. (1992) to monitor atherosclerotic regression in their adult patients undergoing radical dietary modification, are invasive and expensive, and are not used in routine care or research among children. To date, only one study has attempted to relate serum cholesterol and development of atherosclerotic plaque in children (Newman et al., 1986). A few of the children recruited into the Bogalusa

Heart Study have died, primarily from motor vehicle crashes, suicide or homicide, and their bodies were available for autopsy. Among these children, the proportion of the aortic intima covered with aortic streaks (which ranged from 1% to 61%) was correlated ($r=0.67$, $p<0.001$) with both total and low-density lipoprotein cholesterol levels measured while the child was still alive.

CONCLUSIONS—THE ROLE OF CHILDREN'S DIET IN THE DEVELOPMENT OF ATHEROSCLEROSIS

Clear evidence is emerging that dietary habits in childhood do indeed have an impact on several precursor conditions associated in adulthood with increased risk of disease. Excessive energy intake, as evidenced by high relative weight for height, is associated with adverse risk factor profiles (obesity, increased blood pressure) even in young children (Gutin et al., 1989; Shea et al., 1994). Good evidence is available for the relation between saturated fat intake and serum cholesterol level, and between serum cholesterol level and the extent of atherosclerosis. Collectively, studies do not demonstrate a consistent effect of diet on blood pressure in children. There is little direct evidence as to the direct effect of dietary fat intake on atherosclerosis. It is important to remember that although suggestive, the available data do not show that childhood diet affects the risk of clinical disease in adults. The reason is that the studies have not considered the potential for changes in lifestyle between childhood and adulthood, which might attenuate or reverse the development of precursor states. Serum cholesterol in adults, for example, is responsive over weeks to a change in dietary composition (Hegsted, Gandy, Nyers, & Stare, 1965). Similarly, even severe atherosclerosis regresses over a period of 1 to 2 years following radical dietary change (Gould et al., 1992; Ornish, 1993). These dynamic relationships argue against the need for dietary intervention to be started early in childhood. We may also refer to the threshold model described earlier, which suggests that the threshold for overt clinical disease is not likely to be reached until later in life, regardless of childhood diet. This caveat does not apply to children of adults with known premature cardiovascular disease, who may have inherited a particular susceptibility to atherosclerosis, and for whom early screening and risk assessment and reduction are clearly indicated.

MODIFICATION OF DIETARY BEHAVIOR

The feasibility of intervention that modifies children's long-term dietary habits has not been adequately tested. Although children as a whole tend to eat diets similar to those of their parents, it is clear that other influences exist. Children of migrants eat a diet more like that of the host country than their parents, who tend to retain the dietary habits of their home country. Health education and parental guidance are not the only sources of information concerning nutrition and health—children are also exposed to peers and advertising. Furthermore, the choices made available to them in supervised settings such as schools, camp, or sporting events will influence the range of potential foods selected. If low-fat choices are unavailable, they cannot be selected, and even with adequate knowledge and desire, changes in diet may not be feasible.

Several studies designed to assess the effect of education on nutritional behavior and cardiovascular risk-factor status among preschool and school-aged populations are presently under way. In one of these (C. E. Basch, personal communication, June 1995), skim and low-fat milk and milk products are being substituted for their whole-milk equivalents in the diet of Hispanic preschool children whose serum cholesterol is normal. In another, the Child and Adolescent Trial for Cardiovascular Health (CATCH), third grade school classes in four regions of the United States have been randomized to three study groups: in-class nutrition education, in-class nutrition education with parental involvement, and control. A detailed report of the CATCH study has appeared as a special issue of *Preventive Medicine* (Resnicow, Robinson, & Frank, 1996). Intervention schools successfully reduced the fat and sodium content of school meals, and children's awareness of the relation between nutrition and health increased. Physical activity increased, and children reported consuming less total fat and saturated fat. No differences between the intervention and control schools were observed for several cardiovascular risk factors (obesity, blood pressure, serum lipids).

The DISC study, described above, has shown that dietary modification among motivated school-aged children is feasible and can be maintained over the medium term, but that the short-term benefits are small. The effort required to attain these changes is beyond the resources available to clinicians in general practice. Modest intervention alone may not lead to measurable change. Moreover, the effects may not persist over the long term and the trial did not assess the feasibility of dietary intervention among children not motivated by knowledge of their own elevated cholesterol.

POTENTIAL ADVERSE EFFECTS
OF FAT RESTRICTION

There has been concern that restricting fat intake in children may retard child growth (Kaplan & Toshima, 1992). Evidence for this claim comes from studies of populations over time, from studies of migrants, and from case reports of children with growth failure.

Studies in Japan and Europe suggest that trends in age-specific height parallel the per capita availability of food. Growth was slowed during World War II, and increased steadily between 1950 and the mid-1970s. These increases parallel increases in per capita fat and protein consumption. A limitation of these studies is that they do not relate growth of individual children to the children's own energy and nutrient intakes, however.

Migrant studies compare attained height in groups of people who share cultural backgrounds but who have been raised in different environments. In the Ni-Hon-San study, men born and living in Japan were compared with men of Japanese descent, born in Japan and living in Hawaii and San Francisco (Kagan et al., 1974). The men in the U.S. study populations were 1.5–1.75 cm taller than men living in Japan. Although total energy intakes were similar, the men in Japan consumed less fat than their migrant counterparts. Other migrant studies have reported similar findings. This type of migrant study suffers from two limitations: first, there is no direct assessment of nutrient intakes during childhood (when dietary restriction may have its impact), and second, it is possible that there were other differences between the migrant populations and those people who remained in the source country. This limitation can be addressed by considering migrants and children of migrants. Such a design reduces the selection biases somewhat, as both groups have migrated, although at different periods. A study using this approach found Israeli-born Jews (almost all of whom were born to immigrant parents) to be 3.1 cm (males) and 2.1 cm (females) taller than Jews who had immigrated to Israel (Tartakovsky, Carel, & Luz, 1983). It is suggested that the healthier lifestyle in Israel did not restrict childhood growth to the extent that this had been restricted in the countries of origin. The study did not, however, restrict its analysis to comparisons of Jews who had migrated to Israel from the same region, nor did it control for age at migration in the migrating generation.

Several authors have published reports of growth failure attributed to excessive dietary restriction. In none of these reports was severe restriction of fat responsible for the caloric deficits—where reported, fat density exceeded 20% in all, and exceeded 25% in most affected children. Pugliese, Lifshitz, Grad, Fort, and Marks-Katz (1983) evaluated 201 children who presented with short stature, delayed puberty, or both. In 14 the syndrome was attributed to self-imposed dietary restrictions motivated by fear of obesity (in the rest, other causes were ascribed). The major identified deficiency was calories; fat concentration of the diet was not reported. In a second report, Pugliese, Weyman-Daum, Moses, and Lifshitz (1987) described seven infants, aged 7–22 months, that had been referred for growth failure. These children had been calorie-deprived by parents over-concerned with obesity and cardiovascular disease. A third report (Lifshitz & Moses, 1989) described children who were being treated (without medical supervision) for hypercholesterolemia. Of the 40 children in the report, 8 experienced growth failure, which was attributed to deficiency of energy and zinc. All children improved under supervision, once caloric intake was increased.

As these reports make clear, severely restricted diets may be detrimental to child health and growth. Nutrition policies that advocate moderate restriction in childhood of dietary fat intakes need to address the legitimate concern that some parents, in their zeal to provide a healthy diet for their children, may in fact provide inadequate nutrition. Nutritional counseling should stress that children who are not increasing in stature are not receiving enough calories. Although moderate fat restriction tends to reduce total energy intake, as the resulting food mix is less calorically dense, this moderate caloric restriction is unlikely to affect health or growth adversely. Vegans, who consume no animal products, generally have low intakes of fat, whereas vegetarians who consume dairy products often have intakes of fat not much lower than omnivores. Children consuming vegetarian diets throughout their life do not, in general, experience growth failure, although they tend to be slightly lighter (~1kg) and shorter (~2cm) than their omnivorous counterparts. One study found a tendency for growth failure in the weaning period, followed by accelerated catch up growth past the age of 3 years (Dwyer et al., 1983). A British study found a slightly increased tendency for vegan children to be below the 5th percentile of height for age at age 4 (Sanders & Purves, 1981), although this deficit had disappeared when the children became older (Sanders, 1988). Several studies that have compared omnivorous children with differing fat intakes have all reached the conclusion that the moderately reduced fat intakes associated with the Step-1 diet of the National Cholesterol Education Program are not associated with growth failure (DISC Collaborative Research Group, 1995; Friedman & Goldberg, 1976; Shea et al., 1993). The adult step-2 diet, in which total fat is reduced to below 20% of total calories and saturated fat to less than 7% of calories, may not provide enough energy for optimal growth in young children. For this reason, the National Cholesterol Education Program (NCEP) Expert Panel on High Blood Cholesterol Levels in Children and Adolescents did not recommend a full step-2 diet for hyperlipidemic children who fail to respond to the step-1 diet, but suggested that saturated fat be reduced to less than 7% of energy, with total fat maintained at less than 30% of energy. (National Cholesterol Education Program, 1991).

CONCLUSIONS

A moderate reduction in fat intake, to the levels recommended by the National Cholesterol Education Program, the American Academy of Pediatrics, and many other authorities, is safe for children past the age of 2 years, and may have beneficial effects on future cardiovascular risk. In particular, saturated fat intakes are related to serum cholesterol levels. These in turn are related to progression of atherosclerosis, in both childhood and adolescence. Atherosclerosis is reversible in adulthood and the impact of childhood atherosclerosis on adult cardiovascular disease is as yet unknown, however. There is only weak and inconsistent evidence that nutrient intakes play a role in determining blood pressure levels in children, provided that total energy intake is appropriate. Overzealous fat restriction may have the adverse result of unduly restricting total energy intakes, which in some instances may result in failure to thrive.

From the perspective of the practicing public health nutritionist, the question of policy implications remains. Children whose family history suggests elevated risk of cardiovascular disease need to be screened, and if found to be hypercholesterolemic, dietary and pharmacological intervention should be considered by their physician. The majority of children are best reached through their parents and the school system. Screening for growth failure and excessive weight gain are both useful. Educational activities to encourage a heart-healthy diet could be targeted at schools in the CATCH model. However, allocation of major resources to such a program needs to await the results of further studies, to assess whether the educational components indeed have an impact on the children's cardiovascular risk factors. Until then, parents should be encouraged to ensure that their children consume a diverse diet that provides adequate calories for growth. An additional role for the nutrition officer is the identification and recruitment of a cadre of influential role models from the community. Finally, reducing the prevalence of overweight and maintaining energy balance through increased physical activity and modest restriction of dietary fat intakes may be the safest way to ensure that children enter adulthood with a low initial risk of premature atherogenic disease.

REFERENCES

American Academy of Pediatrics Committee on Nutrition. (1986). Prudent lifestyle for children: Dietary fat and cholesterol. *Pediatrics, 78,* 521–525

Basch, C. E., Shea, S., & Zybert, P. (1992). Food sources and dietary behavior patterns that determine Latino children's dietary saturated fat intake. *American Journal of Public Health, 82,* 810–815.

Berenson, G. S., Srinivasan, S. R., Hunter, S. M., Nicklas, T. A., Freedman, D. S., Shear, C. L., & Webber, L. S. Risk factors in early life as predictors of adult heart disease: The Bogalusa Heart Study. *American Journal of Medical Science, 298,* 141–51.

Berenson, G. S., Blonde, C. V., Farris, R. P., Foster, T. A., Frank, G. L., Srinivasan, S. R., Voors, A. W., & Webber, L. S. (1979). Cardiovascular disease risk factor variables during the first year of life. *American Journal of Diseases of Children, 133,* 1049–1057.

Birch, L. L., Johnson, S. L., Andresen, G., Peters, J. C., & Schulte, M. C. (1991). The variability of young children's energy intake. *New England Journal of Medicine, 324,* 232–235.

Dwyer, J. T., Andrew, E. M., Berkey, C., Valadian, I., & Reed, R. (1983). Growth in 'new' vegetarian preschool children using the Jenss-Bailey curve-fitting technique. *American Journal of Clinical Nutrition, 37,* 815–827.

DISC (Dietary Intervention Study in Children) Collaborative Research Group. (1995). Efficacy and safety of lowering dietary intake of fat and cholesterol in children with elevated low-density lipoprotein cholesterol: the Dietary Intervention Study in Children (DISC). *Journal of the American Medical Association, 273,* 1429–1435.

Enos, W. F., Holmes, R. H., & Beyer, J. (1995). Coronary disease among United States soldiers killed in action in Korea: Preliminary report. *Journal of the American Medical Association, 152,* 1090–1093.

Farris, R. P., Frank, G. C., Webber, L. S., Sringivason, S. R., & Berenson, G. S. (1982). Influence of milk source on serum lipids and lipoproteins during the first year of life, Bogalusa Heart Study. *American Journal of Clinical Nutrition, 35,* 42–49.

Feld, L. G., & Springate, J. E. (1988). Hypertension in children. *Current Problems in Pediatrics,* 323–373.

Food and Nutrition Board, National Academy of Sciences. (1980). *Recommended daily allowances* (9th ed.). Washington DC: National Academy Press.

Food and Nutrition Board, National Academy of Sciences. (1989). *Recommended daily allowances* (10th ed.). Washington DC: National Academy Press.

Friedman, G., & Goldberg, S. J. (1976). An evaluation of the safety of a low-saturated fat, low-cholesterol diet beginning in infancy. *Pediatrics, 58,* 655–657

Geleijnse, J. M., Drobbee, D. E., & Hofman, A. (1990). Sodium and potassium intake and blood pressure change in childhood. *British Medical Journal, 300,* 899–902.

Gibson, R. S. (1990). *Principles of nutritional assessment.* New York: Oxford University Press.

Gillman, M. W., Oliviera, S. A., Moore, L. L., & Ellison, R. C. (1992). Inverse association of dietary calcium with systolic blood pressure in young children. *Journal of the American Medical Association, 267,* 2340–2343.

Gould, K. L., Ornish, D., Kirkeeide, R., et al. (1992). Improved stenosis geometry by quantitative coronary arteriography after vigorous risk factor modification. *American Journal of Cardiology, 69,* 845–853.

Gutin, B., Basch, C., Shea, S., Contento, I., DeLozier, M., Rips, J., Irigoyen, M., & Zybert, P. (1990). Blood pressure, fitness and fatness in 5- and 6-year old children. *Journal of the American Medical Association, 264,* 1123–1127.

Hegsted, D. M., Gandy, R. B., Nyers, M. L., & Stare, F. J. (1965). Quantitative effects of dietary fat on serum cholesterol in man. *American Journal of Clinical Nutrition, 17,* 281–295.

Hofman, A., Hazebrouk, A., & Valkenburg, H. A. (1983). A randomized trial of sodium intake and blood pressure in newborn infants. *Journal of the American Medical Association, 250,* 370–373.

Holman, R. L., McGill, H. C. Jr, Strong, J. P., & Geer, J. C. (1958). The natural history of atherosclerosis: The early aortic lesions as seen in New Orleans in the middle of the 20th century. *American Journal of Pathology, 34,* 209–235.

Kagan, A., Harris, B. R., Winkelstein, W. Jr., Johnson, K. G., Kato, H., Syme, H. L., Rhoads, C. G., Gay, M. L., Nichaman, M. E., Hamilton, H. B., & Tillotson, J. (1974). Epidemiologic studies of coronary heart disease and stroke in Japanese men living in Japan, Hawaii, and California: Demographic, physical, dietary, and biochemical characteristics. *Journal of Chronic Disease, 27,* 345–363.

Kaplan, R. M., & Toshima, M. T. (1992). Does a reduced fat diet cause retardation in child growth? *Preventive Medicine, 21,* 33–52.

Keys, A. (1980). *Seven countries: A multivariate analysis of death and coronary heart disease.* Cambridge MA: Harvard University Press.

Levine, R. S., Hennekens, C. G. H., Klein, B., Ferrer, P. L., Gourley, J., Cassady, J., Gelband, H., & Jesse, M. J. (1979). A longitudinal evaluation of blood pressure in children. *American Journal of Public Health, 69, 11,* 1175–1177.

Lifshitz, F., & Moses, N. (1989). Growth failure: A complication of dietary treatment of hypercholesterolemia. *American Journal of Diseases of Child, 143,* 537–542

McDowell, M. A., Briefel, R. R., Alaimo, K., Bischof, A. M., Caughman, C. R., Canoll, M. D., Loria, C. M., & Johnston, C. C. (1994). Energy and macronutrient intakes of persons ages 2 months and over in the United States: Third National Health and Nutrition Examination Survey, Phase 1, 1989–91. *Advance data from vital and health statistics;* No 255. Hyattsville, MD: National Center for Health Statistics.

McNamara, J. J., Molot, M. A., Stremple, J. F., & Cutting, R. T. (1971). Coronary artery disease in combat casualties in Vietnam. *Journal of the American Medical Association, 216,* 1185–1187.

Miller, J. Z., Kimes, T., Hui, S., Andon, M. B., & Johnston, C. C. (1991). Nutrient intake variability in a pediatric population: Implications for study design. *Journal of Nutrition, 121,* 265–274.

National Cholesterol Education Program. (1991). *Report of the expert panel on high blood cholesterol levels in children and adolescents.* Rockville, MD: National Heart, Lung, and Blood Institute.

National Research Council. (1989). *Diet and health: Implications for reducing chronic disease risk.* Washington DC: National Academy Press.

Nelson, M., Black, A. E., Morris, J. A., & Cole, T. J. (1989). Between- and within-subject variation in nutrient intake from infancy to old age: Estimating the number of days required to rank dietary intakes with desired precision. *American Journal of Clinical Nutrition, 50,* 155–167.

Nestel, P. J., Poyser, A., & Boulton, T. J. (1979). Changes in cholesterol metabolism in infants in response to dietary cholesterol and fat. *American Journal of Clinical Nutrition, 32,* 2177–82.

Newman, W. P. III, Freedman, D. S., Voors, A. W., Gard, P. D., Srinivasan, S. R., Cresanta, J. L., Williamson, G. D., Webber, L. S., & Berenson, G. S. (1986). Relation of serum lipoprotein levels and systolic blood pressure to early atherosclerosis: The Bogalusa heart study. *New England Journal of Medicine, 314,* 138–144

Nicklas, T. A., Farris, R. P., Smoak, C. G., Frank, G. C., Srinivasan, S. R., Webber, L. S., & Berenson, G. S. (1988). Dietary factors relate to cardiovascular risk factors in early life. Bogalusa Heart Study. *Arteriosclerosis, 8,* 193–199.

Nicklas, T. A., Farris, R. P., Major, C., Frank, G. C., Webber, L. S., Cresanta, J. L., & Berenson, G. S. (1987). Dietary intakes (Bogalusa Heart Study). *Pediatrics, 80,* (Suppl.), 797–806.

Nicklas, T. A., Koschak, M. L., Webber, L. S., & Berenson, G. S. (1992). Nutrient adequacy of low fat diets for children: Bogalusa Heart Study. *Pediatrics, 89,* 221–228.

Nishio, T., Mori, C., Watanabe, K., Haqneda, N., Kishida, K., Hayashi, Y., & Horino, N. (1989). Quantitative analysis of systolic blood pressure tracking during childhood and adolescence using a tracking index: The Shimane Heart Study. *Journal of Hypertension, 7,* (Suppl.), S35–S36.

Ornish, D. (1993). Can lifestyle changes reverse coronary heart disease? *World Reviews of Nutrition and Dietetics, 72,* 38–48

Palti, H., Gofin, R., Adler, B., Grafstein, O., & Belmaker, E. (1988). Tracking of blood pressure over an eight-year period in Jerusalem school children. *Journal of Clinical Epidemiology, 41,* 731–735.

Pugliese, M. T., Lifshitz, F., Grad, G., Fort, P., & Marks-Katz, M. (1983). Fear of obesity: A cause of short stature and delayed puberty. *New England Journal of Medicine, 309,* 513–518.

Pugliese, M., Weyman-Daum, M., & Moses, N., (1987). Parental health beliefs as a cause of non-organic failure to thrive. *Pediatrics, 80,* 187–192.

Resnicow, K., Robinson, T., & Frank, E. (Eds.). (1996). Special issue: The Multicenter Child and Adolescent Trial for Cardiovascular Health (CATCH): Promoting cardiovascular health through schools. *Preventive Medicine, 25,* 377–494.

Sanders, T. A. B. (1988). Growth and development of British vegan children. *American Journal of Clinical Nutrition, 48,* S822–S825.

Sanders, T. A. B., & Purves, R. (1981). An anthropometric and dietary assessment of the nutritional status of vegan preschool children. *Journal of Human Nutrition, 35,* 349–357.

Shea, S., Stein, A. D., Basch, C. E., & Zybert, P. (1992). Variability and self-regulation of energy intake in young children in their everyday environment. *Pediatrics, 90,* 542–546.

Shea, S., Basch, C. E., Stein, A. D., Contento, I. R., Irigoyen, M., & Zybert, P. (1993). Is there a relationship between dietary fat and stature or growth in children three to five years of age? *Pediatrics, 92,* 579–586.

Shea, S., Basch, C. E., Gutin, B., Stein, A. D., Contento, I. R., Irigoyen, M., & Zybert, P. (1994). Changes in aerobic fitness and obesity are related to the rate of increase in blood pressure in children 5 years of age. *Pediatrics, 94,* 465–470.

Shea, S., Basch, C. E., Irigoyen, M., Zybert, P., Rips, J. L., Content, I., & Gutin, B. (1991). Relationships of dietary fat consumption to serum total and low density lipoprotein-cholesterol in Hispanic preschool children. *Preventive Medicine, 20,* 237–49.

Shear, C. L., Burke, G. L., Freedman, D. S., & Berenson, G. S. (1986). Value of childhood blood pressure measurements and family history in predicting future blood pressure status: Results from 8 years of follow-up in the Bogalusa heart study. *Pediatrics, 77,* 862–869.

Sigman-Grant, M., Zimmerman, S., & Kris-Etherton, P. M. (1993). Dietary approaches for reducing fat intake of preschool children. *Pediatrics, 91,* 955–960.

Stein, A. D., Shea, S., Basch, C. E., Contento, I. R., & Zybert, P. (1991). Variability and tracking of nutrient intakes of preschool children based on multiple administrations of the 24-hour dietary recall over three years. *American Journal of Epidemiology, 134,* 1427–1437.

Stein, A. D., Shea, S., Basch, C. E., & Zybert, P. (1995). *A prospective study of intakes of energy, sodium, potasssium, calcium, magnesium and fiber in relation to change in blood pressure among young children.* Presented at the Society for Epidemiologic Research, Snowbird, UT.

Strong, J. P., & McGill, H. C. Jr. (1962). The natural history of coronary atherosclerosis. *American Journal of Pathology, 40,* 37–49.

Tartakovsky, M. B., Carel, R. S., & Luz, Y. (1983). A comparison of the body height of the Israeli-born and immigrants to Israel. *Human Heredity, 33,* 73–78.

Trieber, F. A., Leonard, S. B., Frank, G. C., Musante, L., Davis, H., Strong, W. B., & Levy, M. (1990). Dietary assessment instruments for pre-school children: Reliability of parental responses to the 24-hour recall and a food frequency questionnaire. *Journal of the American Dietetic Association, 90,* 814–820.

Watson, R. L., Langford, H. G., Abernethy, J., Barnes, T. Y., & Watson, M. J. (1980). Urinary electrolytes, body weight and blood pressure: pooled cross-sectional results among four groups of adolescent females. *Hypertension, 2* (Suppl. I), 193–198.

Zhu, K., He, S., Pan, X., Zheng, X., & Gu, Y. (1987). The relation of urinary cations to blood pressure in boys aged seven to eight years. *American Journal of Epidemiology, 126,* 658–663.

CHAPTER 15

Nutrition Policy for the Elderly

David Rush, Robert Russell, and Irwin Rosenberg

I n economically developed societies, the proportionate increase of older people is greater than that of any other age group. This will peak in the next century, as the "baby boomer" generation ages. Thus, these societies will be faced with unprecedented challenges in helping old people sustain their health and quality of life. Meeting nutritional needs is essential to maintaining health, preventing disease, and sustaining function.

SPECIAL CHARACTERISTICS OF OLD PEOPLE

Social and Demographic Changes

There are many social and demographic differences between the elderly and other adults, differences that become more extreme with increasing age.

Increased Proportion of Women

Where no artificial constraints are placed on the well-being of women (unequal resources or opportunities) they live, on average, considerably longer than men. Thus, with increasing age, the proportion of women increases.

Isolation

Among the elderly, with loss of companionship, and with decreased mobility and functional ability, there is increased likelihood of isolation, and consequent feelings of hopelessness. This can initiate a spiral of decreased ability to cope with what are often difficult challenges. Men who live into old age, especially if they survive their spouses or companions, may be less well able to cope with their life situations, particularly in terms of housekeeping and meal preparation.

Depression

The incidence of clinical depression and attempts at suicide increase with advancing age.

Poverty

Although costs of health and nursing homes increase steeply with age, the individual's resources, on average, decrease. Only some of these costs are paid in the United States by Medicare, and there is pressure in the U.S. Congress to cut current Medicare benefits. Nursing home care is only covered by Medicare for limited periods of time, and if long-term nursing home care becomes necessary, the elderly person may have to exhaust economic resources in order to become eligible for Medicaid reimbursement of nursing home care. Approximately half of all nursing home care in the United States is paid by Medicaid, a large part for those who became poor primarily because of their health and nursing home costs ("spend down"). Thus the economic, social, and physical aspects of aging are interrelated and declining economic resources and social supports can compound the physical frailty and social isolation of old age.

Functional Changes

Decreased Ability to Carry out Activities of Daily Living   Activities of daily living (ADLs), and the more basic Instrumental Activities of Daily Living (IADLs) are standard indices of how old people function. The decline in function with aging is variable: the needs of those with markedly eroded function are far greater than those whose abilities remain relatively intact. ADLs are impaired by increased fragility and lack of mobility, by decreased strength, and also by decreased cognitive ability, depression, and loneliness. Nutritional status affects and is affected by all of these.

Cognition and Dementia   Some cognitive functions tend to decrease with aging, such as short-term memory or reaction time. The most dramatic impact of aging is the exponentially increasing proportion of those who become moderately to profoundly impaired from age-associated dementia. There have been estimates of dementia as high as 40% in the population aged 80 and over (Hebert al., 1995). Thus, in planning for nutritional support services, it is essential for public health planners to estimate the numbers of demented old people for whom they must care, and to identify those with this problem, especially those with profound deficits, who are particularly vulnerable to nutritional problems.

Institutionalized Elderly

With increasing age a growing proportion of old people are institutionalized. The primary reasons are physical frailty, immobility, and deterioration in cognitive function. The institutionalized elderly are particularly vulnerable to nutritional problems and these problems must be addressed differently from problems of those who dwell at home. The institutionalized require continuous surveillance and scrutiny, and minimum standards for their care must be set and met.

NUTRITION AND AGING

Our current knowledge of the value of diet and nutrition in disease prevention and health maintenance mandates that nutrition assessment and planning be integral to care for the elderly. Studies of the institutionalized elderly have demonstrated that calorie, protein, and micronutrient malnutrition are common, reflecting and adding to the burden of concurrent chronic disease, as well as to social and economic deprivation (Baker, Frank, Thind, Jaslow, & Louria, 1979; Vir & Love, 1979). In contrast, the prevalence of undernutrition in noninstitutionalized, free-living old people is modest (de Groot, van Staveren, & Hautvast, 1991; Garry, Goodwin, Hunt, Hooper, & Leonard, 1982; Hartz, Russell, & Rosenberg, 1992). Beyond the prevention of poverty and undernutrition, we are also concerned with the role of diet and nutritional factors in the preservation of functional ability and health.

Optimum nutrition for the aging adult, whether well or afflicted with disease, should lessen the risk and/or progression of degenerative disease (cardiovascular, nervous, musculoskeletal, visual, and gastrointestinal) and minimize the negative impact of chronic disease on nutritional status and function.

CHANGING NUTRITIONAL REQUIREMENTS WITH AGING

The physiologic changes of aging affect nutritional needs and requirements. Past dietary recommendations for older adults (e.g., the Recommended Dietary Allowances [RDA] in the United States) have depended on data extrapolated from the young and middle-aged. Now, more concrete information on dietary requirements in the elderly is available. Table 15.1 presents some of the changes in body composition and physiological function with age that influence changing nutritional requirements.

BODY COMPOSITON; LOSS OF LEAN BODY AND MUSCLE MASS (SARCOPENIA)

Body composition changes dramatically with age. Figure 15.1 plots the decline in lean body mass with age (Frontera, Hughes, Lutz, & Evans, 1991). In women, these changes accelerate after menopause, and in both sexes lean body mass declines beyond the age of 80. When pathologic, this has been called "sarcopenia," deficiency of flesh or muscle (Rosenberg, 1989). Loss of muscle mass leads to decreased strength and mobility, and increased severity and frequency of falls.

With age, muscle mass declines more than lean body mass. A study of 959 healthy men aged 20 to 97 years used 24-hour creatinine excretion as a measure of muscle mass (Tzankoff & Norris, 1977) and found dramatically lower levels among men over age 60. At the level of the mid-thigh, muscle accounts for 90% of the cross-sectional area in active young men, but for only 30% in frail elderly women (Fiatarone et al., 1991).

These changes in body composition have nutritional implications. Energy requirements decrease about 100 calories per decade, reflecting the reduction in the amount of lean (metabolizing) body tissue. With decreasing

Table 15.1 Age-Related Changes in Physiologic Function that
Influence Nutrient Needs

- Energy requirements decline as the muscle mass of the aging person decreases: fewer calories are used in physical activity.

- Peripheral tissues of older persons take up fat-soluble vitamins at slower rates, thus vitamin A intake in elderly people results in higher circulating levels of vitamin A.

- There is a decline in immune function with age that may be responsible in part for the increased susceptibility to conditions such as infection and malignancy. At the same time there is evidence that increased vitamin and mineral intake including zinc may counteract this age-related change.

- Although the efficiency of nutrient absorption is relatively well maintained during aging, intestinal absorption of calcium declines.

- Skin synthesis of vitamin D diminishes.

- Metabolic utilization of vitamin B_6 in older subjects is less efficient.

- One-third of individuals over age 70 lose entirely or have significantly diminished capacity to secrete stomach acid. The effect of lower stomach acid on the absorption of vitamin B_{12}, calcium, iron, folic acid, and possibly zinc appears to explain some of the increased tendency for depletion of some of those nutrients with age and the possible need for increased intake by diet or supplement use.

- Both smell and taste decline with age.

---

energy intake micronutrient requirements are less easily met; nursing home residents classified as "sarcopenic" had intakes of vitamin D, magnesium, calcium, and zinc substantially below the RDA (Fiatarone et al., 1990). Sawaya et al. (1996) have recently shown that energy intakes are substantially underestimated in elderly people using classical dietary techniques. In addition, they demonstrated a peculiar inability of the elderly to readapt after a period of low or high energy intake (Roberts et al., 1994). Thus, after a period of enforced over- or underfeeding, elderly people do not readily return their caloric intakes to baseline levels; rather, they continue to over- or underfeed when fed ad libitum. This is in contrast to younger people who immediately return to their former caloric intakes, quickly readapting their energy balance. This observation has important

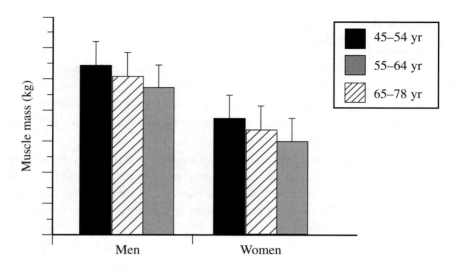

Figure 15.1 Declining muscle mass with increasing age.

clinical implications for elderly people who have been sick and have not eaten adequately during the period of illness. They may need help to return to their optimal calorie intakes.

The amount of muscle is functionally important. In a study of resistance training and nutritional supplementation in frail nursing home residents, aged 72 to 99 years, lean body mass was found to be strongly related to both function and mobility (Fiatarone et al., 1991).

Frontera et al. (1991) found that strength in all muscle groups decreases with increasing age. Although women's strength was only about half that of men, these differences became trivial when adjusted for muscle mass. Thus, preservation of muscle mass into old age is an attractive strategy for preserving strength.

Exercise is an important determinant of body composition and muscle function. Resistance training (i.e., against weight) affects both muscle mass and especially strength; therefore resistance training may prevent or reverse the effects of sedentary living. This was true in frail institutionalized women as old as 100 years (Fiatarone et al., 1990). Among previously sedentary nonagenarians enrolled in a resistance-training program for the lower extremities, the cross-sectional muscle area of their mid-thigh went up by 9% and maximal muscle strength increased by 174% (Fiatarone et al., 1991).

The amount of body muscle is of metabolic importance: skeletal muscle is the largest site for glucose disposal and muscle mass is correlated with glucose tolerance. Moreover, if lean body mass is maintained (or even enhanced) by exercise, energy, micronutrient intake, and basal metabolic rate can be sustained with advancing age (Shock, 1972; Tzankoff & Norris, 1978).

DECLINING BONE DENSITY AND SKIN SYNTHESIS OF VITAMIN D

Inadequate vitamin D intake can lead to bone loss and increased risk of fracture (see Chapter 10). Levels of 25-hydroxyvitamin D, the best clinical index of adequacy of available vitamin D, decline with age (Tsai et al., 1987) and are low in the winter and spring because of lower exposure to sunlight (Stamp & Round, 1974). Reduced levels of 25-hydroxyvitamin D in the elderly reflect declining intake, decreased sun exposure, and perhaps most important, less efficient skin synthesis of vitamin D (Webb, Kline, & Holick, 1988). Krall, Sahyoun, Tannenbaum, Dallal, and Dawson-Hughes (1989) have reported that among healthy postmenopausal women, 25-hydroxyvitamin D levels were lower in winter only in those whose vitamin D intakes were below 220 I.U. daily. Treatment with a vitamin D supplement of 400 I.U. prevented significant seasonal variation in 25-hydroxyvitamin D and, more important, reduced winter bone loss from the spine (Dawson-Hughes et al., 1991).

Those with seasonal bone changes (increases in summer/fall, decreases in winter/spring) also had parallel seasonal changes of similar magnitude in lean tissue mass; this suggests that vitamin D may also have a role in preserving muscle mass.

Two studies have challenged these results, however (Aloia et al., 1994; Reid, Ames, Evans, Gamble, & Sharpe, 1993). In one study beneficial effects on lumbar spinal bone density were seen in elderly people taking a calcium supplement of 1,000 mg/day, even though mean dietary intake of the calcium supplement group was in the range of 800 mg/day (the present RDA). It is not known what amounts of calcium are required in the medical management of women with established osteoporosis, that is, whether greater amounts of dietary calcium may be needed than recommended by the National Institutes of Health (NIH) Consensus Panel. However, difficulty may arise from a very high calcium dietary intake; there may be interference with the absorption of other minerals. This needs further study before strong recommendations for further increases in calcium intake can be made. In addition, exercise in the elderly might reduce bone loss, which could further moderate calcium need.

A recent study in which normal human volunteers were purposely depleted of vitamin K appears to show that elderly people are more resistant to acute vitamin-K deficiency than younger subjects (Ferland, Sadowski, & D'Brien, 1993). The best way to judge vitamin K deficiency is uncertain, however. In the past, blood-coagulation parameters have been used, but it has recently been suggested that carboxylation of bone protein is more susceptible to vitamin K deficiency than are various coagulation factors (Shearer, 1995). Thus, a functional test (carboxylation of vitamin K dependent protein) could be more useful for defining vitamin K deficiency than standard tests of vitamin K adequacy.

IMMUNITY, NUTRITION, AND AGING

Beginning with the involution of the adenoids and the thymus, there is a continuing decline of the relative mass of immune tissue over the life cycle; this is associated with some decline in immune function (Thomas & Weigle, 1989). Increased susceptibility to infection and certain cancers in old age may be related to declining immune function, and adequate protein, vitamin, and mineral intake is essential to the integrity of immune function. Immune function may also be influenced by dietary lipids that are precursors of eicosanoids, prostaglandins, and leukotrienes; eicosanoid synthesis can be modified by dietary antioxidants, such as vitamin E, selenium, vitamin C, and copper. The age-associated decline in T-cell mediated immune function has been attributed to defective interleukin II production and responsiveness, and healthy elderly subjects supplemented with 800 I.U. of vitamin E for 30 days had significantly greater production of interleukin II than those consuming a placebo (Meydani et al., 1989). Chandra (1992) found that a multivitamin, multimineral supplement improved in vitro lymphocyte function, and led to lowered incidence of infections.

Vitamin B_6 depletion in healthy elderly subjects causes significant reduction in interleukin II production, which returns to baseline following vitamin B_6 repletion (Meydani et al., 1990a). Zinc deficiency in rats (Dowd,

Kelleher, & Guillou, 1986) and humans is associated with impaired T-cell mediated function. Thus, protein malnutrition, zinc deficiency, vitamin B_6 deficiency, and inadequate antioxidant intake, all conditions for which the elderly are at greater risk, may negatively influence the function of the immune system. It is reasonable to suppose that some of the age-related decline in immune function may be preventable by dietary modification (Chandra, 1989).

NUTRITION AND THE AGING VASCULAR SYSTEM

The associations among dietary fat, cholesterol, and heart disease are attenuated, but do not disappear, with age. Also, high blood levels of homo-cysteine, a nonprotein-forming sulfur amino acid, are related to vascular disease. The moderate elevations in circulating homocysteine that are associated with aging (Selhub, Jacques, Wilson, Rush, & Rosenberg, 1993) may increase risk of coronary heart disease, stroke (Clark et al., 1991; Ueland & Refsum, 1989), and peripheral occlusive vascular disease (Boers et al., 1985). Blood homocysteine levels are inversely related to folate, vitamin B_{12} and vitamin B_6 intake and blood levels: high homocysteine levels are due, in part, to subclinical vitamin deficiency (Selhub et al., 1993). Low vitamin B_{12} stores, with resulting high homocysteine levels, can be caused by atrophic gastritis. The incidence of atrophic gastritis rises with age: approximately 40% by age 80 (Krasinski et al., 1986). The resulting achlorhydria impairs the intestinal absorption of food-bound vitamin B_{12} by lowering gastric acid-peptic activity.

Some deficits in neurocognitive function in the elderly are probably caused by moderate elevations in homocysteine. Lindenbaum et al. (1988) have shown that vitamin B_{12} therapy, which reduces homocysteine levels, also improves function of some neurologically impaired individuals, often in the absence of hematologic signs of vitamin deficiency and even with vitamin B_{12} blood levels in the lower end of the normal range.

NUTRITION AND COGNITIVE FUNCTION

The central nervous system (CNS) is exquisitely sensitive to its nutrient supply. In turn, the CNS has profound effects on dietary intake. The

Table 15.2 Neurological and Behavioral Effects of Vitamin Deficiencies

Vitamin	Presentation
1. Thiamin (B_1)	Beri-Beri, Wernicke-Korsakoff's psychosis
2. Niacin (B_3)	Pellagra, dementia
3. Pantothenic Acid	Myelin degeneration
4. Pyridoxine (B_6)	Peripheral neuropathy, convulsions
5. Folate	Irritability, depression
6. Cobalamin (B_{12})	Peripheral neuropathy, subacute; combined system degeneration, dementia
7. Vitamin E	Spinocerebellar degeneration, peripheral axonopathy

number and function of brain receptors for cholecystokinin, opioidlike endorphins (Morley, Levine, Yim, Yim, & Lowy, 1983), and serotonin decline with age in laboratory animals, but the importance of these observations for humans is uncertain. In addition, there are well-documented declines in olfactory function and less dramatic declines in taste that may influence eating behavior in the elderly (Schiffman, Hornack, & Reilly, 1979).

Table 15.2 describes nutrients required for central nervous system function. Although overt vitamin and mineral deficiencies are uncommon, milder, subclinical vitamin deficiencies may play a role in the pathogenesis of declining neurocognitive function with age (Rosenberg & Miller, 1992). Healthy elderly subjects with low blood levels of certain vitamins score less well on tests of memory and nonverbal abstract thinking (Goodwin, Goodwin, & Garry, 1983). Vitamin B_{12} treatment can reverse cognitive and peripheral nervous-system deficits, even in the absence of the hematologic abnormalities of vitamin B_{12} deficiency (Lindenbaum et al., 1988). Twenty percent of the Framingham Heart Study cohort (age 69–96) have elevated homocysteine levels, and most of these high levels are associated with low circulating levels of folate, vitamin B_{12}, or vitamin B_6 (Selhub et al., 1993). Elevated blood levels of homocysteine are strong predictors of occlusive carotid arteriosclerosis (Selhub et al., 1995). Homocysteine levels may be lowered by increasing dietary levels of folic acid or vitamin B_6; however, in the case of vitamin B_{12} it is not certain how best to treat elderly people with B_{12} deficiency or borderline B_{12} deficiency, due to the high prevalence of atrophic gastritis in this population. Food-bound vitamin B_{12} is not well absorbed in hypochlorhydria, but crystalline B_{12} (which is used in vitamin supplements) appears to be easily absorbed (Suter, Golner, Goldin, Morrow, & Russell, 1991). At the present time most practitioners continue to give vitamin B_{12} by injection to elderly people who are B_{12} deficient. It is probable that oral supplements of crystalline B_{12} in relatively low doses (e.g., 15–25 mg) constitute adequate treatment for B_{12} deficiency in the elderly with atrophic gastritis, however. Given the potentially devastating effects of vitamin B_{12} deficiency on the nervous system and the high prevalence of atrophic gastritis, the 1989 RDA for vitamin B_{12} for the elderly should not have been decreased from 3.0 mg to 2.0 mg: 3.0 mg is more prudent, given our present state of knowledge.

NUTRITION AND VISION

Visual deficit is the commonest functional impairment in old people. Nearly half of the population between age 75 and 85 has significant visual loss because of cataracts (Kahn et al., 1977). Fortunately, loss of vision due to cataracts can be corrected by surgery; cataract removal has become the most common operation performed in the elderly. There is growing evidence that onset of cataracts can be retarded by attention to behavioral and nutritional factors (Taylor, 1992). Smoking and excessive light exposure both cause cataracts. Antioxidant nutrients (vitamin C, vitamin E, and beta-carotene) in and around the lens may be protective (Jacques & Chylack, 1991; Taylor, Jacques, & Dorey, 1993). It has been recently demonstrated that the carotenoids leutein and zeaxanthin are present in the lens (Seddon et al., 1994); however, it is uncertain that these antioxidants play a role in cataract prevention. Several observational and case-control studies have documented lower rates of cataract among those with high antioxidant intake and serum levels (Jacques & Chylack, 1991). Intervention studies that are now under way should provide better information about the optimum levels of intake.

Antioxidant nutrients may protect against macular degeneration, the most common irreversible cause of blindness in the elderly (Taylor et al., 1991). Zeaxanthin and leutein are both concentrated in the macular region of the retina and these carotenoids may play a role in preventing senile macular degeneration. Seddon et al. (1994) showed that there is an inverse relationship between senile macular degeneration and the intake of vegetables (especially spinach), which are high in leutein and zeaxanthin . Until further studies are available, universal dietary supplementation with antioxidants is not recommended. However, it is prudent to recommend generous intakes of green, yellow, and orange fruits and vegetables.

THE ROLE OF ORGANIZED PUBLIC HEALTH IN NUTRITIONAL WELL-BEING OF THE ELDERLY

Public Health Education and the Attempt to Affect Health Behavior

Public health authorities are necessary participants in the health education of both the community and professionals, aiming to optimize nutritional behavior and status among the elderly. There are many strategies available: dissemination of written and audiovisual materials, promoting health fairs for the public, meetings and symposia for professionals, supporting and organizing community programs to promote exercise and better dietary habits, and so on. The aim is to raise the level of nutritional knowledge and improve nutritional behaviors of old people in the community, as well as in institutions. These educational efforts should address the following issues.

Weight and Obesity

Although much emphasis is focused on the importance of avoiding and treating obesity, the more serious problem among the elderly is the avoidance of wasting. On average, weight stops rising in the 60's and decreases thereafter, simultaneous with an increase in the proportion of body fat and a decrease in the proportion of bone and muscle. There is no direct evidence from trials, but prudence dictates that, except for those with specific pathologies (e.g., diabetes, hypertension), weight loss programs are inappropriate for people after the age of 65 or 70. Rather, sustaining body weight, and avoiding consequent loss of muscle and bone mass should be the objectives for the individual and the community. Change in the body mass index (BMI; kg/m^2) is a strong predictor of morbidity and mortality.

Increased mortality is associated with extremes in BMI (U.S. Department of Agriculture, 1990). (However, many studies have shown that levels of BMI in old people vary enormously from community to community, as well as within communities [de Groot et al., 1991] and that the mean BMI of people in their 70's may be as high as 29 or 30, with no obvious adverse effects.)

Physical Activity

Another element essential to continued well-being in old age is adequate and vigorous exercise, both aerobic and against weight resistance. There is now clear evidence that aerobic physical activity is associated with reduced risk of cardiovascular disease and overall mortality (Helmrich, Ragland, Leung, & Paffenbarger, 1991; Blair, Kohl, Barlow, & Gibbons, 1991; Paffenbarger, Hyde, Wing, & Hsieh, 1986) and that in spite of what was considered to be inevitable muscle wasting with age, systematic programs to maintain and increase muscle strength are successful in sustaining and even increasing muscle and bone mass, and strength. It has not yet been established whether exercise affects the incidence of osteoporotic fractures, the incidence and severity of falls, and the preservation of functional capacity. Prudence dictates, however, the promotion of individual and community exercise programs.

Exercise in the free-living population, even among the oldest old, can be promoted in a variety of ways by those in public health, through educational efforts, and by directly promoting programs, such as the state of Massachusetts' "Keep Moving" program, which helps groups of old people in the community organize themselves for regular, vigorous walking.

Thus, *all* old people should, to the limits of their mental and physical ability, engage in both aerobic exercise and strength training. This should be in the forefront of any public health program and policy for nutritional support in the elderly. Any place and organization where older people congregate or meet on a regular basis should consider implementation of exercise programs: churches, senior centers, retirement communities, and so on. The more accessible and less forbidding such programs become, the more likely they will be implemented and used. A new generation of exercise support professionals may be ultimately required, but dietitians, social workers, nurses and public health personnel, including the health officer, should become the vanguard in this aspect of preventive care for the elderly.

Diet

The public health messages for diet are not radically different for the elderly from those for other adults, but there are high-risk nutrients, and it is essential that energy, protein, fiber, calcium, vitamin D, vitamin B_{12}, folate, vitamin B_6, and several other nutrients be ingested in adequate amounts. In the past, RDAs were grouped for all of those who are 50 and over; this can no longer be justified. The Surgeon General recommends that older Americans consume sufficient nutrients and energy and achieve levels of physical activity that maintain desirable body weight and may prevent or delay the onset of chronic disease. It is difficult to maintain adequate nutrient intake on low-calorie diets; this is another reason older people should maintain at least moderate levels of physical activity and sedentary older individuals should be counseled on appropriate methods to increase caloric expenditure. Recommended intakes of calcium for men and women over age 65 are 1500 mg/day and at least 400 I.U. of vitamin D per day. These are higher than for younger adults (NIH Consensus Statement, 1994) and may require dietary supplements.

Older persons who do not (or cannot) consume adequate levels of nutrients from food sources and those who have dietary, biochemical, or clinical evidence of inadequate intake should receive advice about the proper type and dosage of nutrient supplements. Self-prescribed supplementation, especially in large doses, however, may be harmful and should be discouraged. Recent surveys show the importance of vitamin D intake in the range of at least 10 mg (400 I.U.), particularly for individuals living in the extreme north latitude where sunlight-generated vitamin D synthesis in the skin is nearly absent during the winter months. Increased requirements in aging have been defined for riboflavin; however, no clear health benefit has been demonstrated from an increase in dietary riboflavin to an aged population (Boisvert et al., 1993).

The following list includes other topics that should be addressed in public health education efforts:

1. Maintain hydration consciously, especially in hot, dry weather, as thirst in the elderly is not always an adequate guide to fluid needs.
2. Use relatively high fiber diets to avoid constipation, a particular danger with decreased physical activity.
3. Older people who suffer from diet-related chronic diseases should receive dietary counseling from dietitians, and those who take medications should be given professional advice on diets that minimize food–drug interactions.

ISSUES TO CONSIDER WHEN OLD PEOPLE COME IN CONTACT WITH THE HEALTH CARE SYSTEM

Almost all old people come into fairly regular contact with the health care system. It is therefore an attractive strategy to use such contacts as a way of assessing nutritional needs, and then disseminating nutritional information. We recommend counseling diets low in animal fats, high in vegetables, fruits, and whole grains, with sufficient energy and protein. Although there is no general policy on the use of vitamin supplements, supplements that supply the Recommended Daily Allowances are reasonable. A case can be made for supplementation for the following nutrients: vitamin D, vitamin B_{12}, calcium, and vitamin E. As indicated above, Vitamin D supplementation in the range of 400 mg has been recommended for homebound and institutionalized elderly not exposed to sunlight. Supplemental oral vitamin B_{12} may be needed in many elderly people with atrophic gastritis, a condition that interferes with absorption of food-bound vitamin B_{12}. Calcium may be needed by those who cannot increase their dietary sources of calcium, particularly if they avoid dairy products. Finally, vitamin E supplementation in pharmacologic amounts may have a protective effect against coronary artery disease due to inhibition of low-density lipoprotein oxidation (Rimm et al., 1993). The doses that are required for such an effect appear to be well out of the range that is possible in a healthy diet, however. Beneficial effects of vitamin E supplementation have also been reported on immune function; however, the quantities required are beyond the range that can be achieved in the ordinary, healthy diet (400–800 I.U./day) (Meydani et al., 1990b). Clark et al. (1996) found a halving of serious cancer incidence in a double-blinded trial of supplementation with selenium. This is extremely provocative, but the study needs to be replicated before a definitive policy recommendation can be made: This finding was for a secondary outcome of the trial.

ASSESSING NUTRITIONAL NEEDS IN THE HEALTH CARE SETTING

Medical History

A carefully performed history is central to defining nutrition risk and possible deficiency. Some of the findings in the medical history suggesting

Table 15.3 Findings in the Medical History that Suggest Increased
Risk of Nutrient Deficiency

Recent weight loss

Restricted dietary intake
    limited variety
    food avoidances

Psychosocial situation
    depression, cognitive impairment
    isolation, economic difficulties

Problems with eating, chewing, swallowing

Previous surgery

Increased losses due to gastrointestinal disorders, such as
    malabsorption and diarrhea

Systemic disease interfering with appetite or eating
    (chronic lung, liver, heart and renal disease, abdominal angina,
    cancer)

Excessive alcohol use

Medications that interfere with appetite and/or nutrient metabolism

---

increased risk of nutrient deficiency are listed in Table 15.3. Unintentional
loss or gain of 5 to 10 pounds or more of body weight in the past 6 months
to a year is a strong indication of likely coexistent morbidity.

The history should include a qualitative assessment of diet, including a
description of the usual dietary pattern; problems in eating, chewing, swallowing, or bowel function; and description of food avoidances as well as
drug use that may influence appetite or nutrient utilization. The number of
daily servings of breads, cereals, legumes, and fruits and vegetables, along
with frequency of intake of meat, fish, and poultry will provide an overview
of dietary pattern. The frequency and content of dietary supplements should
be noted.

Weight and Height

Although weight is an essential part of any nutritional evaluation,
height is also important, as height can decrease with age due to spinal
compression.

Laboratory Measures

Low serum albumin level (below 3.5 g/dL) is associated with protein depletion and subsequent morbidity and mortality. Except in starvation, however, dietary intake of protein is unrelated to serum albumin levels. Very low cholesterol levels are correlated with increased mortality in the institutionalized elderly, but are probably unrelated to diet. A total lymphocyte count under 1500 per cm^3 may also reflect calorie-protein malnutrition.

The risk of folate and B$_{12}$ deficiency is increased with age: 20% of those over age 65 may have borderline or low vitamin B$_{12}$ levels.

With age, there is increased fat deposition in the muscles, therefore standard anthropometric measures such as arm circumference and fatfold thickness give underestimates of body fat content. More sophisticated techniques such as bioelectric impedance measurements do not provide as valid results in old people as in younger subjects (Roubenoff, Dallal, & Wilson, 1995).

PUBLICLY FUNDED OR SPONSORED NUTRITIONAL PROGRAMS FOR THE ELDERLY

Inevitably, the public health authorities will be involved in planning, targeting, and monitoring scarce public resources for nutritional programs for the elderly. These include home-delivered meals, homemaker and other community-based home services for the frail elderly, provision of congregate meals, and participation in such ventures as food pantries and other private or voluntary activities. Typically, private agencies or church groups lack the staffing and background to evaluate who is at greatest need, and what the optimal meal content might be. Burt (1993) showed that the majority of those who might profit most from senior meals programs are not receiving them and that the majority of those receiving congregate meals often are not those at greatest nutritional or economic risk. As pressure for the accountability of public or private funds aimed at helping the needy increases, the public health officer will be one of several professionals called on to help set the criteria for such programs and to see whether these criteria have been met.

The public health officer must take into account the age and gender distribution of the population at risk, its economic, ethnic and social status, the likely levels of disability, and the proportion that is institutionalized. The incidence of the various risk factors for nutritional deficit varies strongly with each of these factors, as will the likely efficacy of strategies to respond to such needs.

Food Stamps

Given the general reduction in income among those no longer active in the work force, it is important that old people use available mechanisms for increasing food supply, when eligible. The elderly should therefore be regularly assessed for eligibility for food stamps and other public-assistance programs.

Congregate Meals Programs

The proportion of federal funds going to congregate versus home delivered meals has been falling progressively, although the eligibility criteria for congregate meals are very inclusive (self-declared age) and have not changed. Recipients must only state that they are at least 60 years of age; there is no means test. Health and social professionals caring for old people should encourage participation in these programs, but as currently constituted, the programs are limited and cannot provide for all who are eligible.

The central criteria for meals programs for the ambulatory elderly will be economic and social: the justification for these programs is to get adequate amounts of a well-balanced diet to the poorest elderly, and to promote the social experience of those who are most likely to live in isolation. Thus, evaluation is essential for congregate meals programs: they ought to be where the poor elderly are concentrated. Moreover effective relationships need to be established between these programs and other social service program, so that those in greatest need are directed to and have relatively easy access to them.

Home-Delivered Meals and Other Services for the Homebound Elderly

There has been a marked growth in the United States in home-delivered meals programs over the last decades. Typically, these programs have been financed jointly by federal, state, and voluntary sources, and have involved significant volunteer time and effort. The programs are appealing because they aim to improve the independence and nutritional well-being of the recipients. Unfortunately, the results of available studies do not clearly demonstrate that nutritional status has been improved or that institutionalization has been deferred as a result of the provision of home-delivered meals and other home-based services.

OTHER COMMUNITY FOOD AND MEALS PROGRAMS

Food pantries and many meals programs for the poor and homeless have tended to be run by churches and other charitable groups, but public health authorities can be of great help to these community efforts by assisting in the design, placement, and content of the programs, and by helping with some minimal data gathering to see whether the programs meet goals.

SETTING STANDARDS AND MONITORING THE NUTRITIONAL NEEDS OF THE INSTITUTIONALIZED ELDERLY

Public health authorities will inevitably have some jurisdiction over those institutions in which old people are being cared for, either temporarily or permanently. These include the hospital and the nursing home and are likely to include, at least in the future, other facilities for old people, such as retirement communities, old age homes, and so on.

A large and well-documented literature exists on the importance of nutritional status for both medical and surgical outcomes. The techniques for improving preoperative nutritional status are often complex and take skilled intervention and monitoring. Although nutritional status is strongly related to surgical outcome, it is less clear that intensive nutritional rehabilitation of individuals with poor nutritional status can achieve major improvements in lowering morbidity and mortality.

On the other hand, setting standards for, and monitoring the care of the chronically institutionalized elderly, especially those who are most debilitated, the nursing home population, is an essential part of public health activity. Two-thirds of nursing home residents do not meet the

Recommended Daily Allowance for energy and protein intakes (Abassi & Rudman, 1994). Inadequate dietary intake can be caused by depression, physical disability, cognitive deficit, unmet needs for assistance with eating, poor dentition, and anorexic effects of inactivity, illness, and medication. Chronic illness interacts with nutritional status: needs are increased, just as intake may be decreased by such conditions as decubitus ulcers, urinary tract infection, chronic bronchitis, congestive heart failure, rheumatoid arthritis, and so on. Nursing home staffing may be inadequate fully to care for patients who are unable to monitor and sustain their own diets, not only those with chronic illness, but especially those with cognitive deficit.

Over the next several years, standards of nutritional care and monitoring will become a part of certification and will be required for continued public and private nursing-home care reimbursement. It is likely that semiquantitative measurement and plotting of food intake and body weight will be required with urgent attention to those with acute, unintentional weight loss (i.e., 5–10 pounds over a 6-month to 1-year period).

In summary, residential institutions for the elderly should pay special attention to meeting their clients' caloric and other nutrient needs. Nutritional assessment and guidance should be undertaken at admission or enrollment in, and discharge from, institutional or community-based services for older adults (for example, acute- and long-term care inpatient services, hospital-based outpatient services, alcohol and drug treatment programs, community health services, and home-delivered meals programs).

SUMMARY, AND LIKELY FUTURE TRENDS

As we write, it becomes more likely that the American elderly enrolled in Medicare will be receiving a higher proportion of their health care from health maintenance organizations (HMOs) and other centralized providers of health care. As health care becomes more centralized, and as a higher proportion of payment comes from the government or other third-party sources, it is likely that there will be stringent minimum standards of nutritional care. The elderly use health care facilities more regularly and intensively than do any other age group except infants. Thus, minimum standards of care for the ambulatory elderly are likely to fall more and more into the purview of public health (and the public health officer). Burt (1993) found that in poor communities up to 30% of old people may present some evidence of compromised access to food or nutritional stress. Although the rates in the general community are lower (somewhere in the range of 5%–10%), this still represents a large group of very vulnerable old people.

Several schemes have been developed for community assessment of nutritional status. The Nutrition Screening Initiative is the best known (Posner, Jette, Smith, & Miller, 1993). However, there is little or no empirical evidence that broad-based population screening is an effective mechanism for identifying and intervening among old people (Rush, 1993). It has not been established that current screening instruments have adequate levels of sensitivity and specificity to identify those likely to profit from intervention, and we do not know if screening is cost-beneficial, that is, better than other strategies in terms of results achieved. Although this assessment tool has yet to be shown to be useful, the thrust is clear: attention to diet, weight, and exercise, as well as to economic resources and a general psychosocial well-being will inevitably become part of obligated health care for old people. Although this seems clear, how to carry out such goals is not. We lack proven interventions and estimates of their relative costs and benefits; further, there are no validated risk assessments to identify those who are likely to profit from such interventions.

What little work has been done on health screening in the elderly has not been encouraging. A study of population screening for high blood pressure in one county of Norway showed that very few new cases not already identified and involved in the health care system were uncovered by a large and expensive population survey for hypertension (Holmen et al., 1991). Other studies of less than optimal health behaviors and of the presence of cardiovascular risk factors, such as high cholesterol levels, have yielded such high rates of those at risk that health care services would be overwhelmed and unable to cope with all those who are identified as being at risk (Gibbins, Riley, & Brimble, 1993).

EVALUATION

We cannot stress strongly enough that evaluation is a necessity for new and, indeed, ongoing public health programs. Without such evaluation, resources cannot be efficiently allocated and programs cannot be modified to function better. In the political arena they cannot be defended on the basis of actual performance. Program evaluation should be built into programs at their inception, and appropriate and adequate data should be collected as part of the routine process of carrying out the program. Resources should be allocated in the program's budget to make sure that these data are collected, and effectively used and disseminated. Without such evaluation, programs will not be optimally managed and will be vulnerable to attack.

REFERENCES

Abassi, A. A., & Rudman, D. (1994). Undernutrition in the nursing home: Prevalence, consequences, causes and prevention. *Nutrition Reviews, 52,* 113–122.

Aloia, J. F., Vaswani, A., Yeh, J. K., Ross, P. L., Flaster, E., & Dilmanian, F. A. (1994). Calcium supplementation with and without hormone replacement therapy to prevent postmenopausal bone loss. *Annals of Internal Medicine, 120,* 97–103.

Baker, H., Frank, O., Thind, I. S., Jaslow, S. P., & Louria, D. B.(1979). Vitamin profiles in elderly persons living at home or in nursing homes versus profiles in healthy subjects. *Journal of the American Geriatric Society, 29,* 444–450.

Boers, G. H. J., Smals, A. G. H., Trijbels, F. J. M., Fowler, B., Bakkeren, J. A. J. M., Schoonderwaldt, H. C., Kleijer, W., & Kloppenborg, P. W. C. (1985). Heterozygosity of homocysteinuria in premature peripheral and cerebral occlusive vascular disease. *New England Journal of Medicine, 313,* 709–715.

Boisvert, W. A., Mendoza, I., Castaneda, C., De Portocarrero, L., Solomons, N. W., Gershoff, S. N., & Russell, R. M. (1993). Riboflavin requirement of healthy elderly humans and its relationship to macronutrient composition of the diet. *Journal of Nutrition, 123,* 915–925.

Burt, M. R. (1993). *Hunger among the elderly: Local and national comparisons.* Washington, DC: Urban Institute.

Blair, S. N., Kohl, H. W. III, Barlow, C. E., & Gibbons, L. W. (1991). Physical fitness and all-cause mortality in hypertensive men. *Annals of Medicine, 23,* 307–312.

Chandra, R. K. (1989). Nutritional regulation of immunity and risk of illness in old age. *Immunology, 67,* 141–147.

Chandra, R. K. (1992). Effect of vitamin and trace-element supplementation on immune responses and infection in elderly subjects. *Lancet, 340,* 1124–1127.

Clark, L. C., Combs, G. F. Jr., Turnbull, B. W., Slate, E. H., Chalker, D. K., Chow, J., Davis, L. S., Glover, R. A., Graham, G. F., Gross, E. G., Krongrad, A., Lesher, J. L. Jr., Park, H. K., Sanders, B. B. Jr., Smith, C. L., & Taylor, R. (for

the Nutritional Prevention of Cancer Study Group). (1996). Effects of selenium supplementation for cancer prevention in patients with carcinoma of
the skin. A randomized controlled trial. *Journal of the American Medical
Association, 276,* 1957–1963.

Clarke, R., Daly, L., Robinson, K., Naughton, E., Cahalane, S., Fowler, B., &
Graham, I. (1991). Hyperhomocysteinemia: An independent risk factor for
vascular disease. *New England Journal of Medicine, 324*(17),1149–1155.

Dawson-Hughes, B., Dallal, G. E., Krall, E. A., Harris, S., Sokoll, L. J., &
Falconer, G. (1991). Effect of vitamin D supplementation on wintertime and
overall bone loss in healthy postmenopausal women. *Annals of Internal
Medicine, 115,* 505–512.

de Groot, L. C. P. G. M., van Staveren, W. A., & Hautvast, G. A. J. (Eds.). (1991).
Euronut-Seneca: Nutrition and the Elderly in Europe. *European Journal of
Clinical Nutrition, 45*(Suppl.), 3 Dec.

Dowd, P. S., Kelleher, J., & Guillou, P. J. (1986). T-lymphocyte subsets and inter-
leukin-2 production in zinc deficient rats. *British Journal of Nutrition, 55,*
59–69.

Ferland, G., Sadowski, J. A., & O'Brien, M. E. (1993). Dietary induced subclinical vitamin K deficiency in normal human subjects. *Journal of Clinical
Investigation, 91,* 1761–1768.

Fiatarone, M. A., Marks, E. C., Ryan, N. D., Meredith, C. N., Lipsitz, L. A., &
Evans, W. J. (1990). High-intensity strength training in nonagenarians.
Effects on skeletal muscle. *Journal of the American Medical Association,
263,* 3029–3034.

Fiatarone, M. O'Neill,E., Ryan, N., Joseph, L., Roberts, S., Kehayias, J., Lipsitz,
L., & Evans, W. (1991). Body composition and muscle function in the very
old. *Medicine and Science in Sports Exercise, 23,* S20.

Frisancho, A. R. (1981). New norms of upper limb fat and muscle areas for
assessment of nutritional status. *American Journal of Clinical Nutrition, 34,*
2540–2545.

Frontera, W. R., Hughes, V. A., Lutz, K. J., & Evans, W. J. (1991). A cross-sectional
study of muscle strength and mass in 45- to 78- yr-old men and women.
Journal of Applied Physiology, 71 (2), 644–650.

Garry, P. J., Goodwin, J. S., Hunt, W. C., Hooper, E. M., & Leonard, A. G. (1982).
Nutritional status in an elderly population: Dietary and supplemental status.
American Journal of Clinical Nutrition, 36, 313–319.

Gibbins, R. L., Riley, M., & Brimble, P. (1993). Effectiveness of programme for
reducing cardiovascular risk for men in one general practice. *British Medical
Journal, 306,* 1652–1656.

Goodwin, J. S., Goodwin, J. M., & Garry, P. J. (1983). Association between nutritional status and cognitive functioning in a healthy elderly population.
Journal of American Medical Association, 249, 2917–2921.

Hartz, S. C., Russell, R. M., & Rosenberg, I. H. (1992). *Nutrition in the elderly:*

The Boston nutritional status survey. New York: Smith-Gordon.

Hebert, L. E., Scherr, P. A., Beckett, L. A., Albert, M. S., Pilgrim, D. M., Chown, M. J., Funkenstein, H. H., & Evans, D. A. (1995). Age-specific incidence of Alzheimer's disease in a community population. *Journal of the American Medical Association, 273,* 1353–1359.

Helmrich, S. P., Ragland, D. R., Leung, R. W., & Paffenbarger, R. S. (1991). Physical activity and reduced occurrence of non-insulin-dependent diabetes mellitus. *New England Journal of Medicine, 325,* 147–152.

Holmen, J., Forsen, L., Hjort, P. F., Midthiell, K., Waaler, H. T., & Bjorndal, A. (1991). Detecting hypertension: Screening versus case finding in Norway. *British Medical Journal, 302,* 219–222.

Jacques, P. F., & Chylack, L. T., Jr. (1991). Epidemiologic evidence of a role for the antioxidant vitamins and carotenoids in cataract prevention. *American Journal of Clinical Nutrition, 53,* 352S–3525S.

Kahn, H. A., Leibowitz, H. M., Ganley, J. P., Kini, M. M., Colton, T., Nickerson, R. S., & Dowber, T. R. (1977). The Framingham Eye Study I. Outline and major prevalence findings. *American Journal of Epidemiology, 106,* 17–32.

Krall, E. A., Sahyoun, N., Tannenbaum, S., Dallal, G. E., & Dawson-Hughes, B. (1989). Effect of vitamin D intake on seasonal variations in parathyroid hormone secretion in postmenopausal women. *New England Journal of Medicine, 321,* 1777–1783.

Krasinski, S. D., Russell, R. M., Samloff, M., Jacob, R. A., Dallal, G. E., McGandy, R. B., & Hartz, S. C. (1986). Fundic atrophic gastritis in an elderly population. Effect on hemoglobin and several serum nutritional indicators. *Journal of the American Geriatrics Society, 34,* 800–806.

Lindenbaum, J., Healton, E. B., Savage, D. G., Brust, J. C., Garrett, T. J., Podell, E. R., Marcell, P. D., Stabler, S. P., & Allen, R. H. (1988). Neuropsychiatric disorders caused by cobalamin deficiency in the absence of anemia or macrocytosis. *New England Journal of Medicine, 318,* 1720–1728.

Meydani, S. N., Barklund, M. P., Liu, S., Meydani, M., Miller, R. A., Cannon, J. G., Morrow, F. D., Rocklin, R., & Blumberg, J. B. (1990b). Vitamin E supplementation enhances cell-mediated immunity in healthy elderly subjects. *American Journal of Clinical Nutrition, 52,* 557–563.

Meydani, S. N., Meydani, M., Barklund, P. M., Liu, S., Miller, R. A., Cannon, J. C., Rocklin, R., & Blumberg, J. B. (1989). Effect of vitamin E supplementation on immune responsiveness of the aged. *Annals of the New York Academy of Sciences, 510,* 283–290.

Meydani, S. N., Ribaya-Mercado, J. D., Russell, R. M., Sayhoun, N., Morrow, F. D., & Gershoff, S. N. (1990a). Effect of vitamin B_6 on immune responses of healthy elderly. *Annals of the New York Academy of Sciences, 587,* 303–306.

Morley, J. E., Levine, A. S., Yim, G. K. W., Yim, G. K., & Lowy, M. T. (1983). Opioid modulation of appetite. *Neurosciences and Biobehavioral Reviews, 7,* 281–305.

Optimal Calcium Intake. (1994). *NIH consensus statement, 12*(4), 1–31.

Paffenbarger, R. S., Hyde, R. T., Wing, A. L., & Hsieh, C-C. (1986). Physical activity, all-cause mortality, and longevity of college alumni. *New England Journal of Medicine, 314,* 605–613.

Posner, B. M., Jette, A. M., Smith, K. W., & Miller, D. R. (1993). Nutrition and health risks in the elderly: The Nutrition Screening Initiative. *American Journal of Public Health, 83,* 972–978.

Reid, I. R., Ames, R. W., Evans, M. C., Gamble, G. D., & Sharpe, S. J. (1993). Effect of calcium supplementation on bone loss in postmenopausal women. *New England Journal of Medicine, 328,* 460–464.

Rimm, E. B., Stampfer, M. J., Ascherio, A., Giovannucci, E., Colditz, G. A., & Willett, W. C. (1993). Vitamin E consumption and the risk of coronary heart disease in men. *New England Journal of Medicine, 328,* 1450–1456.

Roberts, S. B., Fuss, P., Heyman, M. B., Evans, W. J., Tsay, R., Rasmussen, H., Fiatarone, M., Cortiella, J., Dallal, G. E., & Young, V. R. (1994). Control of food intake in older men. *Journal of the American Medical Association, 272,* 1601–1606.

Rosenberg, I. H. (1989). Summary Comments: Epidemiological and methodological problems in determining nutritional status of older persons. *American Journal of Clinical Nutrition, 50,* 1231–1233.

Rosenberg, I. H., & Miller, J. W. (1992). Nutritional factors in physical and cognitive function in the elderly. *American Journal of Clinical Nutrition, 55,* 1237S–1243S.

Roubenoff, R., Dallal, G. E., & Wilson, P. W. F. (1995). Predicting body fatness: The Body Mass Index vs estimation by bioelectrical impedance. *American Journal of Public Health, 85,* 726–728.

Rush, D. (1993). Editorial: Evaluating the Nutrition Screening Initiative. *American Journal of Public Health, 83,* 944–945.

Sawaya, A. L., Tucker, K, Tsay, R., Willett, W., Saltzman, E., & Roberts, S. B. (1996). Evaluation of four methods for determination of energy intake in young and older women: Comparison with doubly labeled water measurements of total energy expenditure. *American Journal of Clinical Nutrition, 63,* 491–499.

Schiffman, S. S., Hornack, K., & Reilly, D. (1979). Increased taste thresholds of amino acids with age. *American Journal of Clinical Nutrition, 32,* 1622–1627.

Seddon, J. M., Ajani, U. A., Sperduto, R. D., Hiller, R., Blair, N., Burton, T. C., Farber, M. D., Gragoudas, E. S., Haller, J., Miller, D. T., Yannuzzi, L. A., & Willett, W. (1994). Dietary carotenoids, vitamins A, C, and E, and advanced age-related macular degeneration. *Journal of the American Medical Association, 272,* 1413–1420.

Selhub, J., Jacques, P. F., Wilson, P. W. F., Rush, D., & Rosenberg, I. H. (1993). Vitamin status and intake as primary determinants of homocysteinemia in the elderly. *Journal of the American Medical Association, 270,* 2693–2698.

Selhub, J., Jacques, P. F., Boston, A. G., D'Agostino, R. B., Wilson, P. W. F., Belanger, A. J., O'Leary, D. H., Wolf, P. H., Schaefer, E. J., & Rosenberg, I. H. (1995). Association between homocysteine concentrations and extracranial carotid-artery stenosis. *New England Journal of Medicine, 332,* 286–291.

Shearer, M. J. (1995). Vitamin K. *Lancet, 345,* 229–234.

Shock, N. W. (1972). Energy metabolism, caloric intake and physical activity of the aging. In L. A. Carson (Ed.), *Nutrition in old age, X Symposium Swedish Nutrition Foundation.* Uppsala: Almqvist & Wiksell.

Stamp, T. C., & Round, J. M. (1974). Seasonal changes in human plasma levels of 25-hydroxyvitamin D. *Nature, 247,* 563–565.

Suter, P. M., Golner, B. B., Goldin, B. R., Morrow, F. D, & Russell, R. M. (1991). Reversal of protein-bound vitamin B_{12} malabsorption with antibiotics in atrophic gastritis. *Gastroenterology, 101,* 1039–1045.

Taylor, A. (1992). Role of nutrients in delaying cataracts. *Annals of the New York Academy of Sciences, 669,* 111–123.

Taylor, A., Jacques, P. F., Nadler, D., Morrow, F., Sulsky, S. I., & Shepard, D. (1991). Relationship in humans between ascorbic acid consumption and levels of total and reduced ascorbic acid in lens, aqueous acid in lens, aqueous humor, and plasma. *Current Eye Research, 10,* 751–759.

Taylor, A., Jacques, P. F., & Dorey, K. (1993). Oxidation and aging: Impact on vision. *Toxicology Industrial Health, 9,* 349–371.

Thomas, M. L., & Weigle, W. O. (1989). The cellular and subcellular basis of immunosenescence. *Advances in Immunology, 46,* 221–261.

Tsai, K. -S., Wahner, H. W., Offord, K. P., Melton, L. J. III, Kuman, R., & Riggs, B. (1987). Effect of aging on vitamin D stores and bone density in women. *Calcified Tissue International, 40,* 241–243.

Tzankoff, S. P., & Norris, A. H. (1978). Longitudinal changes in basal metabolism in man. *Journal of Applied Physiology, 45,* 536–539.

Tzankoff, S. P., & Norris, A. H. (1977). Effect of muscle mass decrease on age-related BMR changes. *Journal of Applied Physiology, 43,* 1001–1006.

U.S. Department of Agriculture, U.S. Department of Health and Human Services. (1990). *Nutrition and your health. Dietary guidelines for Americans.* (3rd ed., p. 9). Washington, DC: U.S. Government Printing Office.

Ueland, P. M., & Refsum, H. (1989). Plasma homocysteine, a risk factor for vascular disease: plasma levels in health, disease, and drug therapy. *Journal of Laboratory and Clinical Medicine, 114*(5), 473–501.

Vir, S. C., & Love, A. G. H. (1979). Nutritional status of institutionalized and non-institutionalized aged in Belfast, Northern Ireland. *American Journal of Clinical Nutrition, 32,* 1934–1947.

Webb, A. R., Kline, L., & Holick, M. F. (1988). Influence of season and latitude on the cutaneous synthesis of vitamin D_3. Exposure to winter sunlight in Boston and Edmonton will not promote vitamin D_3 synthesis in human skin. *Journal of Clinical Endocrinology and Metabolism, 61,* 373–378.

PART 4

Nutrition Policy Perspective

Opportunities and Challenges of New Nutrition Environments: International Experiences and Implications for U.S. Policymaking

Nancy Milio

T he best-designed nutrition policies will not be effective if they do not fit the settings in which they are to operate. Today more than ever, policymaking environments are complex: they are affected by world conditions, as well as by national and local policies. Conditions change rapidly and with apparent unpredictability. Yet, policy decisions in governments and corporate board rooms continue to be made that affect nutrition and the prospects for better nutrition policies. Those who have public and professional responsibility for the health of Americans must be more than mere bystanders in this challenging social arena. They must take account of the environments as they design and promote nutrition policies that underly population health.

Effective nutrition policymaking is more than sound substantive goals designed to improve population nutrition and health. Impressive science-based documents exist, like the U.S. Dietary Guidelines (U.S. Department of Agriculture [USDA]/Department of Health and Human Services [DHHS],

1990), the recent plan of the Association of State and Territorial Health Officers and Nutrition Directors (ASTHO, 1993), and other widely lauded reports (DHHS, 1988; Institute of Medicine, 1991; National Research Council, 1989). Most recently, work is under way to create Public Health practice guidelines on community-wide prevention for such major problems as cardiovascular disease (Council on Linkages, 1995).

In addition to sound science, policy action must also have a strategic plan whose goals and means can propel the policy to adoption and implementation. Accordingly, the aims and instruments of this twin substantive and strategic process must have timeliness—relevance to the conditions of today and tomorow; it must be pursued with special energy at timely moments in political, bureaucratic and social arenas; and it must recognize that it will take time, not only to gain acceptance and use, but also to protect the gains that have been made. To do this, an adequately financed strategic management vehicle(s) is essential to act as an organized "policykeeper," "champion," and "watchdog" to monitor, promote, coordinate, evaluate, and publicly report on progress toward strategic and substantive objectives.

These are among the lessons that can be gleaned from the experiences of European countries in recent decades as they have attempted to guide their nations toward healthier food and nutrition patterns through policies intended to affect both food supply and consumer demand.

This chapter provides examples of recent policymaking from the author's on-site case studies and other international experiences. The major case centers on Finland's efforts to develop a comprehensive food and nutrition policy (FNP) to stem the health effects of its animal-fat-rich diet. This case is briefly compared with a similar and earlier attempt by Norway. From these and other analyses, implications will be suggested for nutrition policy development in the United States in light of the changing social, economic, and political climate.

FINLAND

The demographics of an aging, affluent, well-educated population and the imperatives of global economic integration brought about new political and national priorities in Finland in the early 1980s. Unlike Norway, it looked toward closer ties with Europe and eventual membership in the European Union. Overall objectives emphasized economic and bureaucratic efficiency, deregulation consistent with environmental and welfare goals, and decentralization, with corresponding fiscal and administrative responsibility by local governments and industry. These social, economic, and political conditions influenced FNP development and implementation.

Diet-Related Health Status

Although Finnish life expectancy and infant mortality rates are more favorable than in the United States, Finland's adult mortality and morbidity were higher than that of its Scandinavian partners, especially with respect to deaths attributed to high-animal-fat diets. The decline in cardiovascular disease had slowed, attributed to a slowing of the decline in serum cholesterol levels; 80% had a higher than desirable serum cholesterol (Vartiainen et al., 1988). By international standards, Finns were overweight, the men increasingly so.

POLICY GOALS

Finland's Food and Nutrition Policy was approved by Parliament in 1985 with goals and instruments similar to Norway's: "The goal . . . is to ensure a sufficient, balanced, and varied diet based primarily on domestic production and pure raw materials . . ." (p. 4) through increasing consumption of fish, cereals, potatoes, vegetables, berries, and low-fat meat and dairy products. Sugar- and salt-dense foods were to be reduced through:

- information and education in schools, mass media, and voluntary organizations;
- meal services in day-care centers, educational facilities, and other public and private workplaces;
- new product development of low-fat, low-salt, low-sugar, high-fiber foods;
- food pricing changes through modified farm prices, excise duties, value-added tax, price control, and government subsidies;
- quality requirements.

Finland's National Nutrition Council (NNC, 1989) developed "A Programme for the Implementation of Nutrition Recommendations" in 1989. The scope covered food production and marketing, regulation, education, meal services, and research aimed at improvements by the end of the century. It placed its objectives with the context of political priorities and related economic policy shifts in agriculture, trade, and retailing, as well as previous nonbinding recommendations from such groups as the Finnish Heart Association.

The plan noted the uncoordinated nature of nutrition planning and follow-up activities and advised "further coordinating measures." Other strategic and capacity-building points included the need for closer cooperation between local public health and regulatory authorities to encourage restaurants and other food services to follow the dietary guidelines; nutrition training for health, social welfare, elder, and child care, and educational personnel through continuing education and basic education programs; additional nutrition staff in health care settings, with coverage by health insurance, and development of information systems on food production and marketing, as well as research on the macronutrient content and sales of food services.

Substantive policy objectives called for food pricing that encouraged purchase of recommended types of food relative to their high-fat, low-fiber, high-sugar and high-salt counterparts. Incentives were to be available to food manufacturers that developed foods according to the national dietary guidelines. Improvements in food labeling and ingredient regulations were also proposed.

Strategic Management

The NNC succeeded in raising social and political awareness of food and nutrition policy issues, and facilitated implementation of some recommendations. But it had also blurred some issues and deterred implementation. As an advisory body with 23 members, it had no staff, no budget, and met at the discretion of the Minister of Agriculture and the interests of its members.The NNC had no capacity to act as a strategic planning, coordinating, or monitoring body. Its member ministries did not seek new funds or earmark staff to implement the FNP. Monitoring tended to be personal, and the policy "self-administering."

The NNC recognized that it did not have the institutional capacity to act as a strategic planning body, yet it was the pivotal advisory and intersectoral body charged with policy coordination and development. Further, it may have been housed in the fox's lair, the Ministry of Agriculture, cochaired by the Ministry of Social Affairs and Health, and heavily endowed with food industry members.

POLICY IMPLEMENTATION: INSTRUMENTS FOR GUIDED CHANGE

Economic Instruments

Economic policies in the mid-1980s affected food production, availability, and prices. They were to harmonize with Economic Community and General Agreement on Trades and Tariff (GATT) arrangements. This meant the end of tariff and food taxes that favored full-fat dairy products in order to reduce Finland's surplus milkfat production.

To assist and preserve farm communities, low-cost loans, subsidies, and incentive contracts were encouraged in order to allow shifts to forestry, fur, and organic farming, and sideline farm-based businesses like tourist, light processing, horticulture, aqua-culture enterprises. To deter surpluses taxes were assessed on fertilizers, feed, landclearing, and over-quota milk.

At the same time, access to new imports would expose Finns to less desirable food choices (energy-, fat-, sugar-, salt-dense, low-fibre products) at competitive prices. Moreover, decentralization would mean that FNP implementation would be deferred in some communities in competition with other priorities. Still, cheaper fish and fresh produce would also enter from the European market. Economic priorities also brought certain anti-nutrition actions, such as continuing subsidies for sugar production and "freeing" alcoholic drinks from taxation to eliminate trade barriers.

Regulation

The food industry began to restructure, adjusting to a shrinking farm economy and responding to the new food concerns of the domestic market, while expanding in the rest of Europe. The growing concentration of both national and foreign industry showed evidence of a lack of responsiveness to small and less profitable (e.g, rural) markets, reducing food choices for some subgroups.

The Food Industry Federation (comprising 95% of food processing and marketing), as a member of the NNC, sought voluntary overmandated FNP changes, gaining *voluntary* food labeling, while keeping price advantages for butter over margarine, whole over skim milk, and full control over labeling. The bakery industry succeeded in getting wheat pricing based on higher protein content to improve baking quality, bringing both industry and nutrition benefits.

A new streamlined regulatory structure was set up in 1990 capable of altering the macronutrient quality of the food supply from production to the retail level. Whether it would do so would depend on how it defined "quality" beyond specific food safety and labelling restrictions; the types of research and data it sought; and how broadly it chose to educate food inspectors about NNC nutrition guidelines. Incentives arising from international standards emphasized hygiene, toxins, additives, quantity, and minimal labeling rather than macronutrient composition.

The main industry actors on the NNC were the largest value-added sectors (meat, dairy, bakery, brewery, and sugar), which in traditional terms had the least to gain from FNP implementation. At the same time, advertising and promotions to consumers and retailers succeeded in increasing sales of milk, cream, cheese, snacks, soft drinks, and beer throughout the 1980s.

Provision of Direct Services: Meals at Public and Private Sites

Away-from-home eating continued to expand in the 1980s, especially at private sites. At the same time the government provided or subsidized the majority of meals at inpatient institutions, workplaces, schools, child day care, the military, and prisons. Several sets of guidelines consistent with FNP goals were developed for many of these sites, but monitoring and follow-up were weak or absent.

Decentralization and deregulation raised concerns by nutrition and health leaders that local school budgets would be reduced along with their capacity for providing school meals. Monitoring subsidized food programs as to food actually eaten was limited and was not used for improving food availability or consumer choices. Occasional site-specific studies suggested that school meals were high in fat, as were some meals for elders.

Whether and to what extent kitchen staff, health and welfare officials, education, health and safety worker delegates, supervisors, and local environment officials and staff were familiar with the Dietary Guidelines was unknown and not monitored. Most of the nutrition services provided to clients by local health centers were limited in practice to counseling, following risk-factor screening of most age groups, rather than focusing on developing healthier local food options for the total population. This would have required collaboration with local and regional producers, suppliers, retailers, media and voluntary groups by health center staff or by their environmental health counterparts.

Nutrition Information

Finns were increasingly exposed to many diverse and sophisticated sources of information on food and nutrition. This was especially true for young people, who received "messages" and incentives from outside traditional family–school–health channels, mainly the globalized mass media. Studies showed that most nutrition materials approved for teens (1967–85) did not reflect NNC Guidelines, nor take account of actual eating patterns. Over half of teen food ads were for sugared products, and advertising provided little if any nutritional information. Nordic youth (9–24 years) watched more foreign TV, exposing them to increased advertising and new lifestyles. Adding to their patterns of away-from-home eating, snacking, peer-group priorities, proclivity for hamburgers and ice cream, advertising was more likely to influence the nutrition and health habits of the young than of adults.

Food-industry advertising explicitly attempted to shed a "fatty" image and create a "healthy-lifestyle" image, based on consumer surveys and sales data that showed "no promise of profits" in fat. Finns (38%) reported the most common reason for changing their diet was to lose weight. The majority of those who seriously and successfully attempted to lose weight or eat less fat did so without the influence of physicians or family—especially women, more highly educated people, and those with a high serum cholesterol. Although Finns viewed physicians as the most reliable health information sources, only 15% (of the 60% who sought a checkup) were advised to reduce dietary fat; as were just one-quarter to one-third of high-risk patients.

The Finns' sources of knowledge, incentive, and support—as in many industrialized populations—derived from the media; the availability of alternative food products; affordable prices; convenient eating sites and times influenced the work world and peer priorities and values (Milio, 1989).

Education, Training, and Research

Improvements in nutrition instruction were made in general education, in vocational training for some occupations, and in higher education for nutrition and medicine. Generally, however, the full scope and implications of the FNP were not addressed. Food and nutrition concepts based on NNC dietary guidelines were integrated into the national curriculum framework through home-economics courses in at least two grades, textbooks were adopted, based on whether they adhered to the dietary guidelines. Course content for continuing education was determined locally, within the national curricular framework, but no data systems for monitoring or evaluation existed.

In contrast to extensive Finnish research on diet-related issues, there were information gaps in organizational and policymaking processes. This dearth of "how-to" knowledge became increasingly significant as education and persuasion replaced governmental regulatory powers in addressing food and nutrition issues.

SUMMARY

Some progress was made in each aspect of Finland's Food and Nutrition Policy: access to nutritional information and education increased; improvements were made in food-service menus; an increase in healthier food products was seen; as was nutritionally favorable pricing in some commodities, and improvements were made in food-quality requirements and labeling. The eating patterns of Finns also improved in relation to some recommended foods and macronutrients.

The structural changes in farm and food production are largely the result of new political and economic realities in Finland and internationally, resulting in the government's focus on fiscal efficiency, decentralization, and a more competitive, consumer-oriented market. The new environment created pressures to reduce surplus animal-fat production and to expand markets in new foods to Finns and other Europeans whose demographic, health, work, and living arrangements demanded new, and sometimes healthier (or "healthy-image") foods. Some national public health leaders grasped this new environment and were able to design and work for proposals that were consistent with political and economic imperatives, as well as nutrition and health needs.

Major problems in policy implementation persisted. Although much was done in research and demonstration, and in the development of national guidelines for food services and labeling, there was a gap in transfering such "soft [how-to-do-it] technology" to sites for action and monitoring their implementation in order to develop correctives at the operational level. This gap could increase with decentralized budget control and a less regulated market, where "listening to the consumer" (whether individuals or retailers) would not necessarily result in healthier products or more accurate consumer information, especially as more foreign products and global media attracted Finnish youth.

Rapid progress in economic and farm-policy development and food enterprises could lead to conditions that are supportive of nutrition goals, if health interests are taken into account to avoid potential untoward changes. This would require initiative, clarity of strategic purpose, and organization by health and nutrition leaders. Such an effort requires a leading strategic body able authoritatively to assess and anticipate problems in policy development and implementation, address them, and coordinate and monitor necessary actions.

NORWAY

Norway's policy predated that of Finland by 10 years. It had comparable dietary goals, although initially it sought fat reduction to 35% of food energy rather than Finland's goal of 30% or less. In the 1990s, it adopted the lower goal, having reached the first. Norway placed more emphasis on food self-sufficiency, on development of less-advantaged agricultural regions, and on world food security; in 1994 it voted not to join the European Economic Union (EU), but nonetheless to be active in EU economic and other pursuits, requiring a *somewhat* less outward-oriented economy than Finland's.

Norway entered the 1980s with a relatively more controlled foreign and domestic food system, derived from long-time statutory authority given to the agricultural system. Thus many changes required by its Food and Nutrition Policy were effectively resisted or slowed when powerful farm organizations perceived them not to be in their interests. For example, although consumer subsidies were granted to skim and low-fat milks to lower the price, the long-term price changes in the 1980s continued to favor foods high in animal fat. Phasing out consumer subsidies allowed flour, bread, and fish prices to rise faster than the consumer price index, contrary to dietary goals. At the same time, however, farm price measures included incentives for producing higher protein milk, improved potatoes, leaner meat, more fish, and controls on animal food surplus. These were mainly in response to government budget limitations—protested by farmers but supported by the public—and a growing awareness of the possibility of freer trade with Europe.

The Norwegian NNC's 15-year efforts to become involved in government-farm-food economics met with little success. The Consumer Affairs Ministry, responsible for subsidies and income policies, did not give priority to nutritional issues over those affecting prices and wages, neither did the Agriculture Ministry, although the latter claimed to speak to nutritional concerns.

The NNC attempted to solve the central government–local community linkage problem by focusing on collaboration with local public health services, schools, and food businesses. In support of this, the 1990's National Health Plan defined "environmental health" broadly and included nutrition. Several local projects were funded accordingly, including one to promote the use of the Dietary Guidelines in Oslo's eating places and work sites, incorporating nutritional evaluation in the training of local food inspectors. To improve the public's nutrition information, the NNC systematically reviewed and revised all public and voluntary health agency materials to make them consistent with the Guidelines during the 1970s.

Strategic Management

Norway's counterpart to the Finnish strategic management body, the NNC, was its Interministerial Coordinating Committee (IMC) composed of 10 ministries and chaired by the Health Ministry. Its resource base was comparably meager, and it has met infrequently. By all accounts, including those of its members, inaction preserved the interests of its ministries and, with rare exception, was ineffective in promoting the implementation of Norwegian Food and Nutrition Policy.

Recognizing such structural and political realities shortly after Parliament's adoption of the FNP in 1976, however, Norway's NNC took the initiative to reconstitute itself as an independent expert body rather than as an IMC appendage, as initially planned. As such, it obtained a limited budget and small staff (4–6) to conduct a variety of education, information, evaluation, reporting, and advisory activities, taking action as resources allowed. Coordination to some extent was possible, but strategic planning and research on policy implementation were not.

Norway met many of its food goals, mainly those closely tied to agricultural interests, that is, food self-sufficiency, rural development, and contributions to world food security. Health objectives made slower progress. This was due to both the power of agricultural interests and a lack of leadership by high-level health authorities. Nutritional progress was spurred by a variety of information, education, assessment, negotiation, and sometime advocacy activities by the NNC. Some advances were also made in basic and medical education and in research development.

In summary, what is common to Finland and Norway, both of whose exports were growing, was the emerging national and global economic picture. This required a rethinking of goals and priorities in food production and consumption in light of open and competitive markets, high farm input and environmental costs, government deficits and health costs, and social changes. Common too was an awareness by farm leaders of this "handwriting on the wall," the need to change—although not admitted publicly. Within this context Finland appeared to have made relatively fast progress in placing nutrition and health issues on the agendas of relevant public and private sectors, perhaps because high-level health professionals took initiatives outside the traditional health services bureaucracy. Both countries moved only slowly and unevenly toward meeting their dietary goals and both had problems in policy organization, however, impairing their strategic capacity for effective policy implementation.

Finland and Norway were selectively successful in meeting both substantive (farm, food, dietary, and health) and strategic ("how to get from here to there" through target organization commitments and capacity-building) policy goals. They were most effective when the policies (a) had the best fit with (or were shaped to fit) changing facets of the environment—political, bureaucratic, economic, social, demographic; (b) when policy design took account of the changing interests of target public and private stakeholder organizations without compromising the public's health interests; and (c) when strategic management was adequate to the tasks at hand.

THE CHANGING NUTRITION ENVIRONMENT
IN EUROPE

Despite west European experience with an impressive array of nutrition policies, programs, and projects, governments and peoples in the region face in the 1990s and beyond even greater challenges to nutrition policy-making and the health of their populations. The emerging European Union (EU) will have increasing impact on national policies and on the availability of and access to new types of food, nutrition, and on resource and health gaps between countries and populations. This will be further complicated by the reconfiguration of the Eastern and Central European countries and Russia.

A broadbrush picture of nutrition and health in Europe shows northern Europe with high rates of diet-related disease that are beginning to decline and dietary patterns high in animal fat, sugar, and sodium that are slowly improving. Eastern and central Europe has high and rising disease rates, and dietary patterns are becoming increasingly adverse. In southern Europe, diet-related diseases are increasing to some extent and certain aspects of diet are becoming less favorable as the South gains easier access to northern and other new foods, and as incomes of its people grow (Food and Agriculture Organization, 1990a, b). In large part, the extent and strength of EU and national food and nutrition policies will determine whether economic and other changes in the Mediterranean area will be allowed to reproduce the relatively less healthy aspects of northern diets, and whether eastern and central countries' economic liberalization and linkage to the EU will compound their already nutritionally burdensome animal-based national diets.

Eastern and Central Europe

In these emerging economies, as income gaps widen, nutritious food becomes less affordable because of measures to privatize markets and reduce government deficits. The results, for example, are unemployment rates of 15%–20%, while governments are removing consumer, producer, and housing subsidies, and providing only sparse if any, unemployment insurance (Blanchard, Commander, & Corelli, 1994; Gupta & Hagemann, 1994).

Previously, the food sector was guided by Communist ideology rather than by market forces. Food was generously subsidized and there was strong demand; many countries had a high caloric supply. Recent reforms lowered food production; food costs rose faster than wages; the food basket became less diverse, and a growing gap occurred between the dietary patterns of rich and poor.

Agriculture plays a large part in these national economies, absorbing up to a third of employment, whereas agriculture employs less than 3% of the population in the United States. In eastern Europe, agriculture is being increasingly turned toward export markets to bolster the economies. This redirection provides incentives for intensive high-animal-fat production, including heavy use of pesticides. These practices tend to bring the highest producer prices but augur poorly for the nutrition and health prospects of the populations (Brooks, 1993).

Many vulnerable groups, such as the elderly and disabled, have experienced a drop in energy intake by up to 10% (World Health Organization [WHO], 1992). Large majorities of children in the cities are less than "fully healthy." Life expectancy is declining in several countries, mainly due to infections, suicide, and substance abuse in younger men, and from chronic diseases in older persons, especially heart disease, attributed to very high-fat diets, tobacco, and obesity (Feshbach, 1993).

Western Europe

Nutrition and health authorities in western Europe have voiced concern over the new environment throughout Europe, including the effects of multicountry trade agreements, worldwide competition, deregulation, transnational corporate mergers, and global telecommunications and advertising. They are wary of Europe-wide policies limiting the strength of their national nutrition efforts (Bletz, Dorcksen, & Van Paridon, 1993); of food and labeling deregulation being done in consultation with multinational corporations in the EU; and of governments offering inducements to food-industry giants with a reduction of nutrition priorities, loosening of controls on pesticides and other farming-intensive practices to the detriment of the environment, the workforce and consumer health (National Nutrition Council, 1992), They also fear less vigilance about incorrect or misleading consumer nutrition information and advertising and are intensifying educational efforts accordingly to shift dietary habits toward the national dietary goals (Sweden, 1992).

American health officials face parallel issues. The United States is moving rapidly into the world economy through GATT and the North American Free Trade Agreement (NAFTA), especially in agriculture and food. International and domestic competitive pressures are incentives to skillful, if not wholly accurate, marketing information to achieve short-term, bottom-line success (Levine, 1986, 1989; Peterson et al., 1986), and new cable, video, and computer technologies provide ever-growing marketing access to every age group. This new economic environment, combined with shifts in political priorities toward major federal and state government budget cuts in nutrition and health programs and enforcement capacity; deregulation, decentralization, and block grants, and growing gaps in income and health (Bureau of the Census, 1994), create prospects for a smaller and weaker nutrition and health safety net (Service Employees International Union, 1995) and growing health risks.

PUBLIC POLICYMAKING, NUTRITION, AND HEALTH IN THE U.S.

By definition, public policy is simply a guide to government action, including the ways government uses to guide the actions of other parts of society: for-profit and nonprofit organizations, other jurisdictions, and citizens. These instruments include economic subsidies and taxes; regulation of food standards, labeling and advertising; provision of direct services (e.g., nutrition counseling, meals-on-wheels, food services); training and education of personnel and the public; research and evaluation of consumer and organizational behavior (Milio, 1988b).

As the case studies and other evidence suggest, effective policy requires careful analysis of social reality and informed judgment about the direction of health-supporting changes. Nutrition policy thus requires more than the creation of nutrition and dietary guidelines. It also requires decisions by policymakers, farm organizations, food corporations, retailers, advertisers, and educators. If these decisions conform to the guidelines, then consumers will be offered healthful choices in eating places, workplaces, institutional, and home-based dining.

Individual and public health information, per se, tends to have a limited effect on personal behavior change, varying in different groups and for different health risks. These limits of health or lifestyle counseling, teaching, and "advertising" are seen in the slowing decline in teen smoking (Nelson et al., 1995), in the lessening of physical activity (Center for Disease Control, 1993) and of the consumption of healthy diets (Serdula et al., 1995) and the increase in obesity (Louis Harris, & Association, 1994).

Healthful practices are improved more widely and long term when environmental incentives are created and public policy measures are initiated and enforced, like tobacco taxes (National Cancer Institute, 1991), regulation of public food-service meal preparation and menu offerings (IOM,

1991). Such community-wide environmental and policy changes demand public health leadership, community mobilization, and policy advocacy.

If food and nutrition policies are to be effective, they will have to take account of changes in economic currents and political priorities at the global and national levels, and address specifically the conflict and confluence of economic interests and nutrition–health priorities. Nutrition proponents will need to be better acquainted with large-scale changes. Just as the U.S. Department of Agriculture and Congress have monitored for years the effect of food and nutrition policy changes abroad and at home, so nutrition proponents must be able to assess the potential impacts on U.S. farming (Economics Statistics and Cooperative Service, 1980; General Accounting Office, 1988, 1990; Langley, 1987; O'Brien, 1993).

Farm-Food Economics

As cosponsor of the Dietary Guidelines, the USDA's economic policy responses can only be termed, generously, anomalous. For example, facing the imperative of GATT and federal budget deficit reduction, the USDA was forced to cut costly dairy subsidies that have led to large stocks of dry milk as American families age and shrink. The milk can only be sold at a loss and the plan is to promote dairy exports and domestic sales in value-added forms, such as premium, high-fat ice creams and butter and butter-based processed foods. The target foreign markets are mainly newly industrializing nations (e.g., Brazil, Mexico, South Korea) where USDA uses market-promotion funds on behalf of U.S. producers. Also the USDA continues to use about $250 million each year to promote a marketing program mainly for dairy products, eggs, and beef, designed and managed by industry Boards. Its nutrition unit is not involved in these programs (General Accounting Office, Dec., 1993, 1994).

The consumer side of food economics is also changing and must be taken into account in an effective nutrition strategy. The new food market to which food systems must adapt is shifting from stable national markets to small specialized market segments, on the one hand, and to large foreign markets, on the other.The consumer too has changed, splitting between group providers and new families and individuals. There are away-from-home food services, both public and private, which in many countries now shape one-third to one-half of the typical diet. And there is the customary individual/family food buyer who is no longer the typical woman with children and an employed husband. Rather, as populations age, as more women and youth enter the work force, as solo living, smaller families, single-parenthood, and widowhood increase, the foods that buyers need, want, and can afford and where they eat them is also changing (Milio, 1989).

Telecommunications, Marketing, and Nutrition Information

Another critical aspect of the food and nutrition environment is the growing role of the mass media in information, education, and consumer behavior, especially for younger people. Coming mainly from commercial sources, messages about nutrition are conveyed explicitly (e.g., advertising, sensationalist news reports) and implicitly (e.g., modeling behavior) in the press and in the electronic media. These may be misleading or inaccurate, and often few countervailing perspectives are provided. This new fact of global telecommunications technologies needs to be faced at the policy level by nutrition proponents and at the local level by nutrition officers in health departments.

Options for action include media monitoring and content analysis with public reporting of findings, and media literacy education. Both of these have to some extent been practiced in Finland and Norway. Other options include the use of "countercommercials," and joint educational seminars and collaboration among journalists, nutrition and health personnel, as in Germany. There, where over 80% of all premature deaths are thought to be due to nutrition-related diseases, nutritional knowledge is not widespread, high general educational standards notwithstanding. The ministries of health and of food and agriculture jointly administer nutritional counseling and coordination programs of all agencies that disseminate nutrition information, for example, voluntary societies, professional associations, and public agencies. The impetus here was a 1989 law that required health insurance societies (to which 95% of people belong) to provide services that promote health. Thus dietary counseling is now a financially covered health service (National Report, 1992).

Nutritional Profile of Local Food

Corporate competition in farm and food production internationally and at home has as its result that producers pay little attention to supplying healthier and affodable food to small and low-income communities. Ever-multiplying new, "market-grabbing" products are aimed at upscale consumers (Freimuth et al., 1988; Levine, 1986). Another element in local food availability is that as national bureaucracies retain less fiscal and regulatory control over local public and private organizations, the local infrastructure that assures food quality and security becomes increasingly important.

To address this situation, Norway's NNC has given more attention to integrating the national nutrition and food agenda through the health services system. For example, together with the Oslo environmental health authorities it designed a program in which inspection and education concerning quality of food in public and private eating places was made part of the training program. A similar program has been in operation in Wales for several years (Milio, 1990b). Similar, continuing education to expand the nutrition-effectiveness of other personnel such as public health and welfare staff, education, and child care workers, would support local work with farmers, grocers, local media, schools, and food services at work sites and in public eating places (Toronto Food Policy Council, 1994).

Several collaborating cities in seven countries across Europe are also attempting to get beyond just "immunizing" consumers against misleading ads with sound nutrition information (Vaandrager, 1994). Using local government funds and links to universities and health departments, coalitions of community groups (e.g., social work, neighborhood groups, local schools, health centers) and local food shops are promoting nutrition activities, such as cooking courses, food demonstrations, and in-store food promotions. After 2 years, there were only minor differences in consumption patterns, although two-thirds of the population were aware of the activities. The major problems were the unwillingness of retailers and other stakeholders to commit resources to ongoing changes, for example, to alter food prices or use valuable shelf space to promote healthier foods. This underscores the necessity to take account of stakeholders' material interests and plan strategies that will induce them to adopt long-term changes.

A few local food policy councils in the United States, acting as voluntary bodies, often in cooperation with local government, have attempted to change the amount and nutritional quality of their food supply. They have promoted community gardening and greenhouses, set up farmers' markets, assisted grocers' associations in developing cooperative buying agreements, and lobbied for city-based food policies to improve the healthfulness and equity of the local food supply (Yeatman, 1994).

Taking account of the strong interest of food producers and retailers in safe and expanding markets (Kendall, 1993; Peterson et al., 1986), local and national governments and community organizations can use their considerable market power to influence the proportion of macronutrients in local food supply and, at the same time, to "practice what they preach," that is, buy, prepare, and offer foods that follow the Dietary Guidelines.

This exercise at the policy level of the modeling and market power of public agencies in just local city and county jurisdictions and school districts, numbering about 35,000 (Bureau of the Census, 1993), led by health departments, would have several public benefits (Hovey, 1989). The work force, that is, clients, patients, and inmates of public agencies (e.g., government services, schools, hospitals, child care and military sites, prisons) would have healthier food choices; health and nutrition policy officials could lead and educate by example; and, with an overall increase in the local supply of more nutritious food, the prices may become more affordable for the entire population.

In addition, promotion of local ethnic food markets of many Asian, Middle Eastern, and Latin countries, as well as farmers' markets, would afford access to fresh, lower fat, higher fiber products and expand markets for local farmers and retailers, supporting the local economy. This enhanced local self-sufficiency would also reduce the economic and environmental costs of transportation and packaging (Milio, 1991).

The recent USDA requirement that school food services move toward implementing the Dietary Guidelines offers a ready opportunity for schools to join with local food suppliers to promote children's health, especially if public health agencies promote such arrangements.

Another emerging opportunity to improve the nutrition environment is the use of new information technologies by health agencies (Milio, 1996). Electronic networks now make possible closer links between health-supporting, public and private, voluntary, and grass roots organizations (Baker et al., 1994; Bauman, 1995). These connections can serve not only communication, information, education, and data-analysis purposes. They also can support collaboration in program development, community mobilization, and advocacy for improved nutrition policies.

Organization for Action

Public policy is an attempt to bring a degree of coherence to the otherwise often chaotic and inequitable competition for resources in society; it requires coordinated activity. To develop effective nutrition policy, as the Scandinavian cases suggest, a source of stability must emerge in the universe of contending organizations and other social forces; that is, some unit or linked groups with shared views must first form, around which political and social momentum can grow. Whether this unit begins in or outside government, whether it is a single entity or a network, and whether its shape changes over time as its tasks change is not of primary importance. The crucial element is its purpose: the management of policy development to ensure momentum in policymaking, that is, to make policymaking effective (Milio, 1988b). This calls for collaboration among health officials in national and local jurisdictions, and, increasingly, transnational cooperation.

Evidence suggests that continued effectiveness of health-supporting policies in nutrition, or alcohol and tobacco, cannot depend only on the strength of scientific evidence, or only on the impact of individual local programs (Pietinen et al., 1989; Vartiainen et al., 1989). Of themselves, these will neither sustain healthful national trends nor remedy inequalities in health. What is essential is constant organized policy management that is sensitive to changing environments and adjusts strategy accordingly, emphasizing monitoring and enforcement, accountability, advocacy, and the maintenance of political and public support. This includes defining policy problems and goals; selecting and implementing policy instruments that can meet the goals; devising the strategic framework and processes to do these things and evaluate their impacts; and ensuring a political and social climate that enables these activities to move forward.

Much of the information in this chapter is based on separate on-site studies commissioned by WHO, Copenhagen, pursuant to evaluating its Health for All Programme. Each study involved analysis of over 100 documents, media content analysis, and 1–2-hour interviews with officials from all social and governmental sectors in Finland (50 from 38 organizations in 1990) and Norway (72 from 49 organizations in 1980 and 1987). Detailed information is available in the original reports, which are the principal sources drawn on in this account (Milio, 1988a, 1989, 1990a, 1990b).

REFERENCES

Association of State and Territorial Health Officers and Association of State and Territorial Public Health Nutrition Directors. (1993). *The national project to develop a strategic plan for changing the American diet to prevent cancer, heart disease, and other chronic diseases.* Atlanta, GA: Centers for Disease Control and Prevention.

Baker, E. L., Melton, R. J., Stange, P. V., Fields, M. L., Koplan, J. P., Fernando, A. G., & Satcher, D. (1994). Health reform and the health of the public: Forging community health partnerships. *Journal of the American Medical Association, 272,* 1276–1275.

Bauman Foundation. (1995) *Agenda for access: Public access to federal information on sustainability through the information superhighway.* A report prepared for the Office of Management and Budget. Washington, DC: Author.

Blanchard, O., Commander, S., & Corelli, F. (1994, December). Unemployment in Eastern Europe. *Finance & Development*, pp. 6–13.

Bletz, F., Dercksen, W., & Van Paridon, K. (1993). *Shaping factors for the business environment in the Netherlands after 1992.* The Hague: Netherlands Scientific Council.

Brooks, K., & Lerman, Z. (December, 1994). Farm reform in the transition economies. *Finance & Development*, pp. 25–28.

Bureau of the Census. (1993). *Census of governments.* Washington, DC: Department of Commerce.

Bureau of the Census. (1994). *The earnings ladder.* Stat. Brief. Washington, DC: Department of Commerce.

Centers for Disease Control and Prevention. (1993). Prevalence of sedentary lifestyle-behavioral risk factor surveillance system, United States. *Morbidity Mortality Weekly Report, 42,* 576–579.

Council on Linkages between Academia and Public Health Practice. (1995). *Guidelines development project for public health practice.* Baltimore: Johns Hopkins University Press.

Department of Health and Human Services. (1988). *Surgeon General's report on nutrition and health.* Washington, DC: U.S. Government Printing Office.

Economics, Statistics and Cooperatives Service. (1980). *Agricultural and food policy review.* AFPR-3. Washington, DC: U.S. Department of Agriculture.

Feshbach, M. (1993). Health crisis in Russia. *Central European Health & Environment Monitor, 1*(2), 1–6.

Food and Agriculture Organization. (1990a). *Policy changes affecting European agriculture.* Background report, ERC/90/IND/4. Rome: Author.

Food and Agriculture Organization. (1990b). *Balanced diet: A way to good nutrition.* Background Report, ERC/90/4. Rome: Author.

Freimuth, V. et al. (1988). Health advertising: Prevention for profit. *American Journal of Public Health, 78,* 557–561.

General Accounting Office. (1988, June). *California dairy production, sales and product disposition.* Washington, DC: U.S. Congress.

General Accounting Office. (1990, February). *Alternative agriculture: Federal incentives and farmers' opinions.* Washington, DC: U.S. Congress.

General Accounting Office. (1993, December). *Agriculture commodities research and promotion programs.* Washington, DC: U.S. Congress.

General Accounting Office. (1994, January). *Dairy marketing.* Washington, DC: U.S. Congress.

Gupta, S., & Hagemann, R. (1994, December). Social protection during Russia's economic transformation. *Finance & Development,* pp. 14–17.

Hovey, H. (1989). Analytic approaches to state-local relations. In E. Liner (Ed.), *A decade of devolution: Perspectives on state-local relations.* Washington, DC: Urban Institute Press.

Institute of Medicine. (1991). *Improving America's diet and health.* Washington, DC: National Academy Press.

Kendall, A. (1993). *Supermarket nutrition education in New York State.* Albany: New York State Department of Health.

Langley, J. (1987, July). The policy web affecting agriculture. *ERS Bulletin,* No. 524. Washington, DC: U.S. Department of Agriculture.

Levine, J. (1986). Hearts and minds: The politics of diet and heart disease. In R. Sapolsky (Ed.). *Consuming fears* (pp. 42–79). New York: Basic Books.

Levine, J. (1989, June). Grocery line typecasting. *World & I,* 275–280.

Louis Harris and Associates. (1994). *The prevention index.* Rodale, PA: Rodale Press.

Goggin, M. (1987). *Policy design and the politics of implementation.* Knoxville, TN: University of Tennessee Press.

Milio, N. (1988, March). *An analysis of the implementation of Norwegian nutrition policy, 1981–87.* Background document prepared for the World Health Organization, WHO Regional Office for Europe. 1990 Conference on Food and Nutrition Policy, Copenhagen.

Milio, N. (1988b). Making healthy public policy: Developing the science by learning the art: An ecological framework for policy studies. *Health Promotion International, 2,* 87–93.

Milio, N. (1989). Nutrition and health: Patterns and policy perspectives in food-rich countries. *Social Sciences and Medicine, 29*(3), 413–423.

Milio, N. (1990, June). *Finland's food and nutrition policy: Progress, problems, and recommendations. Report to the World Health Organization.* Copenhagen: WHO Regional Office for Europe.

Milio, N. (1990b). *Nutrition policy for food-rich countries: A strategic analysis.* Baltimore, MD: Johns Hopkins University Press.

Milio, N. (1991). Sustainable nutrition and health: Ecological dimensions and policy issues. In V. Brown (Ed.), *Health and the quality of life* (pp. 175–192). Canberra: Australian National University Press.

Milio, N. (1996). *Engines of empowerment: Using information technology to create healthy communities and challenge public policy.* Chicago, IL: Health Administration Press.

National Cancer Institute. (1991). *Strategies to control tobacco use in the United States: A blueprint for public health action in the 1990s.* Smoking and Tobacco

Control Monographs 1. (National Institute of Health, Publication No. 92-3316). Bethesda, MD: U.S. Department of Health and Human Services.

National Nutrition Council. (1989). *A programme for the implementation of nutrition recommendations.* Helsinki: Ministry of Agriculture.

National Nutrition Council. (1992, December). *Nutrition, food and health in the Netherlands.* International Conference on Nutrition, Rome, Amsterdam, The Netherlands: Author.

National Report of the Federal Republic of Germany. (1992, December). *Food and nutrition: Policy and practice in Germany.* International Conference on Nutrition, Rome.

National Research Council. (1989). *Diet and health.* Washington, DC: National Academy Press.

Nelson, D., Giovino, G. A., Shopland, D. R., Mowery, P. D., Mills, S. L., & Eriksen, M. P. (1995). Trends in cigarette smoking among US adolescents, 1974 through 1991. *American Journal of Public Health, 85*(3), 34–40.

O'Brien, P. (1993, June). *Diet, health, and agriculture.* Washington, DC: U.S. Department of Agriculture, Economic Research Service.

Peterson, G., Elder, J. P., Knisley, P. M., Colby, J. C., Beaudin, P., DeBlois, D., & Carleton, R. A. (1986). Developing strategies for food vendor intervention: The first step. *Journal of the American Dietetic Association, 86,* 659–661.

Pietinen P., Vartianen, E., Korhonen, H. J., Kartovaara, L., Uusitalo, U., Tuomilehto, J., & Puska, P. (1989). Nutrition as a component in community control of cardiovascular disease (the North Karelia Project). *American Journal of Clinical Nutrition, 49,* 1017–1024.

Serdula, M., Coates, R., Byers, T., Simoes, E., Mokdad, A. H., & Subar, A. F. (1995). Fruit and vegetable intake among adults in 16 states. *American Journal of Public Health, 85*(3), 236–239.

Service Employees International Union. (1995). *Block grants: A state-by-state analysis of the fiscal impacts of program consolidation.* Washington, DC: Author.

Sweden's Country Paper to the FAO/WHO International Conference on Nutrition. (1992). Stockholm: Swedish ministeries of health and social affairs, and of agriculture.

Toronto Food Policy Council. (1994, June). *If the health care system believed you are what you eat: Strategies to integrate our food and health systems.* Toronto: TFNC Discussion Paper Series.

USDA/DHHS. (1990). *Nutrition and your health. Dietary guidelines for Americans.* (3rd. ed.). Washington, DC. Author.

Vaandrager, L. (1994). *European food and shopping research network.* (SUPER). Wageningen, The Netherlands: Wageningen Agricultural University.

Vartiainen E., et al. (1988). *Changes in cardiovascular risk factor patterns in treated and untreated hypertensive Finnish men and women during 1982-1987.* Helsinki: National Institute of Public Health.

World Health Organization. (1992, April). *Regional conference on food and nutrition problems in central and eastern Europe.* 1–4, Report. Copenhagen: WHO Regional Office for Europe.

Yeatman, H. (1994). *Food policy councils in North America.* Research Report. NSW, Australia: University of Woolongong.

Author Index

Subject Index

Chronic toxicity tests, 42
Clostridia, 59, 100
Clostridium perfringens, 59, 101
Cocci, 54
Collective health:
 motivation for individual pursuit of,
 25–29
 outcomes, 19–25
Color Additive Amendments of 1960
 (CCA), 49–50
Color additives, regulation of, 49–50
Commercialized agriculture, 121–123
Commodity Supplemental Food Program,
 257
Congregate meal programs, 304
Consumer activists, 14–15, 29
Consumer satisfaction, 5–6
Convenience foods, 11, 94–95
Cooking methods, nutritive losses, 103
Copper, dietary impact of, 294
Coronary artery disease, 158, 161
Coronary heart disease (CHD):
 dietary change, impact on, 164–165,
 167–169
 diet–heart disease hypothesis, 160–164
 early precursors of, 160
 mortality trends from, 158–159
 risk factors, 165
 serum cholesterol and, 161
 types of, 157–158
Cyanobacteria, 61

Death:
 from cancer, 174, 183
 coronary heart disease and, 158–159
 dental caries and, 207
 diet-induced, 17–18, 103, 106, 138
Delaney Amendment/Clause, 10–11, 15,
 47–48, 73, 84–85, 176
Dental caries prevention:
 antifluoride movement, 222–224
 community water fluoridation:
 alternatives to, 218, 220–222
 cost aspects of, 215–216
 individual rights, infringement of,
 225–226

 purpose of, 210–212
 epidemiology of, 218, 220
 fluoridation:
 antifluoride movement, 222–224
 of community water, *see* community
 water fluoridation
 defined, 208–209
 impact of, 212–214
 review of, 214–215
 safety issues, 216–218
 history of, 209–210
 political issues, 224–225
DETERMINE checklist, nutritive care for
 cancer patients, 186
Developmental toxicity tests, 41–42
Dexfenfluramine, 153
Diabetes, generally, 147
Diabetes mellitus, 236–237
Dietary guidelines, *see* Recommended
 Daily Allowance (RDA)
 fat consumption, 170
 purpose of, 154–155, 167, 315
Dietary habits, impact of, 270–272
Dietary Intervention Study in Children
 (DISC), 275, 278
Dietary Supplement Act (DSA), 82–83
Dietary Supplement Health and Education
 Act (DSHEA), 83–84, 86
Dietary supplements, regulation of,
 77–79, 86. *See also specific vita-
 mins*
Diet–cancer relationship, 173–176
Diet–heart disease hypothesis:
 fat consumption, 163, 167–169
 overview, 160–161
 serum cholesterol, 161, 274–275
Direct food additives, *see* Intentional food
 additives
Disadvantaged population, poor nutrition
 and, 18
Diseases, nutrition-related, *see* Nutrition-
 related conditions/diseases
Drying technology, 99

Eating disorders, 142–143. *See also*
 Obesity

$) Springer Publishing Company

International Perspectives in Environment, Development, and Health: Toward a Sustainable World

Gurinder S. Shahi, PhD, MBBS, MPH,
Barry S. Levy, MD, MPH, **Al Binger,** PhD,
Tord Kjellstrom, MD, and **Robert Lawrence,** MD

This comprehensive text is a collaborative initiative of the World Health Organization, the United Nations Development Programme, and the Rockefeller Foundation, and examines health and development issues on a global scale. The volume addresses the broad range of approaches necessary to deal with environment and development-related concerns across various fields of endeavor and geographical regions.

Topics include:
- Epidemiology
- Comparative Health Risk Assessment
- Environmental Risk Transition
- Population Growth
- Sanitation
- Food Security
- Lifestyle
- Poverty and Global Economics
- Gender
- Species Extinction
- Climate Change
- Vector-Borne Diseases
- Coastal Management
- Military Impact
- Global Migration and Hazardous Industries
- Workers' Health
- Urban and Rural Planning
- Child Development

International Perspectives on
Environment,
Development,
and Health
Toward a Sustainable World
A collaborative initiative of the World Health Organization, the United Nations Development Programme, and the Rockefeller Foundation.

Gurinder, S. Shahi, PhD, MBBS, MPH
Barry S. Levy, MD, MPH
Al Binger, PhD
Tord Kjellstrom, MD
Robert Lawrence, MD
Editors

$) Springer Publishing Company

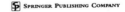

1997 744pp 0-8261-9190-8 *hardcover*

536 Broadway, New York, NY 10012-3955 • (212) 431-4370 • Fax (212) 941-7842